theclinics.com

INFECTIOUS DISEASE CLINICS OF NORTH AMERICA

Bioterrorism and Bioterrorism Preparedness

GUEST EDITOR
Nancy Khardori, MD, PhD

CONSULTING EDITOR
Robert C. Moellering, Jr, MD

June 2006 • Volume 20 • Number 2

SAUNDERS

An Imprint of Elsevier, Inc.
PHILADELPHIA LONDON TORONTO MONTREAL SYDNEY TOKYO

W.B. SAUNDERS COMPANY
A Division of Elsevier Inc.

Elsevier, Inc., 1600 John F. Kennedy Blvd., Suite 1800, Philadelphia, PA 19103-2899.

http://www.theclinics.com

INFECTIOUS DISEASE CLINICS OF NORTH AMERICA
June 2006
Editor: Rachel Glover

Volume 20, Number 2
ISSN 0891–5520
ISBN 1-4160-3510-9

Infectious Disease Clinics of North America (ISSN 0891–5520) is published in March, June, September, and December (For Post Office use only: volume 20 issue 1 of 4) by W.B. Saunders, 360 Park Avenue South, New York, NY 10010-1710. Business and Editorial Offices: 1600 John F. Kennedy Blvd., Suite 1800, Philadelphia, PA 19103-2899. Accounting and Circulation Offices: 6277 Sea Harbor Drive, Orlando, FL 32887-4800. Periodicals postage paid at New York, NY and additional mailing offices. Subscription prices are $170.00 per year for US individuals, $285.00 per year for US institutions, $85.00 per year for US students, $200.00 per year for Canadian individuals, $345.00 per year for Canadian institutions, $225.00 per year for international individuals, $345.00 per year for international institutions, and $110.00 per year for Canadian and foreign students. To receive student rate, orders must be accompained by name of affiliated institution, date of term, and the *signature* of program/residency coordinator on institution letterhead. Orders will be billed at individual rate until proof of status is received. Foreign air speed delivery is included in all *Clinics* subscription prices. All prices are subject to change without notice. **POSTMASTER**: Send address changes to *Infectious Disease Clinics of North America*, Elsevier Periodicals Customer Service, 6277 Sea Harbor Drive, Orlando, FL 32887-4800. **Customer Service: 1-800-654-2452 (US). From outside of the US, call 1-407-345-4000. E-mail: hhspcs@wbsaunders.com**.

Infectious Disease Clinics of North America is also published in Spanish by Editorial Inter-Médica, Junin 917, 1er A 1113, Buenos Aires, Argentina.

Reprints. For copies of 100 or more, of articles in this publication, please contact the Commercial Reprints Department, Elsevier Inc., 360 Park Avenue South, New York, New York 10010-1710. Tel. (212) 633-3813, Fax: (212) 462-1935, email: reprints@elsevier.com.

Infectious Disease Clinics of North America is covered in *Index Medicus, Current Contents/Clinical Medicine, Science Citation Alert, SCISEARCH, and Research Alert.*

Printed in the United States of America.

CONSULTING EDITOR

ROBERT C. MOELLERING, Jr, MD, Herrman L. Blumgart Professor of Medical Research, Harvard Medical School; and Physician-in-Chief and Chairman, Department of Medicine, Beth Israel Deaconess Medical Center, Boston, Massachusetts

GUEST EDITOR

NANCY KHARDORI, MD, PhD, Professor of Medicine and Microbiology/Immunology; Chief, Division of Infectious Diseases, Department of Internal Medicine, Southern Illinois University School of Medicine, Springfield, Illinois

CONTRIBUTORS

ALYS ADAMSKI, BS, Researcher, Division of Infectious Diseases, Department of Internal Medicine, Southern Illinois University School of Medicine, Springfield, Illinois

NIKOLAOS AKRITIDIS, MD, Director, Internal Medicine Department, General Hospital "G. Hatzikosta," Ioannina, Greece

ERIK BÄCK, MD, PhD, Department of Infectious Diseases, Örebro University Hospital, and Department of Clinical Medicine, Örebro University, Örebro, Sweden

STEPHANIE M. BORCHARDT, PhD, MPH, Division of Infectious Diseases, Illinois Department of Public Health, Chicago, Illinois

TINA BROMAN, DVM, PhD, Department of NBC Analysis, Swedish Defence Research Agency, Umeå, Sweden

BRUCE BUDOWLE, PhD, Federal Bureau of Investigation, Laboratory Division, Quantico, Virginia

LEONIDAS CHRISTOU, MD, Assistant Professor of Medicine, Internal Medicine Department, University Hospital, Ioannina, Greece

DENNIS J. CLERI, MD, Professor, Department of Medicine, Seton Hall University School of Graduate Medical Education, South Orange; Program Director, Internal Medicine Residency, Department of Medicine, Seton Hall University School of Graduate Medical Education at St. Francis Medical Center, Trenton, New Jersey

BURKE A. CUNHA, MD, Chief, Infectious Disease Division, Winthrop-University Hospital, Mineola; Professor of Medicine, State University of New York School of Medicine, Stony Brook, New York

CHESTON B. CUNHA, Pennsylvania State University College of Medicine, Hershey, Pennsylvania

KAREN M. DAVENPORT, MD, Assistant Professor of Clinical Pediatrics, Department of Pediatrics and the Steele Children's Research Center, Section of General Pediatrics, University of Arizona Health Sciences Center, Tucson, Arizona

MARK S. DWORKIN, MD, MPHTM, Division of Infectious Diseases, Illinois Department of Public Health, Chicago, Illinois

MOHAMED EL-AZIZI, PhD, Assistant Professor, Department of Medicine, Division of Infectious Diseases, Southern Illinois University, School of Medicine, Springfield, Illinois

HENRIK ELIASSON, MD, Department of Infectious Diseases, Örebro University Hospital, Örebro, Sweden

SEAN P. ELLIOTT, MD, Associate Professor of Clinical Pediatrics, Department of Pediatrics and the Steele Children's Research Center, Section of Pediatric Infectious Diseases, University of Arizona Health Sciences Center, Tucson, Arizona

MATS FORSMAN, PhD, Department of NBC Analysis, Swedish Defence Research Agency, Umeå, Sweden

NANCY KHARDORI, MD, PhD, Professor of Medicine and Microbiology/Immunology; Chief, Division of Infectious Diseases, Department of Internal Medicine, Southern Illinois University School of Medicine, Springfield, Illinois

JANAK KOIRALA, MD, MPH, FACP, Associate Professor, Division of Infectious Diseases, Department of Internal Medicine, Southern Illinois University School of Medicine, Springfield, Illinois

DEMETRIOS N. KYRIACOU, MD, PhD, DTM&H, Associate Professor, Department of Emergency Medicine and Department of Preventive Medicine, Northwestern University Feinberg School of Medicine, Chicago, Illinois

STEPHEN A. MORSE, MSPH, PhD, Bioterrorism Preparedness and Response Program, Centers for Disease Control and Prevention, Atlanta, Georgia

ADNAN MUSHTAQ, MD, Senior Fellow, Department of Medicine, Division of Infectious Diseases, Southern Illinois University, School of Medicine, Springfield, Illinois

PARASKEVI PANAGOPOULOU, MD, MPH, Institute for Continuing Medical Education of Ioannina, Ioannina, Greece

GEORGIOS PAPPAS, MD, Institute for Continuing Medical Education of Ioannina, Ioannina, Greece

RICHARD B. PORWANCHER, MD, Clinical Associate Professor, Department of Medicine, UMDNJ-Robert Wood Johnson Medical School, New Brunswick; Chief, Division of Infectious Diseases, Department of Medicine, St. Francis Medical Center, Trenton, New Jersey

LUZ S. RAMOS-BONNER, MD, Chief Medical Resident, Department of Medicine, St. Francis Medical Center, Trenton, New Jersey

ANTHONY J. RICKETTI, MD, Assistant Professor, Department of Medicine, Seton Hall University School of Graduate Medical Education, South Orange; Chairman, Department of Medicine, Seton Hall University School of Graduate Medical Education at St. Francis Medical Center, Trenton, New Jersey

KATHLEEN A. RITGER, MD, MPH, Division of Infectious Diseases, Illinois Department of Public Health, Chicago, Illinois; Epidemic Intelligence Service, Centers for Disease Control and Prevention, Atlanta, Georgia

ZAKIR HUSSAIN A. SHAIKH, MD, MPH, CPE, Attending Physician, Department of Infectious Diseases, Methodist Dallas Medical Center; Hospital Epidemiologist and Medical Director, Infection Control, Methodist Health System, Dallas, Texas

JOHN R. VERNALEO, MD, Chief, Division of Infectious Diseases, Wycoff Heights Medical Center, Brooklyn, New York

RODRIGO G. VILLAR, MD, Associate Professor of Clinical Pediatrics, Department of Pediatrics and the Steele Children's Research Center, Section of General Pediatrics, University of Arizona Health Sciences Center, Tucson, Arizona

CONTENTS

Preface xiii
Nancy Khardori

Bioterrorism and Bioterrorism Preparedness: Historical Perspective and Overview 179
Nancy Khardori

The epidemics and pandemics of natural infectious diseases caused by communicable agents have changed the course of human history frequently. In the context of bioterrorism, infectious diseases are not only a public health issue, but also an issue of national and international security. Because most bioterrorism events would be covert, health care providers would be the "first responders" by diagnosing and reporting the event to public health authorities. This response would lead to immediate involvement of security and law enforcement agencies. This article provides an overview and historical perspective of bioterrorism and bioterrorism preparedness.

Categorization, Prioritization, and Surveillance of Potential Bioterrorism Agents 213
Stephanie M. Borchardt, Kathleen A. Ritger, and Mark S. Dworkin

Critical biologic agents with potential for use in a bioterrorism attack have been prioritized into three categories based on their ability to cause illness and death, their capacity for dissemination, public perception as related to plausible civil disruption, and special needs required for effective public health intervention. Health care providers, public and private laboratories, local and state health departments, and public health officials from several agencies share the responsibility of disease surveillance. Surveillance for bioterrorism-related illness is dependent on a system that promptly collects, analyzes, and reports data to public health officials. Syndromic surveillance may augment the reporting of unusual or suspicious illness by informed health care providers and laboratorians, improving preparedness for potential bioterrorist attacks by enhancing timeliness of infectious disease surveillance.

Anthrax: From Antiquity and Obscurity to a Front-Runner in Bioterrorism **227**
Demetrios N. Kyriacou, Alys Adamski, and Nancy Khardori

Anthrax infection is caused by *Bacillus anthracis*, a large gram-positive, rod-shaped bacterium found in soil around the world. Although anthrax is usually a disease of grazing animals, human contact with animal products, such as hides, hairs, and wool that are contaminated with anthrax endospores can result in clinical infection with cutaneous, inhalational, gastrointestinal, and neurologic manifestations. Anthrax has recently become a front-runner in potential bioterrorism weapons. This article presents a brief history of anthrax, discusses different clinical presentations of anthrax, reviews the clinical characteristics that can be used to recognize inhalational anthrax victims, discusses current diagnostic and treatment modalities, and provides an overview of emerging and investigational therapies and vaccines.

Impact of Plague on Human History **253**
Cheston B. Cunha and Burke A. Cunha

Plague was first described among the Philistines in the Book of Samuel in 1320 BC and was thought to be related to rodents. The Justinian plague of 42–590 AD was definitely caused by *Yersinia pestis* and was the first plague pandemic. The second pandemic, from the early 1300s to the late 1600s, was known as the "Black Death" in Europe. In the modern era, the third pandemic began in 1894 in China and spread by ships to port cities. Plague epidemics continue to occur in endemic areas. Plague was used in biological warfare in World War II with limited success. This article reviews plague pandemics and the use of plague as a biological weapon from an historical perspective.

Plague: Disease, Management, and Recognition of Act of Terrorism **273**
Janak Koirala

Plague is a zoonosis caused by *Yersinia pestis* that classically presents in bubonic, septicemic, or pneumonic form. Aerosolized *Y pestis* is the most likely method used in a bioterrorist attack, which can lead to a rapidly fatal pneumonic plague. Plague should be suspected when the clinical picture is consistent and bipolar staining gram-negative rods are present. Because vaccines are not currently available in the United States, pre-exposure and postexposure chemoprophylaxis should be used. Recent advances in genomic research on *Y pestis* should help in better understanding the epidemiology and the development of rapid diagnostic tests, and safer and more effective vaccines.

Tularemia: Current Epidemiology and Disease Management 289
Henrik Eliasson, Tina Broman, Mats Forsman, and Erik Bäck

Tularemia, caused by the gram-negative bacterium *Francisella tularensis*, a zoonosis with a complex epidemiology, is transmitted to humans by vectors, direct contact, inhalation, or the alimentary route. Increasing knowledge, on the subspecies level, of pathogenicity, ecology, and epidemiology is being elucidated as a result of intensified research. A low infective dose of the bacterium in combination with a high attack rate via the respiratory route causes concern over its possible use as a bioterrorism agent. Fluoroquinolone therapy is an alternative to aminoglycoside treatment.

Botulism: The Many Faces of Botulinum Toxin and its Potential for Bioterrorism 313
Rodrigo G. Villar, Sean P. Elliott, and Karen M. Davenport

The neurotoxins produced by *Clostridium botulinum* are among the most potent poisons known. Awareness of the botulism syndromes is critical to allow prompt identification of cases and rapid delivery of antitoxin that may alleviate disease severity and to provide supportive care. This article describes the microbiology, pharmacology, and epidemiology of *C botulinum* and its toxins; the recognized botulism syndromes; modes of transmission; and treatment. Additionally, it focuses on the potential use of botulinum toxin as a biological weapon, reviewing potential modes of toxin delivery; recognition of intentional attacks; laboratory methods for toxin detection; and possible methods for prevention, treatment, and control of botulism in the event of an intentional attack.

Smallpox as a Bioterrorist Weapon: Myth or Menace? 329
Dennis J. Cleri, Richard B. Porwancher, Anthony J. Ricketti, Luz S. Ramos-Bonner, and John R. Vernaleo

Smallpox, also known as variola, is a highly contagious, often lethal disease (30–50% mortality) unique to humans. Infection confers near lifelong immunity in survivors. The clinical presentation (ordinary, modified, flat [malignant], hemorrhagic, or visceral) depends on the individual's innate and acquired immunity. The World Health Organization's aggressive containment program of early case identification, isolation, and ring vaccination of contacts eliminated all naturally occurring disease by 1977. Routine smallpox vaccination ceased 20 years ago because the risks associated with vaccination no longer could be justified for a likely nonexistent illness. Because the world's population now has either waning or no immunity to variola, this highly feared pathogen could become a significant bioterrorist threat.

Viral Hemorrhagic Fevers: Current Status of Endemic Disease and Strategies for Control 359
Dennis J. Cleri, Anthony J. Ricketti, Richard B. Porwancher, Luz S. Ramos-Bonner, and John R. Vernaleo

Hemorrhagic fever viruses are ubiquitous in nature and largely live as commensal organisms in rodent and arthropod hosts. Their clinical presentations overlap with other viral illnesses and serious bacterial infections, complicating diagnosis. Their potential for weaponized aerosol spread, person-to-person transmission in select species, a high case-fatality rate, and the relative lack of effective prophylaxis and treatment make these viruses attractive agents for bioterrorism. A vigorous public health program should include plans for large-scale triage and selective quarantine; regional coordination of emergency responses and use of inpatient resources; and education in effective infection control practices for both health care providers and the public at large.

Category B Potential Bioterrorism Agents: Bacteria, Viruses, Toxins, and Foodborne and Waterborne Pathogens 395
Georgios Pappas, Paraskevi Panagopoulou, Leonidas Christou, and Nikolaos Akritidis

Category B of potential biologic weapons encompasses a wide spectrum of pathogens, including bacteria transmitted by inhalation; toxins; arthropod-borne bacteria and viruses; and foodborne and waterborne bacteria, viruses, and protozoa. The particular characteristics of each pathogen important for their bioterrorism potential, and the relative risk projected, underline the need for further stratification of this diverse group of pathogens.

Category C Potential Bioterrorism Agents and Emerging Pathogens 423
Adnan Mushtaq, Mohamed El-Azizi, and Nancy Khardori

The threat of using weaponized forms of biologic agents against civilian populations through bioterrorism attacks has emerged, and with advances in biotechnology, category C bioterrorism agents and emerging pathogens may become attractive weapons for bioterrorists. Category C bioterrorism agents and emerging pathogens have many advantages over conventional weapons and other biologic agents listed under categories A and B, including their relatively low costs; their relative accessibility; and the relative ease with which they could be produced, be delivered, and avoid detection. Their use, or even threatened use, is capable of producing widespread social disruption. Although biotechnology is a tool by which bioterrorists could develop weapons of mass destruction, it also should be used to improve the methods of fighting such weapons.

Practical Aspects of Implementation of a Bioterrorism Preparedness Program in a Hospital setting **443**
Zakir Hussain A. Shaikh

Although it is important to worry about preparedness for novel bioterrorist agents, potential devastation from naturally occurring possibilities, including pandemic influenza, severe acute respiratory syndrome, and H5N1 avian influenza, is more likely. These real threats make it imperative to ensure a hospital's continued readiness and ability to identify cases based on clinical and epidemiologic presentation. For effective implementation of a biologic disaster or bioterrorism preparedness program, multiple practical aspects need to be addressed to achieve the goal of minimizing the morbidity and mortality associated with the event and to provide continued quality care to patients already receiving care in the hospital. This article addresses these practical aspects.

Microbial Forensics: Application to Bioterrorism Preparedness and Response **455**
Stephen A. Morse and Bruce Budowle

To prepare for the next bioterrorist attack or biocrime and to deter a future event, a strong microbial forensics program is being developed. For the purpose of this article, microbial forensics is considered as an evolving subdiscipline of forensic science, which combines several scientific disciplines (eg, molecular biology, microbiology, genomics, bioinformatics, biochemistry) to analyze evidence from a bioterrorism act, biocrime, hoax, or inadvertent release, for the purpose of attribution. This article describes the field of microbial forensics, the challenges to consider, and how this emerging field is integrated into the preparedness and response of the United States to a bioterrorist attack.

Index **475**

FORTHCOMING ISSUES

September 2006

Fungal Infections
Thomas F. Patterson, MD, FACP
Guest Editor

December 2006

Infections of the Head and Neck
Anthony W. Chow, MD, *Guest Editor*

March 2007

Antiviral Therapy
Clyde S. Crumpacker, MD, *Guest Editor*

RECENT ISSUES

March 2006

Hepatitis
Robert C. Moellering, Jr, MD
Consulting Editor

December 2005

Update on Musculoskeletal Infections
John J. Ross, MD, *Guest Editor*

September 2005

Pediatric Infectious Disease
Jeffrey L. Blumer, MD, PhD
and Philip Toltzis, MD, *Guest Editors*

ELSEVIER
SAUNDERS

Infect Dis Clin N Am
20 (2006) xiii–xv

INFECTIOUS
DISEASE CLINICS
OF NORTH AMERICA

Preface

Bioterrorism and Bioterrorism Preparedness

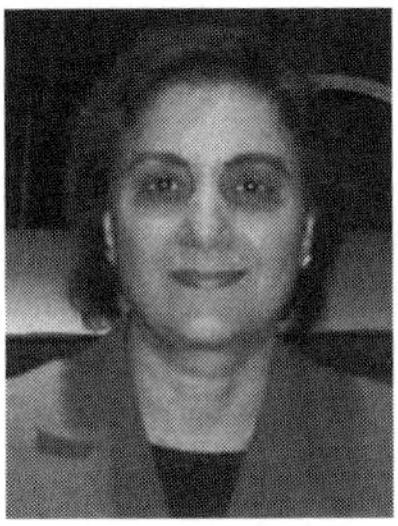

Nancy Khardori, MD, PhD
Guest Editor

On September 9, 2001, the world witnessed the most graphic and dastardly display of how modern technology can be put to evil use. This was followed by the intentional use of microbiology technology to harm humans. We proudly watched as a practicing colleague, Larry Bush, of Florida, made a diagnosis of anthrax from an uncommon presentation of the disease.

Around this time, our team was in the process of convening an educational program on behalf of the Association of Practitioners in Infection Control. West Nile virus was new in our area, and the number of patients with hepatitis C being sent to us was increasing rapidly. These were the topics originally included in our program planned for November 15, 2001. While working on the brochure, I looked up the Centers for Disease Control and Prevention's Categories of Bioterrorism Agents. As I scanned the list of category A agents with the highest potential for causing mass casualties, I realized that at one point or another in my professional career as an infectious diseases clinician and a microbiologist spanning across two different continents, I had seen or diagnosed them all. I had seen cutaneous anthrax and woolsorter's disease as a medical student in the sheep raising and wool carding area of Kashmir, India; smallpox as a young village physician in the early 1970s; Kyasanur Forest disease, a viral hemorrhagic fever, during my post–medical school doctoral training in microbiology; botulism during the outbreak in Peoria, Illinois, from home-canned mushrooms, while I was an ICU resident at Southern Illinois University School of Medicine in Springfield, Illinois; plague during the last outbreak in Gujarat, India, in 1994; and

doi:10.1016/j.idc.2006.03.006

tularemia cases scattered through the last 2 decades from central and southern Illinois. Diseases caused by pathogens included in categories B and C, although uncommon in the United States, have been encountered by most infectious disease clinicians and are of particular importance in returning international travelers.

I suggested to other faculty members of the continuing medical education team that we include bioterrorism-related topics in the upcoming program. They all agreed readily, and the program was very well received. We saw all types of physicians including anesthesiologists and radiologists in a standing room–only conference center. They all came on time, requested an additional presentation during the dinner hour, and stayed until the end. We learned later that ours was one of the first formal education programs on bioterrorism. Next, we were invited by the American Society of Microbiology to present a day-long workshop at the 2002 Interscience Conference on Antimicrobial Agents and Chemotherapy (ICAAC) held in San Diego, California. We prepared an extensive original handout for the workshop participants. At the meeting, a representative from Elsevier met with us to discuss converting the handbook material into a printed book. We continued to offer the program to various regional groups through the year and have presented the workshop every year at ICAAC. In the meantime, two of the presenters started publishing bioterrorism-related articles individually, and collectively the team prepared a 300-page book, recently published by Wiley VCH. An invited review on historical perspectives and overview of bioterrorism agents and bioterrorism preparedness appeared in the *Clinical Microbiology Newsletter*. The consulting editor of *Infectious Disease Clinics of North America*, Dr. Robert Moellering, liked the material and the format in which the information was presented. Next came the invitation to guest edit a bioterrorism issue of the *Clinics* in a relatively short time.

I decided to use an objective method to pick an international group of authors based mostly on their original contributions to the mainstream literature related to various areas and diseases being discussed. In keeping with the goal of making this issue of *Infectious Disease Clinics of North America* a complement to the existing literature, rather than producing more of the same, articles on the practical role of various surveillance methods, practical aspects of implementing a bioterrorism preparedness program in the hospital setting, and microbial forensics as an emerging tool for bioterrorism investigation and preparedness were included. As the articles started arriving, most of them well before the deadline, I was truly impressed by the quality of all the contributions. All the authors made my role as an editor easy and in addition to providing excellent manuscripts responded well to all other requests. It has been an absolute pleasure to work with Ms. Rachel Glover, the editor, and the consulting editor, who gave me total freedom in creating this issue.

It is my sincere hope that this issue becomes a useful reference for teaching and formulating preparedness programs and clinical issues related to pathogens included in various categories of bioterrorism agents. Most of all, I hope this issue provides readers with intellectually stimulating materials. Personally, I offer gratitude to all the authors and to Mrs. Nancy Mutzbauer, who, in addition to preparing the manuscripts, has functioned as a liaison with other authors and the publisher.

Nancy Khardori, MD, PhD
Division of Infectious Diseases
Department of Internal Medicine
Southern Illinois University School of Medicine
701 North First Street, Room A480
Springfield, IL 62702, USA

E-mail address: nkhardori@siumed.edu

ELSEVIER
SAUNDERS

Infect Dis Clin N Am
20 (2006) 179–211

INFECTIOUS
DISEASE CLINICS
OF NORTH AMERICA

Bioterrorism and Bioterrorism Preparedness: Historical Perspective and Overview

Nancy Khardori, MD, PhD

Division of Infectious Diseases, Department of Internal Medicine, Southern Illinois University School of Medicine, 701 North First Street, Room A 484, Springfield, IL 62794-9636, USA

Bioterrorism has been defined by the Centers for Disease Control and Prevention (CDC) as "the intentional release of bacteria, viruses or toxins for the purpose of harming or killing civilians" [1]. The intentional use of microbiologic agents dates back to the days before specific etiologies of infectious diseases were known. The epidemics and pandemics of natural infectious diseases caused by communicable agents have changed the course of human history frequently by claiming more lives and creating more social devastation than wars. With continued emergence and spread of previously unrecognized pathogens and reemergence of others in forms resistant to current antimicrobial agents, natural infectious diseases will remain a tool for mass casualties in the foreseeable future. Accepting "Mother Nature" as the most menacing "bioterrorist," the concept of terror associated with biologic agents should encompass bioterrorism, biowarfare, and current and future global infectious diseases with the potential for mass casualties (eg, pandemic influenza) [2].

Epidemiologic principles, diagnostic criteria, and management strategies are common to infectious diseases regardless of the source. Many emerging pathogens are zoonotic in origin. Coordinated and cohesive efforts by scientists, health care providers, veterinarians, and epidemiologists are needed to control the global impact of infectious diseases. In addition, the law has been considered an important tool of public health, an important example being disease-reporting laws. In the context of bioterrorism, infectious diseases are not only a public health issue, but also an issue of national and international security. The authors of the recently drafted Model State

E-mail address: nkhardori@siumed.edu

0891-5520/06/$ - see front matter
doi:10.1016/j.idc.2006.03.007 ***id.theclinics.com***

Emergency Health Powers Act expanded the definition of bioterrorism to "the intentional use of a pathogen or biological product to cause harm to a human, animal, plant or other living organism to influence the conduct of government and to intimidate or coerce a civilian population" [3]. Because most bioterrorism events would be covert, health care providers would be the "first responders" by diagnosing and reporting the event to public health authorities. This would be the "triggering response" and lead to immediate involvement of security and law enforcement agencies.

Historical perspective

Prebacterial cultivation era

The story of Hercules (the superhero of Greek mythology) and the Hydra may be the first description in Western literature of chemical and biological weapons (*New York Times,* October 7, 2003). In the battle against King Eumeneus of Pergarium (184 BC), the Carthaginian soldiers led by Hannibal achieved victory by hurling earthen pots filled with "serpents of every kind" onto the decks of enemy ships [4]. The association between filth, foul odor, decay, and "disease" and "contagion" was made long before the microbial world was discovered. The crude use of filth, cadavers, and human and animal carcasses as weapons was based on this association [5]. Contamination of wells, reservoirs, and other water sources by these avenues has been used to cause disease and devastation among civilian populations and armies since antiquity well into the twentieth century. The Greeks polluted the wells and drinking water supplies of their enemies with animal corpses in 300 BC [6]. Romans and Persians subsequently performed similar arts. The poisoning of potable water was used as a calculated and effective method of gaining advantage in warfare throughout the Classical, Medieval, and Renaissance periods. In more modern times, the bodies of sheep and pigs to pollute drinking water were used during the US Civil War at Vicksburg in 1863. Pungi sticks smeared with excrement were used by Vietcong until the 1960s [7].

During the Middle Ages, military leaders recognized that victims of disease (infection) themselves could be used for transmission. The use of catapults and siege machines was introduced as the new technology for biological warfare [4]. In 1346, the plague-weakened Tartar forces catapulted their victims into the town of Kaffa (now Feodosia, Ukraine) [8]. An epidemic of plague in the defending forces resulted in a retreat of the Genoese and led to the conquest of Kaffa. This event is believed to have contributed to the second plague pandemic when the ships carrying plague-infected refugees and rats sailed to Constantinople, Genoa, Venice, and other Mediterranean ports (Fig. 1). In 1422, bodies of dead soldiers and cartloads of excrement were hurled onto the enemy side at Carolstein, further contributing to the 25 million deaths in Europe during the Black

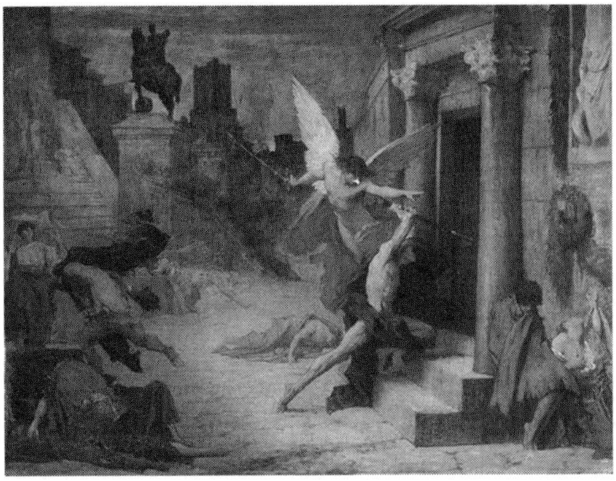

Fig. 1. The Angel of Death (*Peste a Roma*). (The Plague in Rome, Jules-Élie Deluanay, 1869.)

Death. In 1710, during a battle against Swedish forces in Revat, Russian troops resorted to throwing plague victims over the city walls.

The indigenous people of Central and South America were decimated by diseases such as measles and smallpox brought to them by the Spanish conquistadors [4,9]. The use of smallpox victims and their fomites in the New World during the North American Indian wars received notoriety similar to what plague had received in the Old World. During the French and Indian Wars (1754–1767), smallpox-laden blankets were offered to the Indians. The transmission by fomites would have been far less efficient, however, than that by respiratory droplets in the chain of natural transmission. Additionally, the nature of the biologic agents in these materials was largely unknown. These recorded events illustrate the complex nature of disease and epidemiology related to biologic agents. It was and remains difficult to differentiate endemic disease from that caused by deliberate use of infected materials.

Postbacterial cultivation era

The modern era of biological weapons development can be said to have started with the development of the science of bacteriology in the nineteenth century. *Bacillus anthracis* was the first specific microbial agent connected to human disease in 1877, when it was shown by Koch to fulfill his own postulates. Relatively simple cultivation methods started the use of laboratory-grown bacteria, rather than use of the victims of disease or crude infected materials from them. Germany was accused of introducing cholera in Italy and plague in St. Petersburg, Russia, sometime in 1915. Germany developed an ambitious biological warfare program early on during World War I. *B anthracis* and *Burkholderia mallei* were cultivated to infect Romanian sheep for export to Russia [10]. The cultures after being confiscated were identified at the Bucharest Institute of Bacteriology and Pathology.

Neutral trading partners were used to conduct covert operations to infect livestock and contaminate animal feed exported to the Allied Forces. The horror of chemical warfare superseded the impact of biologic agents during World War I. International diplomatic efforts directed at limiting the proliferation and use of weapons of mass destruction culminated in the 1925 Geneva Protocol for Prohibition of the use in war of asphyxiation, poisons or other gases and of biologic methods of warfare [11].

Post–World War I era

Research programs to develop biological weapons were started by many of the parties that ratified the Geneva Protocol at its inception in 1925. These included Belgium, Canada, France, Great Britain, Italy, Netherlands, Poland, and the Soviet Union. Japan conducted its biological weapons program largely under the auspices of Unit 731, a biological warfare research facility. This included 12 large-scale field trials of biological weapons during World War II. *B anthracis, Neisseria meningitidis, Shigella* spp, *Vibrio cholerae,* and *Yersinia pestis* were among the bacteria used [12]. Between 1932 and 1945, an estimated 10,000 prisoners died as a result of experimental infection or postexperimentation execution; 260,000 people died in 11 Chinese cities by contaminated water supplies and food items and spraying of pure cultures of *B anthracis, V cholerae, Shigella* spp, *Salmonella* spp, and *Y pestis*. Large numbers of infected laboratory-bred fleas were released over Chinese cities to initiate epidemic plague. The death and devastation caused by theses attacks attest to the simplicity and the diversity involved in the intentional use of microbial agents. A lesson learned (if it can be called one) was the fact that the perpetrator must be adequately trained and equipped for the hazards of biological weapons. An estimated 10,000 casualties and 1700 deaths occurred among Japanese troops in 1942 mostly as a result of cholera because they had not been trained and equipped adequately for the hazards of biological weapons.

Germany conducted experiments using *Rickettsia prowazekii, Rickettsia mooseri,* hepatitis A virus, and *Plasmodium* spp on prisoners in Nazi concentration camps to study pathogenesis and to develop vaccines. The Weil Felix test was used by the German army to avoid areas with epidemic typhus. Physicians used Proteus Ox-19 as a vaccine to induce false-positive serologic reactions for typhus to save people from deportation.

The Allies developed a biological weapons program for potential retaliatory use in response to the feared German biologic attacks. Experiments using weaponized spores of *B anthracis* were conducted on Gruinard Island near the coast of Scotland [13]. They revealed the extensive longevity of viable anthrax spores in the environment. The US Offensive Biological Program was started in 1942 under the direction of the War Reserve Service, a civilian agency [5]. Under this program, lethal agents such as *B anthracis, Botulinum* toxin, and *Francisella tularensis* and incapacitating agents such as

Brucella suis, Coxiella burnetti, Staphylococcus enterotoxin B, and Venezuelan equine encephalitis. Rice Blast, Rye Stem Rust, and Wheat Stem Rust were stockpiled as anticrop agents, but not weaponized. Aerosolization and dispersal methods were studied using simulants such as *Serratia marcecsens* in cities such as New York and San Francisco. An outbreak of urinary tract infection caused by *S marcescens* occurred at Stanford University Hospital during this period. The *Washington Post* reported a connection between these covert experiments and the outbreak of "Nosocomial Urinary Tract Infection" much later in 1976. The German biological weapons threat during World War II did not materialize [14]. The US Offensive Biological Weapons Program was expanded during the Korean War (1950–1953). Despite allegations, the United States denied using biological weapons against North Korea and China. President Nixon's executive orders in 1969 and 1970 terminated the US Offensive Biological Weapons Program. The ban was extended to include toxins 3 months later. The US Defensive Bioweapons program was maintained at the US Army Medical Research Institute for Infectious Diseases (USAMRIID) at Fort Detrick, Maryland.

The origin of the former Soviet Union's biological weapons program dates back to statements made by Lenin. Experimental work was started in the 1920s; however, post–World War II military building programs ushered in the modern era for biological weapons development [15]. The Soviet Agency Biopreparat was designed to carry out an offensive biological weapons program concealed behind civil biotechnology research. The first visit to the Biopreparat facilities was undertaken by a joint United States and United Kingdom technical team in 1991. Substantial changes occurred within the Biopreparat by the mid-1990s, which led to a concerted effort to help the Russians civilianize former biological weapons research and development establishments. The status of one of Russia's most sophisticated and largest former biological weapons facilities called Vector in Koltsovo is of particular concern. In addition to being one of the two facilities in the world that housed smallpox virus, work on Ebola, Marburg, and other hemorrhagic fever viruses was conducted at Vector [16,17]. It has not been determined with confidence that this is the only storage site for smallpox virus outside of the CDC in the United States. Many scientists from the Soviet facilities have defected to other parts of the world. No one is clear where the others have gone.

Iraq's biological weapons program started in 1974 after the Biological and Toxin Weapons Convention had been signed. In 1995, Iraq confirmed that it had been engaged in producing and deploying bombs, rockets, and aircraft spray tanks containing *B anthracis* and botulinum toxin [18].

The number of countries engaged in biological weapons experimentation grew from 4 in the 1960s to 11 in the 1990s [19]. An estimated 10 and possibly 17 nations possess biological warfare agents [20]. At least five of the seven countries listed by the US Department of State as sponsoring international terrorism are suspected to have biological warfare programs [21–23].

With the ease and low cost of cultivating and transporting microorganisms came threats and actual use of biologic agents by well-financed organizations and dissident groups to accomplish political goals and to make social statements [24,25]. Table 1 summarizes some documented attempts between 1979 and 2001. Although many such attempts do not reach the level of national and international security and response, they do require public health preparedness at the local level. Active surveillance and rapid response at the local level form the cornerstones for preparedness for all types of biologic threats, including natural infectious diseases.

Biological weapons system components

The biological weapons system comprises four components: (1) The biologic material itself consisting of the infectious agent or a toxin produced by bacteria, plants, or animals is the payload. (2) Munitions are the agents that carry, protect, and maintain the virulence of the payload during delivery. (3) The delivery system can range from a missile, a vehicle (aircraft, boat, automobile, or truck), an artillery shell, an expendable soldier or martyr, to everyday postal mail as was the case in the 2001 anthrax incidents. (4) The dispersion system ensures dissemination of the payload at and around the target site among susceptible populations [26–28].

Potential methods of dispersion include aerosol sprays, explosives, and food and water contamination [29]. Aerosol sprays are the most likely method to be used in a potential bioterrorism attack because they are the most effective means of widespread dissemination. Many factors, such as particle size and stability of the agent under prevailing environmental conditions, the wind speed and direction, and atmospheric stability, can alter the effectiveness of a delivery system. Under optimal conditions, the use of hardy organisms would allow clouds of infectious material to travel several hundred kilometers and be delivered to the terminal airways when inhaled. Knowledge of the natural lag time for infection to become disease during the incubation period (3–7 days for most pathogens) would allow planning and safe escape for terrorists before the recognition of the attack. Explosives are likely to inactivate biologic materials from heat and physical stress and are an ineffective means of dispersion. Such a use still would create panic, terror, unnecessary use of resources, and civil disruption, however. Potable water also would be an ineffective dispersal system, unless the agent is introduced after the water passes through the purification facilities or into smaller reservoirs. Effective contamination of large water supplies generally would require an unrealistically large amount of the payload. Foods contaminated immediately before consumption are more effective in transmitting infectious agents, as was the case with the 1984 and 1997 incidents listed in Table 1. The use of the US Post Office mail service to disseminate anthrax spores has revealed the potential of novel delivery and dispersion systems. Biologic agents contained in pellets and flechettes also have been used in incidents involving individuals. Combined with conventional weapons, the mass casualty potential of the payload (biologic agents) can be expected to increase significantly. Categorization, prioritization, and surveillance of potential bioterrorism agents is described in another article in this issue.

Bioterrorism preparedness

Rationale

Infectious diseases, naturally occurring and intentionally disseminated, have been designated as an issue of national security and an issue of major public health concern by the National Intelligence Council for the Central Intelligence Agency. In addition to the rapid mass casualty effect, biologic agents can overwhelm services and the health care system of communities. Most of the civilian population in the United States is susceptible to the infections caused by category A biologic agents, and these agents are expected to cause high morbidity and mortality. The economic impact of a biologic attack involving potential exposure to anthrax has been estimated to be $26.2 billion/100,000 persons exposed [30]. To this would be added the cost and resources needed to decontaminate the environment, depending on the agent. After the 2001 anthrax attacks through the US Postal Service, the estimated cost of decontaminating parts of the Hart Senate building in Washington, DC, was $23 million. The model described by Kaufmann and associates [30] provides justification for programs involving prevention and postattack interventions for potential bioterrorism agents. Improved public health infrastructure and preparedness for potential agents of bioterrorism would add significantly to global defense against infectious disease threats in general.

Obstacles

In most parts of the world, the capacity to detect and respond to epidemics of infectious diseases is still lacking or rudimentary. It would be even more difficult for these localities to respond to and manage potential bioterrorism events [31]. The World Health Organization (WHO) established a community registry of births and deaths and a community-based early warning surveillance and response system for priority infectious diseases in Uganda during the Ebola outbreak [32]. This simple and cost-effective measure subsequently helped in the detection of new cases of hemorrhagic fever by the local staff.

The National Association of Counties in the United States conducted a survey of the Directors of County Public Health Departments about their level of preparedness to respond to a biologic or chemical terrorism event

Table 1
Examples of political attempts at bioterrorism

Year	Group	Attempt	Outcome
1970	Weather Underground	A US revolutionary group intended to obtain agents from Ft. Detrick by blackmail and to incapacitate US cities temporarily to demonstrate the "impotence of the federal government"	Report originated with a US Customs informant. The case later appeared to be apocryphal
1972	R.I.S.E.	A group of college students influenced by ecoterrorist ideology and 1960s drug culture planned to use agents of typhoid fever, diphtheria, dysentery, and meningitis, initially to target the entire world population, but later narrowed the plan to five cities near Chicago	The attack was aborted when cultures were discarded
1978	Unknown	Bulgarian defector Georgi Markov was assassinated in London when a spring-loaded device disguised in an umbrella was used to implant a ricin-filled pellet in his thigh	Similar device used against a second defector in the same area was unsuccessful
1979	Accidental	Accidental release of anthrax spores from a bioweapons facility in Sverdlovsk, Russia, caused an epidemic of inhalational anthrax	At least 77 cases and 60 deaths
1980	Red Army Faction	Members of a Marxist revolutionary ideology group allegedly cultivated botulinum toxin in a safe house in Paris and planned attacks against at least nine German officials and civilian leaders	This probably was an erroneous report, later repudiated by the German government
1984	Rajneeshee Cult	An Indian religious cult headed by Rajneesh plotted to contaminate a restaurant salad bar in Dalles, Oregon, with *Salmonella typhimurium*. The motivation was to incapacitate voters, win local elections, and seize political control of the county	The incident resulted in a large community outbreak of salmonellosis involving 751 patients and at least 45 hospitalizations. The plot was revealed when the cult collapsed and members turned informants

1991	Minnesota Patriots Council	A right-wing "Patriot" movement obtained ricin extracted from castor beans by mail order. They planned to deliver ricin through the skin with dimethyl sulfoxide and aloe vera or as dry aerosol against Internal Revenue Service officials, US Deputy Marshals, and local law enforcement officials	The group was infiltrated by Federal Bureau of Investigation informants
1995	Aum Shinrikyo	A New Age doomsday cult seeking to establish a theocratic state in Japan attempted at least 10 times to use anthrax spore, botulinum toxin, Q fever agent, and Ebola virus in aerosol form	Multiple chemical weapon attacks with sarin, Vx, and hydrogen cyanide in Matsumator and Tokyo and assassination campaigns were conducted. All attempts with use of biological weapons failed. The nerve gas sarin killed 12 and injured 5500 in a Tokyo subway
1997	Disgruntled employee in Texas	Intentional contamination of muffins and donuts with laboratory cultures of *Shigella dysenteriae*	Caused gastroenteritis in 45 laboratory workers, 4 of whom were hospitalized
2001	Unknown	Intentional dissemination of anthrax spores through the US Postal System led to the deaths of 5 people, infection of 22 others, and contamination of several government buildings	Investigation into the attacks so far has not reached a conclusion

Adapted from Khardori N, Kanchanapoom T. Overview of biological terrorism: potential agents and preparedness. Clin Microbiol News 2005;27:1–8; with permission.

[33]. Most reported being partially prepared, and more than 20%, particularly counties with less than 10,000 population, reported not being prepared at all. Insufficient funding, insufficient medical and administrative staff, and insufficient communication networks were cited as obstacles to preparedness. In a study of community reaction to simulated intentional aerosolized release of Rift Valley fever virus in a semirural community, DiGiovanni and colleagues [34] concluded that bioterrorism training should include information management, communications, and public affairs offices. A survey indicated that increased federal funding for state public health preparedness programs has led to an overall improvement in epidemiologic and surveillance capacity for potential bioterrorism agents [35]. There still remains a need for further increase in epidemiologists and other resources to meet federal terrorism preparedness program requirements. The lack of appreciation of just how different biologic attacks are from traditional threats by policy makers is also a serious obstacle. Numerous large-scale, expensive bioterrorism exercises have been conducted in the United States in recent years [36–40] to assess the level of preparedness and the impact of recent upgrading of programs. One of these was Atlantic Storm, an exercise using a simulated smallpox attack on several cities in Europe, the United States, and Canada [41]. The result indicated that no international organization, including NATO, the United Nations, or the European Union, can be relied on to handle the challenges posed by an attack penetrating simultaneously into several nations.

The dual-use capability of advanced biotechnology including genetic engineering is feared to create potential customized biologic agents with enhanced virulence, antibiotic resistance, and evasion from natural or vaccine-induced immunity [42]. Acquisition by terrorist groups of this technology or altered agents created by legitimate research would increase further the spectrum of potential agents of bioterrorism.

Avenues

Public health system

Recognition and training

Because potential bioterrorism attacks are likely to be unannounced and covert, they pose untested challenges to the emergency response system. Most biologic agents would not have an immediate impact, in contrast to bombings and chemical agents. The incubation period would delay the appearance of the first wave of victims, who would need to be recognized and reported by health care providers. The Department of Defense received $36 million in 1996 to initiate the Domestic Preparedness Program to enhance existing first responder training in dealing with terrorist incidents, including incidents involving biological weapons. The program trained responders from fire departments, law enforcement, hazardous materials, and emergency medical systems in the 120 largest cities in the United States [43,44]. The US Epidemic Intelligence Service managed by the CDC has provided training and disease detection expertise for more than 50 years. After the first wave of victims is identified, public health actions would include declaration of an attack, rapid identification of the likely agent, and institution of prevention and management strategies. Clues to a potential bioterrorism attack are listed in Box 1.

Box 1. Clues to a potential bioterrorism attack

Epidemiologic clues

1. Greater caseload than expected of a specific disease
2. Unusual clustering of disease for the geographic area
3. Disease occurrence outside of normal transmission season
4. Simultaneous outbreaks of different infectious diseases
5. Disease outbreak in humans after recognition of disease in animals
6. Unexplained number of dead animals or birds
7. Disease requiring for transmission a vector previously not seen in the area
8. Rapid emergence of genetically identical pathogen from different geographic areas

Medical clues

1. Unusual route of infection
2. Unusual age distribution or clinical presentation of common disease
3. More severe disease and higher fatality rate than expected
4. Unusual variants of organisms
5. Unusual antimicrobial susceptibility patterns
6. Single case of an uncommon disease

Miscellaneous clues

1. Intelligence report
2. Claims of a release
3. Discovery of munitions or tampering
4. Increased numbers of pharmacy orders for antibiotics and symptoms relief drugs
5. Increased number of 911 calls
6. Increased number of visits with similar symptoms to emergency departments and ambulatory health care facilities

---

Adapted from Khardori N. Historical perspective and overview. In: Khardori N, editor. Bioterrorism preparedness—medicine—public health policy. Weinheim: Wiley VCH; 2006. p. 43.

Emergency response capability

The National Disaster Medical System in the United States has voluntary access to approximately 100,000 hospital beds across the country to cope with large-scale medical emergencies [45,46]. Not all are equipped, however, with mechanical ventilators and other specialized supportive care devices that may be needed for critically ill victims. Localities would need to increase their own capability because the current federal plans favor freeing up local bed space for injured and affected individuals [47]. The CDC through its cooperative grant program with states and several large cities is establishing local bioterrorism preparedness programs [48].

Laboratory preparedness

Accurate and rapid identification of biologic agents or their products plays a pivotal role in the response to infectious disease outbreaks caused by known or new agents. Of the 174,000 laboratories operating in the United States, about 2000 are public health laboratories. The public health laboratory network of local, state, and federal laboratories works in an undefined collaboration with private clinical laboratories. The National Laboratory Response Network (LRN) for bioterrorism was started in the United States in 1999 as a part of the CDC's strategic plan for bioterrorism preparedness [49]. The LRN is divided into laboratories at levels A, B, C, and D with increasing stringent levels of safety, containment, and technical proficiency [50,51]. In addition, a rapid response laboratory initially processes samples from suspect cases, provides around-the-clock diagnostic support to bioterrorism teams, and maintains chain of custody of the materials under investigation [48]. All laboratories in the network are equipped with biosafety level 2 facilities. Hospital and other diagnostic laboratories with certified biologic safety cabinets are level A laboratories involved in ruling out or referring the critical agents to the nearest level B or level C laboratory. Levels B, C, and D of LRN have access to the biodetection assays and specialized reagents used in validated protocols for the confirmation of critical agents. The level B laboratories are state and public health laboratories with biosafety level 2 facilities where biosafety level 3 practices are observed. Level C laboratories are public health laboratories with biosafety level 3 facilities or certified animal facilities necessary for performing the mouse toxicity assay for botulinum toxin. Specimens suspected of containing anthrax spores are handled in the level C laboratories. Level D laboratories with biosafety level 4 facilities to handle agents such as smallpox and Ebola are the federal laboratories at the CDC and the USAMRIID. The state and territorial laboratories in the LRN are listed in Appendix A. The procedures and controls for biosafety levels 1 through 4 for microbiology laboratories are available from the CDC [52].

Biohazard containment—personal protective equipment, decontamination and infection control procedures

The Association of Professionals in Infection Control and Epidemiology and CDC prepared a bioterrorism readiness plan for health care facilities [53]. The currently used personal protective equipment in US health care facilities is adequate for dealing with infectious agents with various modes of transmission, including potential bioterrorism agents. Decontamination methods employed in the environmental control of infectious agents must be safe for humans and animals and the materials they are used on [54]. The decontamination methods that can be used for bioterrorism agents include the following: (1) Mechanical decontamination methods remove, but do not neutralize, the agents. Examples include filtration of drinking water, removal of aerosolized organisms by high-efficiency particulate air filters, and washing of skin surfaces with soap and water. (2) Chemical decontamination methods affect the viability of the biologic agents and render them harmless. Hypochlorite is a tested and safe chemical decontaminant for equipment and fabric clothing. A 5% hypochlorite solution with 30-minute contact time is effective. This should be followed by thorough rinsing and oiling of the metal surfaces to prevent corrosion. The standard stock Clorox is a 5.25% solution of sodium hypochlorite. Diluting it with 9 parts of water (1:9) makes a 0.5% solution, which should be prepared fresh to maintain an alkaline pH. For gross contamination of skin surfaces, a 0.5% sodium hypochlorite solution with contact time of 10 to 15 minutes is recommended. Its use is contraindicated for open body cavity wounds because of the risk of adhesion formation and for brain and spinal cord injuries. (3) Physical decontamination methods (eg, heat and radiation) can be employed for decontamination of objects. For sterilization of objects, dry heat at 100°C for 2 hours or autoclaving with steam at 121°C and 15 lb per square inch pressure for 20 to 30 minutes are used. Desiccation and solar UV radiation can be relied on along with oxidation for the natural inactivation of biologic agents in the outdoor environment. Based on simulant studies, secondary reaerosolization is not considered a human health hazard. Chlorine-calcium or lye can be used for environmental decontamination. Dust binding sprays can be used to minimize reaerosolization.

Standard precautions are employed in the care of all patients in health care facilities. The most stringent patient-isolation precautions are needed for agents that can be transmitted person to person by the respiratory route. Isolation precautions other than the standard precautions are applied to infectious agents based on their most likely mode of transmission (Table 2).

Pharmaceutical readiness

The pharmacologic interventions following a bioterrorism event would include the following:

Table 2
Patient isolation precautions[a]

Type	Precautions	Comment
Standard	Wash hands after patient contact. Wear gloves when touching blood, body fluids, secretions, excretions, and contaminated items. Wear a mask and eye protection or a face shield during procedures likely to generate splashes or sprays of blood, body fluids, secretions, or excretions Handle used patient care equipment and linen in a manner that prevents the transfer of microorganisms to people or equipment	Use care when handling sharps, and use a mouthpiece or other ventilation device as an alternative to mouth-to-mouth resuscitation when practical. *Standard precautions are employed in the care of all patients.*
Contact	Standard precautions *plus*: Place the patient in a private room or cohort with someone with the same infection if possible. Wear gloves when entering the room. Change gloves after contact with infective material. Wear a gown when entering the room if contact with patient is anticipated or if the patient has diarrhea, a colostomy, or wound drainage not covered by a dressing. Limit the movement or transport of the patient from the room. Ensure that patient care items, bedside equipment, and frequently touched surfaces receive daily cleaning. Dedicate use of noncritical patient care equipment (eg, stethoscopes) to a single patient or cohort of patients with the same pathogen. If not feasible, adequate disinfection between patients is necessary	Conventional diseases requiring contact precautions: MRSA, VRE, *Clostridium difficile*, RSV, parainfluenza, enteroviruses, enteric infections in the incontinent host, skin infections (SSSS, HSV, impetigo, lice, scabies), hemorrhagic conjunctivitis. Biothreat diseases requiring contact Precautions: viral hemorrhagic fevers and draining anthrax lesions
Droplet	Standard precautions *plus*: Place the patient in a private room or cohort with someone with the same infections. If not feasible, maintain at least 3 ft between patients. Wear a mask when working within 3 ft of the patient. Limit movement and transport of the patient. Place a mask on the patient if he or she needs to be moved	Conventional diseases requiring droplet precautions: Invasive *Haemophilus influenzae* and meningococcal disease, drug-resistant pneumococcal disease, diphtheria, pertussis, mycoplasma, GABHS, influenza, mumps, rubella, parvovirus. Biothreat diseases requiring droplet precautions: pneumonic plague

Table 2 (*continued*)

Type	Precautions	Comment
Airborne	Standard precautions *plus*: Place the patients in a private room that has monitored negative air pressure, a minimum of 6 air changes/hour, and appropriate filtration of air before it is discharged from the room. Wear respiratory protection when entering the room. Limit movement and transport of the patient. Place a mask on the patient if he or she needs to be moved	Conventional diseases requiring airborne precautions: measles, Varicella, pulmonary tuberculosis. Biothreat diseases requiring airborne precautions: Smallpox

Abbreviations: HSV, herpes simplex virus; MRSA, methicillin-resistant *Staphylococcus aureus*; RSV, respiratory syncytial virus; SSSS, staphylococcal scalded-skin syndrome; VRE, vancomycin-resistant enterococci.

[a] A new set of guidelines has been proposed by the CDC, and public comments are being reviewed. The final guideline will be published following revisions.

Adapted from Khardori N, and Kanchanapoom, T. *Overview of biological terrorism: potential agents and preparedness*. Clin Microbiol News, 2005;27:1–8; with permission.

1. Antimicrobial treatment and prophylaxis. The antimicrobial agents of choice for potential bioterrorism agents in a mass casualty setting have been described and discussed extensively [55–58]. These recommendations are based on known patterns of antimicrobial susceptibility and the possibility of genetically altered organisms with resistance to otherwise effective agents. The same agents are recommended for treatment and mass chemoprophylaxis except that only oral agents would be practical for mass prophylaxis. Antibiotic use in large groups of people for extended periods has the inherent disadvantages of side effects, intolerances, noncompliance, and development of resistance.
2. Vaccines. Because diseases caused by potential bioterrorism agents are no longer seen in the US population, routine immunization except in the military personnel is not practiced. Currently, vaccines for human use are available for anthrax and smallpox. The issues pertaining to the civilian use of these two vaccines are discussed in other articles in this issue. Anthrax vaccines with fewer number of injections and better efficacy are under development.
3. Passive immunization (preformed antibody) for immediate protection. Specific antibodies are known to be effective against major potential agents of bioterrorism, including anthrax, smallpox, botulinum toxin, tularemia, and plague [59]. Passive immunization is more effective for prevention and modifying the natural course of infectious diseases than for treatment. The antibody-based therapies are costly, and their development has been hindered by small market size and availability of many antimicrobial agent classes in the recent years. The usefulness

of passive antibody therapy can be enhanced by developing monoclonal antibodies with capability to neutralize virulence factors (eg, anthrax toxin). In addition to providing immediate protection to individuals at the highest risk, this intervention would provide additional time for active immunization against vaccine-preventable diseases.

Stockpiles containing supplies, antimicrobial agents, and vaccines have been created by the Department of Health and Human Services (HHS) and are maintained by the CDC [37]. The national pharmaceutical stockpile is bundled into "push packs" that can be deployed by commercial cargo to the scene of a biologic attack within 12 hours of request by a state. Vendor managed inventory, maintained by pharmaceutical manufacturers, is a follow-up component to the national pharmaceutical stockpile. These materials are shipped to the site of a bioterrorism event within 24 to 36 hours of a request.

Controlled studies in humans evaluating antimicrobial agents and vaccines for bioterrorism-related pathogens are not feasible [60]. The off-label use of therapeutic agents may become necessary, but should be minimized. Infectious diseases specialists and experts at the CDC and the Food and Drug Administration (FDA) should be consulted. The presidential executive order 13,139, issued on September 30, 1999, outlines the conditions under which off-label pharmaceuticals and investigational new drugs can be administered to US servicemen [54]. An informed consent must be obtained from the service member, unless it is not feasible or is contrary to the best interests of the service member or national security. The FDA is part of an interagency group preparing for response in a civilian emergency [61]. The FDA has proposed standards for the use of animal efficacy data as a surrogate for clinical trials when appropriate. The manufacturers still would be expected to provide conventional data to show safety of any agent and immunogenicity of candidate vaccines in humans.

Public health laws

The need for updating state, federal, and international public health laws has come into clear focus because of the potential of speedy transmission and potential of mass casualties related to bioterrorism agents and naturally emerging infectious disease threats. In the United States, the power to act to preserve the public's health is constitutionally an exercise of "Police Powers" by the states. In the aftermath of September 11, 2001, the Model State Emergency Health Powers Act, or the Model Act, was drafted to update the state public health statutes. The modernization of these statutes was designed to avoid problems of inconsistency, inadequacy, and obsolescence [3]. The Model Act is structured to facilitate five basic public health functions: preparedness; surveillance, management of property; protection of persons (including powers to compel vaccination, testing, treatment, isolation, and quarantine when clearly indicated); and communication. Concerns have been raised about the impact of the Model Act on personal rights and civil liberties [62]. As of this writing, 33 states and the District of Columbia have passed bills or resolutions containing provisions from the Model Act.

Some authorities argue that management of response to bioterrorism by federal rather than state authorities would ensure larger financial resources and avoid confusion. The US Defense Against Weapons of Mass Destruction Act (1996) designated the Department of Defense as the lead agency to enhance domestic preparedness for responding to and managing the consequences of intentional use of weapons of mass destruction [37]. The "Select Agent Program" regulations came into effect on April 15, 1997. The act mandates registration of laboratories that possess, transfer, or receive select biologic agents (listed in section 72.6 of Title 42, Code of Federal Regulations) with the CDC [63]. The US Patriot Act was signed into law on October 26, 2001. This act amends the Biological Weapons Statute and criminalizes possession of such materials of a type or the quantity not reasonably justified by bona fide research or peaceful purpose. It also prohibits "restricted persons" from possession in a number of categories set forth in the act. The Public Health Security and Bioterrorism Preparedness and Response Act was signed into law on June 12, 2002. The act is designed to improve coordination of federal antibioterrorism activities, address shortages of specific types of health professionals, protect the nation's food and water supply, and speed up the development of new drugs and vaccines, all with the purpose of improving the health care system's ability to respond to bioterrorism. The American Society for Microbiology worked closely with legislators in drafting Title II of this law to balance public health concerns over safety and security with the need to protect the use of biologic agents in legitimate scientific research and diagnostic testing. The law requires all person possessing biologic agents or toxins deemed a threat to human health to notify the secretary of HHS (HHS select agents and toxins). All persons possessing biologic agents or toxins deemed a threat to animal or plant health or their products are required to notify the Secretary of the US Department of Agriculture (USDA Select Agents and Toxins). Both secretaries are to be notified by persons who possess agents that appear on the HHS and USDA lists—designated as Overlap Select Agents and Toxins (Appendix B). The CDC and the Animal and Plant Health Inspection Service were designated by the HHS and USDA to implement the law [64].

One of the measures of the level of preparedness against infectious disease threats is the quality of, distribution of, and compliance with disease reporting laws [65]. A study of disease reporting laws in the United States commissioned by the CDC pointed to the need for revision or expansion or both of disease reporting requirements to include bioterrorism-associated diseases. The report suggested that the Model Act may be useful to states in readdressing their disease reporting laws. The enactment and enforcement of appropriate disease reporting laws may provide incentive for health care providers to obtain necessary training and skills for diagnosing and managing potential agents of bioterrorism. Because the incidence of disease caused by "critical biologic agents" is low in the United States, each individual case report initially should be considered a sentinel event requiring further investigation [66]. Numerous strategic administrative and legal steps have been recommended to prepare for potential bioterrorism attacks [67]. These steps include the laws and regulations governing the confidentiality of disease surveillance records and developing a legal and administrative procedure for sharing pertinent and relevant information with law enforcement agencies during a bioterrorism attack.

Bioterrorism preparedness—global avenues

With the level and state of global interconnectedness today, the spread of infectious diseases is easier than ever. Most countries where infectious diseases remain the most common cause of morbidity and mortality do not have an effective public health infrastructure or the resources to prepare against bioterrorism. The WHO has more than 50 years of experience providing response to outbreaks and preventing international spread of diseases [32]. The permanently located geographic resources of the WHO include the Geneva Headquarters, 6 regional offices, and 141 country offices. The country offices are primarily in areas with frequent epidemics and likelihood of emergence of new diseases. The WHO has 250 collaborating laboratories and institutions all over the world. The CDC provides direct secondment of staff in addition to a close working relationship with the WHO. Technical support to the WHO is provided by US agencies such as USAID, laboratories in the US Department of Defense Global Emerging Infections Surveillance and Response System, and their counterparts in other WHO member states. The National Institutes of Health through its Fogarty International Center, National Center for Environmental Prediction, NASA–Goddard Space Flight Center, and the State Departments Bureau of Population, Refugees and Migration are other US agencies that provide technical and financial support to the WHO.

The WHO is politically neutral and for many parts of the world the only or the most important source of authoritative advice and technical assistance needed for infectious disease outbreaks. The epidemiologic techniques and laboratory support needed for intentionally used biologic agents is similar to that used for natural outbreaks. WHO coordinates numerous electronic "detective" systems and databases for disease surveillance. The networks operate in real time and watch for known risks and unexpected or unusual disease events. Suspicious reports are investigated each morning by a team responsible for outbreak verification. The supreme governing body of the WHO, the World Health Assembly, adopted a consensus on global health security in May 2001. The WHO is now in a position to investigate and verify rumored outbreaks even before it receives an official notification from the concerned government. The formation of the Global Outbreak Alert and Response Network by the WHO has combined heightened vigilance with rapid response. Guidelines for the assisting foreign nationals during and after field operations in the host country also have been issued. People providing assistance to the WHO have the same privileges and protection in other countries as the WHO staff members.

To help countries strive toward self-sufficiency, the WHO strengthens their epidemiologic and laboratory capacity. Early Warning and Response Networks have been started in partnership with nongovernmental organizations in the field. Training Programs in Epidemiology and Public Health Interventions Network in collaboration with the CDC and a working group on long-term preparedness for outbreak response have been established. The WHO also makes efforts to make improvement in civil administrations with the potential of improving public health infrastructure (eg, the establishment of a community registry of births and deaths). The WHO manuals providing guidance on public health response to biologic and chemical weapons and laboratory safety have been updated recently [68,69]. Global support for vaccine development and equitable distribution to control vaccine-preventable diseases remains a challenge for the WHO.

Similar to state and national efforts, international efforts for protecting global health are governed by laws. These include the humanitarian laws during and after war, international laws and conventions (eg, Biological Weapons Convention) to counteract various types of threats, and the international health laws [70–72]. International Sanitary Regulations, later renamed the International Health Regulations (IHR), are the only legal instrument adapted by the WHO. The original IHR addressed only three diseases (cholera, yellow fever, and plague) and authorized WHO to use information provided by member states only. These regulations were considered outdated and ineffective given the current global infectious disease scene. Consequently, the IHR were revised and adapted by the World Health Assembly in 2005 [73].

Appendix A: State and territorial public health directors

Alabama

Department of Public Health
State Health Officer
Phone No. (334) 206-5200
Fax No. (334) 206-2008

Alaska

Division of Public Health
Alaska Department of Health and Social Services
Director
Phone No. (907) 465-3090
Fax No. (907) 586-1877

American Samoa

Department of Health
American Samoa Government
Director
Phone No. (684) 633-4606
Fax No. (684) 633-5379

Arizona

Arizona Department of Health Services
Director
Phone No. (602) 542-1025
Fax No. (602) 542-1062

Arkansas

Arkansas Department of Health
Director
Phone No. (501) 661-2417
Fax No. (501) 671-1450

California

California Department of Health Services
State Health Officer
Phone No. (916) 657-1493
Fax No. (916) 657-3089

Colorado

Colorado Department of Public Health and Environment
Executive Director
Phone No. (303) 692-2011
Fax No. (303) 691-7702

Connecticut

Connecticut Department of Public Health
Commissioner
Phone No. (860) 509-7101
Fax No. (860) 509-7111

Delaware

Division of Public Health
Delaware Department of Health and Social Services
Director

Phone No. (302) 739-4700
Fax No. (302) 739-6659

District of Columbia

DC Department of Health
Acting Director
Phone No. (202) 645-5556
Fax No. (202) 645-0526

Florida

Florida Department of Health
Secretary and State Health Officer
Phone No. (850) 487-2945
Fax No. (850) 487-3729

Georgia

Division of Public Health
Georgia Department of Human Resources
Director
Phone No. (404) 657-2700
Fax No. (404) 657-2715

Guam

Department of Public Health and Social Services
Government of Guam
Director of Health
Phone No. (671) 735-7102
Fax No. (671) 734-5910

Hawaii

Hawaii Department of Health
Director
Phone No. (808) 586-4410
Fax No. (808) 586-4444

Idaho

Division of Health
Idaho Department of Health and Welfare
Administrator
Phone No. (208) 334-5945
Fax No. (208) 334-6581

Illinois

Illinois Department of Public Health
Director of Public Health
Phone No. (217) 782-4977
Fax No. (217) 782-3987

Indiana

Indiana State Department of Health
State Health Commissioner
Phone No. (317) 233-7400
Fax No. (317) 233-7387

Iowa

Iowa Department of Public Health
Director of Public Health
Phone No. (515) 281-5605
Fax No. (515) 281-4958

Kansas

Kansas Department of Health and Environment
Director of Health
Phone No. (785) 296-1343
Fax No. (785) 296-1562

Kentucky

Kentucky Department for Public Health
Commissioner
Phone No. (502) 564-3970
Fax No. (502) 564-6533

Louisiana

Louisiana Department of Health and Hospitals
Assistant Secretary and State Health Officer
Phone No. (504) 342-8093
Fax No. (504) 342-8098

Maine

Maine Bureau of Health
Maine Department of Human Services
Director

Phone No. (207) 287-3201
Fax No. (207) 287-4631

Mariana Islands

Department of Public Health and Environmental Services
Commonwealth of the Northern Mariana Islands
Secretary of Health and Environmental Services
Phone No. (670) 234-8950
Fax No. (670) 234-8930

Marshall Islands

Republic of the Marshall Islands
Majuro Hospital
Minister of Health and Environmental Services
Phone No. (692) 625-3355
Fax No. (692) 625-3432

Maryland

Maryland Department of Health and Mental Hygiene
Secretary
Phone No. (410) 767-6505
Fax No. (410) 767-6489

Massachusetts

Massachusetts Department of Public Health
Commissioner
Phone No. (617) 624-5200
Fax No. (617) 624-5206

Michigan

Community Public Health Agency
Michigan Department of Community Health
Chief Executive and Medical Officer
Phone No. (517) 335-8024
Fax No. (517) 335-9476

Micronesia

Department of Health Services
FSM National Government
Secretary of Health

Phone No. (691) 320-2619
Fax No. (691) 320-5263

Minnesota

Minnesota Department of Health
Commissioner of Health
Phone No. (651) 296-8401
Fax No. (651) 215-5801

Mississippi

Mississippi State Department of Health
State Health Officer and Chief Executive
Phone No. (601) 960-7634
Fax No. (601) 960-7931

Missouri

Missouri Department of Health
Director
Phone No. (573) 751-6001
Fax No. (573) 751-6041

Montana

Montana Department of Public Health & Human Services
Director
Phone No. (406) 444-5622
Fax No. (406) 444-1970

Nebraska

Nebraska Health and Human Services System
Chief Medical Officer
Phone No. (402) 471-8399
Fax No. (402) 471-9449

Nevada

Division of Health
Nevada State Department of Human Resources
State Health Officer
Phone No. (702) 687-3786
Fax No. (702) 687-3859

New Hampshire

New Hampshire Department of Health and Human Services
Medical Director
Phone No. (603) 271-4372
Fax No. (603) 271-4827

New Jersey

New Jersey Department of Health and Senior Services
Commissioner of Health
Phone No. (609) 292-7837
Fax No. (609) 292-0053

New Mexico

New Mexico Department of Health
Secretary
Phone No. (505) 827-2613
Fax No. (505) 827-2530

New York

New York State Department of Health
ESP-Corning Tower, 14th Floor
Albany, NY 12237
Commissioner of Health
Phone No. (518) 474-2011
Fax No. (518) 474-5450

North Carolina

NC Department of Health and Human Services
State Health Director
Phone No. (919) 733-4392
Fax No. (919) 715-4645

North Dakota

North Dakota Department of Health
State Health Officer
Phone No. (701) 328-2372
Fax No. (701) 328-4727

Ohio

Ohio Department of Health
Director of Health

Phone No. (614) 466-2253
Fax No. (614) 644-0085

Oklahoma

Oklahoma State Department of Health
Commissioner of Health
Phone No. (405) 271-4200
Fax No. (405) 271-3431

Oregon

Oregon Health Division
Oregon Department of Human Resources
Administrator
Phone No. (503) 731-4000
Fax No. (503) 731-4078

Palau, Republic of

Ministry of Health
Republic of Palau
Minister of Health
Phone No. (680) 488-2813
Fax No. (680) 488-1211

Pennsylvania

Pennsylvania Department of Health
Secretary of Health
Phone No. (717) 787-6436
Fax No. (717) 787-0191

Puerto Rico

Puerto Rico Department of Health
Secretary of Health
Phone No. (787) 274-7602
Fax No. (787) 250-6547

Rhode Island

Rhode Island Department of Health
Director of Health
Phone No. (401) 277-2231
Fax No. (401) 277-6548

South Carolina

SC Department of Health and Environmental Control
Commissioner
Phone No. (803) 734-4880
Fax No. (803) 734-4620

South Dakota

South Dakota State Department of Health
Secretary of Health
Phone No. (605) 773-3361
Fax No. (605) 773-5683

Tennessee

Tennessee Department of Health
State Health Officer
Phone No. (615) 741-3111
Fax No. (615) 741-2491

Texas

Department of Health
Commissioner of Health
Phone No. (512) 458-7375
Fax No. (512) 458-7477

Utah

Utah Department of Health
Director
Phone No. (801) 538-6111
Fax No. (801) 538-6306

Vermont

Vermont Department of Health
Commissioner
Phone No. (802) 863-7280
Fax No. (802) 865-7754

Virgin Islands

Virgin Islands Department of Health
Commissioner of Health
Phone No. (340) 774-0117
Fax No. (340) 777-4001

Virginia

Virginia Department of Health
State Health Commissioner
Phone No. (804) 786-3561
Fax No. (804) 786-4616

Washington

Washington State Department of Health
Acting Secretary of Health
Phone No. (360) 753-5871
Fax No. (360) 586-7424

West Virginia

Bureau for Public Health
WV Department of Health and Human Resources
Commissioner of Health
Phone No. (304) 558-2971
Fax No. (304) 558-1035

Wisconsin

Division of Health
Wisconsin Department of Health and Family Services
Administrator
Phone No. (608) 266-1511
Fax No. (608) 267-2832

Wyoming

Wyoming Department of Health
Director
Phone No. (307) 777-7656
Fax No. (307) 777-7439

From USAMRIID's medical management of biological casualties handbook. 5th edition. Fort Detrick (MD): US Army Medical Research Institute of Infectious Diseases; 2004.

Appendix B: Select agents and toxins

HHS select agents and toxins

Abrin
Cercopithecine herpesvirus 1 (herpes B virus)
Coccidioides posadasii

Conotoxins
Crimean-Congo hemorrhagic fever virus
Diacetoxyscirpenol
Ebola viruses
Lassa fever virus
Marburg virus
Monkeypox virus
Ricin
Rickettsia prowazekii
Rickettsia rickettsii
Saxitoxin
Shiga-like ribosome-inactivating proteins
South American hemorrhagic fever viruses
- Flexal
- Guanarito
- Junin
- Machupo
- Sabia

Tetrodotoxin
Tick-borne encephalitis complex (flavi) viruses
- Central European tick-borne encephalitis
- Far Eastern tick-borne encephalitis
- Kyasanur Forest disease
- Omsk hemorrhagic fever
- Russian spring and summer encephalitis

Variola major virus (smallpox virus)
Variola minor virus (alastrim)
Yersinia pestis

Overlap select agents and toxins

Bacillus anthracis
Botulinum neurotoxins
Botulinum neurotoxin–producing species of *Clostridium*
Brucella abortus
Brucella melitensis
Brucella suis
Burkholderia mallei (formerly *Pseudomonas mallei*)
Burkholderia pseudomallei (formerly *Pseudomonas pseudomallei*)
Clostridium perfringens epsilon toxin
Coccidioides immitis
Coxiella burnetii
Eastern equine encephalitis virus
Francisella tularensis
Hendra virus

Nipah virus
Rift Valley fever virus
Shigatoxin
Staphylococcal enterotoxins
T-2 toxin
Venezuelan equine encephalitis virus

USDA select agents and toxins

African horse sickness virus
African swine fever virus
Akabane virus
Avian influenza virus (highly pathogenic)
Bluetongue virus (exotic)
Bovine spongiform encephalopathy agent
Camel pox virus
Classic swine fever virus
Cowdria ruminantium (heartwater)
Foot-and-mouth disease virus
Goat pox virus
Japanese encephalitis virus
Lumpy skin disease virus
Malignant catarrhal fever virus (Alcelaphine herpesvirus type 1)
Menangle virus
Mycoplasma capricolum/M.F38/*M. mycoides capri* (contagious caprine pleuropneumonia)
Mycoplasma mycoides mycoides (contagious bovine pleuropneumonia)
Newcastle disease virus (velogenic)
Peste des petits ruminants virus
Rinderpest virus
Sheep pox virus
Swine vesicular disease virus
Vesicular stomatitis virus (exotic)

USDA plant protection and quarantine (PPQ) select agents and toxins

Candidatus Liberobacter africanus
Candidatus Liberobacter asiaticus
Peronosclerospora philippinensis
Ralstonia solanacearum race 3, biovar 2
Schlerophthora rayssiae var *zeae*
Synchytrium endobioticum
Xanthomonas oryzae pv. *oryzicola*
Xylella fastidiosa (citrus variegated chlorosis strain)

References

[1] Centers for Disease Control and Prevention. US Department of Health and Human Services, the public health response to biological and chemical terrorism, interim planning guidance for state public health officials. 2001. Available at: http://www.be.cdc.gov/Documents/Planning/PlanningGuidance.
[2] Drexler M. Secret agents: the menace of emerging infections. Washington, DC: Joseph Henry Press; 2002.
[3] Gostin LO, Sapsin JW, Teret SP, et al. The model state emergency health powers act: planning for and response to bioterrorism and naturally occurring infectious diseases. JAMA 2002;288:622–8.
[4] Eitzen EM, Takafuji ET. Historical overview of biological warfare. In: Sidell FR, Takafuju EF, Franz DR, editors. Medical aspects of chemical and biological warfare: textbook of military medicine part I: warfare, weaponry and the casualty. Washington, DC: Borden Institute; 1997. p. 415–23.
[5] Christopher GW, Cieslak TJ, Pavlin JA, et al. Biological warfare: a historical perspective. JAMA 1997;278:412–7.
[6] Poupard J, Miller L. History of biological warfare: catapults to capsomers. Ann N Y Acad Sci 1992;666:9–20.
[7] Stubbs M. Has the West an Achilles heel: possibilities of biological weapons. NATO's Fifteen Nations 1962;7:94–9.
[8] Derbes VJ. De Mussis and the great plague of 1348: a forgotten episode of bacteriological warfare. JAMA 1966;96:179–82.
[9] Hopkins DR. Princes and peasants: smallpox in history. Chicago: University of Chicago Press; 1983.
[10] Hugh-Jones M. Wickham Steed and German biological warfare research. Intell Natl Secur 1992;7:379–402.
[11] Geissler E. Biological and toxin weapons: research, development and use from the Middle Ages to 1945. In: SIPRI Chemical and Biological Warfare Studies. No. 16. New York: Oxford University Press; 1986.
[12] Harris S. Japanese biological warfare research on humans: a case study of microbiology and ethics. Ann N Y Acad Sci 1992;666:21–52.
[13] Manchee RJ, Steward R. The decontamination of Gruinard Island. Chem Br 1988;24:690–1.
[14] Nitscherlich A, Mielke F. Medizin ohne menschlichkeit: Dokuments des Nurnberger Arzteprozesses. Frankfurt am Main: Fischer Taxchenbuchverla; 1983.
[15] Davis CJ. Nuclear blindness: an overview of the biological weapons program of the former Soviet Union and Iraq. Emerg Infect Dis 1999;5:509–12.
[16] Henderson DA. Bioterrorism as a public health threat. Emerg Infect Dis 1998;4:488–92.
[17] Henderson DA. Strengthening global preparedness for defense against infectious diseases threats. Hearing on the threat of bioterrorism and the spread of infectious disease, 1st Session, 107th Congress; 2001.
[18] Zalinskas RA. Iraq's biological weapons? The past or future? JAMA 1997;278:418–24.
[19] Rorberts B. New challenges and new policy priorities for the 1990's. In: Biologic weapons; weapons of the future. Washington, DC: Center for Strategic and International Studies; 1993.
[20] Bartlett JG. Update in infectious diseases. Ann Intern Med 1999;131:273–80.
[21] Carus WS. Bioterrorism and biocrimes: the illicit use of biological agents in the 20th century. Washington, DC: Center for Counterproliferation Research, National Defense University; 1999.
[22] Henderson DA. The looming threat of bioterrorism. Science 1999;283:1279–82.
[23] Kortepeter MG, Parker GW. Potential biological weapons threats. Emerg Infect Dis 1999;5:523–7.
[24] Relman DA, Olson JE. Bioterrorism preparedness: what practitioners need to know. Infect Med 2001;18:497–514.

[25] Tucker JB. Historical trends related to bioterrorism: an empirical analysis. Emerg Infect Dis 1999;5:498–504.
[26] Khardori N, Kanchanapoom T. Overview of biological terrorism: potential agents and preparedness. Clin Microb News 2005;27:1–8.
[27] Stewart C. Toxins and biowarfare in biological warfare: preparing for the unthinkable emergency. In: Topics in Emergency Medicine, Vol II. Atlanta: American Health Consults; 2001.
[28] Hawley RJ, Eitzen EM Jr. Biological weapons—a primer for microbiologists. Annu Rev Microbiol 2001;55:235–53.
[29] Richards CF, Burstein JL, Waeckerle J, et al. Emergency physicians and biological terrorism. Ann Emerg Med 1999;34:182–90.
[30] Kaufmann AF, Meltzer MI, Schnid GP. The economic impact of a bioterrorist attack: are prevention and postattack intervention programs justifiable? Emerg Infect Dis 1997;3:83–94.
[31] Obstacles to biodefense [editorial]. Nature 2002;419:1.
[32] Heymann DL. Strengthening global preparedness for defense against infectious disease threats. Committee on Foreign Relations, United States Senate. Hearing on the threat of bioterrorism and the spread of infectious diseases. 1st Session, 107th Congress; 2001.
[33] NACo. County public health preparedness. 2002. Available at: www.naco.org/pubs/surveys/pubhealth/index.cfm.
[34] DiGiovanni C, Reynolds B, Harwell R, et al. Community reaction to bioterrorism: prospective study of simulated outbreak. Emerg Infect Dis 2003;9:708–12.
[35] Boulton MD, Abellera J, Lemmings J, et al. Terrorism and emergency preparedness in state and territorial public health departments—United States, MMWR 2005;54: 459–60.
[36] Lessons learned from a full-scale bioterrorism exercise. Emerg Infect Dis 2000;6:652–4.
[37] Inglesby TV, Grossman R, O'Toole R. A plague on your city: observations from TOPOFF. Clin Infect Dis 2001;32:436–44.
[38] O'Toole T, Mair M, Inglesby TV. Shining light on "Dark Winter." Clin Infect Dis 2002;34: 972–83.
[39] Atlas RM. Bioterrorism: from threat to reality. Annu Rev Microbiol 2002;56:167–85.
[40] Frase-Blunt M. "Operation TOPOFF 2" bioterrorism exercise offers educational lessons. AAMC Reporter; 2003. Available at: www.aamc/org/august03/bioterrorism.html.
[41] Nelson R. Simulation shows lack of readiness for bioterrorism attack. Lancet Infect Dis 2003;5:139.
[42] Dennis C. The bugs of war. Nature 2001;411:232–5.
[43] General Accounting Office. Combating terrorism: need to eliminate duplicate federal weapons of mass destruction training. [GAO/NSAID-00–64]. 2000.
[44] General Accounting Office. Combating terrorism: observations on the Nunn-Lugar-Domenici Domestic Preparedness Program. [GAO/T-NSAID-99–16]. 1998.
[45] Khardori N. Bioterrorism preparedness: historical prespective and overview. In: Khardori N, editor. Bioterrorism preparedness: medicine-public health-policy. Weinheim: Wiley-VCH; 2006.
[46] Siegrist DW. The threat of biological attack: why concern now. Emerg Infect Dis 1999;5: 505–8.
[47] Tonat K. Office of Emergency Preparedness, US Department of Health and Human Services panel discussion at conference "Integrating Medical and Emergency Response." Washington, DC; 1999.
[48] Khan AS, Morse S, Lillibridge S. Public-health preparedness for biological terrorism in the USA. Lancet 2000;356:1179–82.
[49] Centers for Disease Control and Prevention. Biological and chemical terrorism: strategic plan for preparedness and response. MMWR Morb Mortal Wkly Rep 2000;49(RR-4):1–14.
[50] Meyer RF. Bioterrorism preparedness for the public health and medical communities. Mayo Clin Proc 2002;77:619–21.

[51] Khardori N. Preparedness for bioterrorism. In: Meyers RA, editor. Encyclopedia of molecular cell biology and molecular medicine. Weinheim: Wiley-VCH; 2004. p. 507–28.
[52] LRN Network. 2004. Available at: http://www.cdc.gov/od/ohs/pdffiles/Module%202%20-%Biosafety.pdf and http://www.cdc.gov/od/ohs/biosfty/bmbl4bmbl4toc.htm.
[53] English JF, Cundiff MY, Malone JD, et al. Bioterrorism readiness plan: a template for healthcare facilities. APIC Bioterrorism Task Force and the CDC Hospital Infections Program Bioterrorism Working Group; 1999. p. 1–33.
[54] USAMRIID's medical management of biological casualties handbook. 5th edition. Fort Detrick (MD): US Army Medical Research Institute of Infectious Diseases; 2004.
[55] Inglesby TV, O'Toole T, Henderson DA, et al. Anthrax as a biological weapon—updated recommendations for management. In: Henderson DA, Inglesby TV, O'Toole T, editors. Bioterrorism: guidelines for medical and public health management. Chicago: American Medical Association; 2002. p. 66–98.
[56] Inglesby TV, Dennis DT, Henderson DA, et al. Plague as a biological weapon. In: Henderson DA, Inglesby TV, O'Toole T, editors. Bioterrorism: guidelines for medical and public health management. Chicago: American Medical Association; 2002. p. 121–40.
[57] Arnon SS, Schecter R, Inglesby TV, et al. Botulinum toxin as a biological weapon. In: Henderson DA, Inglesby TV, O'Toole T, editors. Bioterrorism: guidelines for medical and public health management. Chicago: American Medical Association; 2002. p. 141–66.
[58] Dennis DT, Inglesby TV, Henderson DA, et al. Tularemia as a biological weapon. In: Henderson DA, Inglesby TV, O'Toole T, editors. Bioterrorism: guidelines for medical and public health management. Chicago: American Medical Association; 2002. p. 167–90.
[59] Casadevall A. Passive antibody administration (immediate immunity) as a specific defense against biological weapons. Emerg Infect Dis 2002;8:833–84.
[60] McKinney WP, Bia FJ, Stewart CS, et al. Bioterrorism: an update for clinicians, pharmacists, and emergency management planners. Emergency medicine consensus reports. Atlanta: American Health Consultants; 2001.
[61] Zoon KC. Vaccines, pharmaceutical products and bioterrorism: challenges for the US Food and Drug Administration. Emerg Infect Dis 1999;5:534.
[62] Annas GJ. Bioterrorism, public health, and civil liberties. N Engl J Med 2002;346:1337–42.
[63] Department of Health and Human Services. Federal Register, 42 CFR 72; 2005.
[64] Centers for Disease Control and Prevention Select Agent Program. FAQ for new regulation. CDC Office of the Director; 2003. Available at: www.cdc.gov/od/sap/addres/htm.
[65] Horton HH, Misrahi JJ, Matthew GW, et al. Critical biological agents: disease reporting as a tool for determining bioterrorism preparedness. J Law Med Ethics 2002;30:262–6.
[66] Chang M, Glynn K, Groseclose SL. Endemic, notifiable bioterrorism-related diseases, United States, 1992–1999. Emerg Infect Dis 2003;9:556–63.
[67] Hoffman RE. Preparing for a bioterrorist attack: legal and administrative strategies. Emerg Infect Dis 2003;9:241–5.
[68] World Health Organization. Public health response to biological and chemical weapons. WHO guidance; 2004. Available at: http://www.who.int/csr/delibepidemics/biochemguide/en/index.html.
[69] World Health Organization. Laboratory biosafety manual. 3rd edition. 2004. Available at: http://www.who.int/csr/resources/publications/biosafety/Biosafety7.pdf.
[70] Laws, war, and public health [editorial]. Lancet 2003;361:1399.
[71] Holdstock D. Reacting to terrorism: the response should be through law not war. BMJ 2001; 323:822.
[72] Fidler DP. Emerging trends in international law concerning global infectious disease control. Emerg Infect Dis 2003;9:285–90.
[73] Sliverman R. Legal preparedness: the modelization of state, national and international public health law. In: Khardori N, editor. Bioterrorism preparedness: medicine-public health-policy. Weinheim: Wiley-VCH; 2006.

ELSEVIER
SAUNDERS

Infect Dis Clin N Am
20 (2006) 213–225

INFECTIOUS
DISEASE CLINICS
OF NORTH AMERICA

Categorization, Prioritization, and Surveillance of Potential Bioterrorism Agents

Stephanie M. Borchardt, PhD, MPH[a],
Kathleen A. Ritger, MD, MPH[a,b],
Mark S. Dworkin, MD, MPHTM[a,*]

[a]*Division of Infectious Diseases, Illinois Department of Public Health, 160 North LaSalle, 7th Floor South, Chicago, IL 60601, USA*
[b]*Epidemic Intelligence Service, Centers for Disease Control and Prevention, 1600 Clifton Road NE, Atlanta, GA 30333, USA*

Think of health surveillance as a set of medical smoke detectors, sounding the alarm before a deadly disease sweeps through an entire community.
Michael T. Osterholm, Washington Post, 2001

In response to global bioterrorism threats, the Centers for Disease Control and Prevention (CDC) created a list of critical biologic agents that have potential for use in bioterrorism [1–3]. This list includes a broad range of biologic agents, prioritized into three categories (A, B, or C) on the basis of their ability to cause illness and death, their capacity for dissemination, public perception as related to plausible civil disruption, and special needs required for effective public health intervention (Table 1) [1,4].

Agents in category A have the greatest potential for major public health impact with a high mortality rate. Most of these agents require special public health preparedness efforts, such as improved surveillance and laboratory diagnostic capability, and require stockpiling of specific medications. Category A agents also have a moderate to high potential for large-scale dissemination through methods such as aerosolization or relatively efficient

This manuscript was supported in part by an appointment to the Applied Epidemiology Fellowship Program administered by the Council of State and Territorial Epidemiologists and funded by the Centers for Disease Control and Prevention Cooperative Agreement U60/CCU007277.

* Corresponding author.
E-mail address: mdworkin@idph.state.il.us (M.S. Dworkin).

doi:10.1016/j.idc.2006.02.005

Table 1
Potential agents of bioterrorism by endemicity in the United States and mortality rate

Disease	Biologic agents	Endemic in United States	Mortality rate
Category A			
Smallpox	*Variola major*	No	30%–100% [8]
Anthrax	*Bacillus anthracis*	Midwest and western	Cutaneous, 5%–20% [9] Gastrointestinal, 25%–60% [8] Inhalational, 85% [8]
Plague	*Yersinia pestis*	Western	Bubonic, 50%–60%[a] Septicemic, 33% [8][a] Pneumonic, 50% [8][a]
Botulism	*Clostridium botulinum* (botulinum toxins)	Sporadic	5%–10% [9]
Tularemia	*Francisella tularensis*	West Central and Mountain regions and localized outbreaks at Martha's Vineyard, Massachusetts	5%–15% [9]
Viral hemorrhagic fevers	Filoviruses and Arenaviruses (eg, Ebola virus, Lassa virus)	No	Ebola, 50%–90% [8] Lassa fever, 15%–25% [8]
Category B			
Q fever	*Coxiella burnetii*	In locations where reservoir animals (eg, sheep, cattle) are present	<1%–2.4% [9]
Brucellosis	*Brucella spp*	In locations where reservoir animals (eg, cattle, swine) are present	≤2% [9]
Glanders	*Burkholderia mallei*	No	>50% [3]
Melioidosis	*Burkholderia pseudomallei*	No	19%–46% [8]
Viral encephalitis	*Alphaviruses* (EEE, VEE, WEE)	EEE, focally along eastern and gulf coasts VEE, no WEE, west of Mississippi river	EEE, 50%–70% [8] VEE, ≤1% [8] WEE, 3%–4% [8]
Typhus fever	*Rickettsia prowazekii*	No	10%–40% [9]
Toxic syndromes	Toxins (eg, Ricin, Staphylococcal enterotoxin B)	Sporadic	Ricin, 2%–6%[b] following ingestion Staphylococcal enterotoxin B, <1% [3]
Psittacosis	*Chlamydia psittaci*	Widespread	20% [8]

Table 1 (*continued*)

Disease	Biologic agents	Endemic in United States	Mortality rate
Foodborne illness	Food safety threats (eg, *Salmonella spp, Escherichia coli* O157:H7)	Widespread	*Salmonella spp,* 1%–21% [5] *E coli* O157:H7, 12% [8] with HUS
Waterborne illness	Water safety threats (eg, *Vibrio cholerae, Cryptosporidium parvum*)	*V cholerae, no* *C parvum*, widespread	*V cholerae,* 1%–> 50% [9] *C parvum,* rare [9]
Category C			
Nipah viral disease, Hantaviral disease	Emerging threat agents (eg, *Nipah virus, hantavirus*)	Nipah viral disease, no Hantaviral disease, mostly western and southwestern regions	Nipah viral disease, 18% [8] Hantaviral disease, 40%–50% [9]

Note: Mortality rates may vary in different populations. Caution should be exercised generalizing published mortality rate ranges as they may represent treated and untreated healthy and unhealthy populations.

Abbreviations: EEE, eastern equine encephalitis virus; HUS, hemolytic uremic syndrome; VEE, Venezuelan equine encephalitis virus; WEE, western equine encephalitis virus.

[a] Source: Perry RD, Fetherston JD. *Yersinia pestis*—etiologic agent of plague. Clin Microbiol Rev 1997;10:35–66.

[b] Source: Franz DR, Jaax NK. Ricin toxin. In: Zajtchuk R, Bellamy RF, editors. Medical aspects of chemical and biological warfare. Washington: Office of the Surgeon General, U.S. Department of the Army; 1997. p. 631–42.

person-to-person transmission. Historically, these agents have been notorious for causing catastrophic illness and might easily cause widespread public fear and civil disruption [1]. For example, anthrax has been referred to as the black bane; "bane" means death, destruction, or murder [5]. During the French and Indian Wars (1754–1767) British soldiers distributed blankets that had been used by smallpox patients with the intent of initiating outbreaks among American Indians. More than 50% of many affected tribes were killed by the resulting epidemics [6]. Furthermore, the recent outbreak of Ebola virus infection in Zaire evoked fear among health care workers given that it was associated with a 79% mortality rate and that health care workers accounted for one third of all cases [7].

Compared with category A agents, most category B agents also have potential for large-scale dissemination resulting in illness, but generally cause less illness and death and are expected to have lower medical and public health impact. These agents also have lower general public awareness than category A agents and require fewer special public health preparedness efforts [1]. Agents in category B require some specific enhancements in public health awareness, surveillance, or laboratory diagnostic capabilities, but present limited additional requirements for stockpiled therapeutics beyond those described for category A agents. Biologic agents that have undergone some development for widespread dissemination but do not otherwise meet the criteria for category A and several foodborne and waterborne agents are included in this category [1].

Category C agents include emerging pathogens not currently believed to present a high bioterrorism risk to public health but that could be engineered for mass dissemination in the future. These agents are addressed nonspecifically through overall bioterrorism preparedness efforts to improve the detection of unexplained illnesses and ongoing public health infrastructure development for detecting and addressing emerging infectious diseases [1].

An example of how these biologic agents are prioritized into categories is illustrated by comparing smallpox (category A) with Q fever (category B). Smallpox is ranked higher than Q fever because of its high mortality (approximately 30% for smallpox [8] compared with <1%–2.4% for Q fever if untreated [9]). Smallpox has a greater capacity for dissemination because of its potential for person-to-person transmission through aerosols expelled from the oropharynx of infected persons or by direct contact with contaminated clothing or bed linens [6]. Smallpox also has special public health preparedness needs that are not required for Q fever. For example, additional vaccine against smallpox must be manufactured, personnel administering the vaccine must be properly trained, and aggressive efforts to identify close contacts of cases must be performed.

Surveillance of infectious diseases

Surveillance provides information for action against infectious disease threats including those related to bioterrorism [10]. In the United States, the responsibility for disease surveillance is typically shared by health care providers, public and private laboratories, local and state health departments, and public health officials from several federal agencies and departments. Examining a flow diagram of where patients may interact with the health care system provides an opportunity to view possible sources of data on infectious diseases at various points of specificity of diagnosis (Fig. 1).

Effective disease surveillance begins with the health care provider [11]. It is the responsibility of the health care provider, with the help of public and private laboratories, to diagnose and report cases of notifiable infectious diseases. In the context of surveillance, the term "health care provider" is defined broadly and may include physicians, nurses, physician assistants, nurse practitioners, infection control practitioners, chiropractors, dentists, and others. Generally, state legislation or regulations require health care providers and laboratories to report confirmed or probable cases of notifiable infectious diseases to their local or state health department [11]. Each state has at least one state public health laboratory to support its infectious disease surveillance activities. On diagnosing a case of a notifiable infectious disease, health care providers and others who report are required to notify

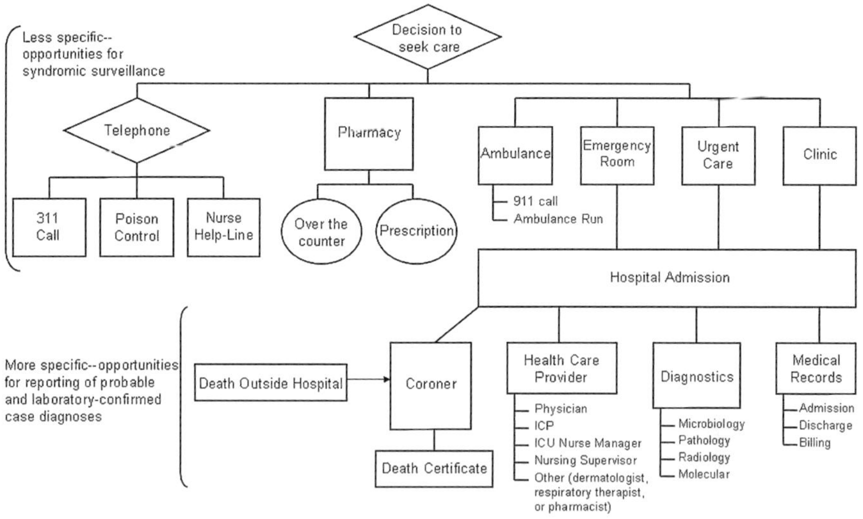

Fig. 1. Flow diagram of health care system demonstrating opportunities for sources of data for surveillance of infectious diseases in humans with variable specificity. ICP, infection control practitioner; ICU, intensive care unit. (*Adapted from* Minnesota Department of Public Health. Available at: http://www.health.state.mn.us/bioterrorism/episurv/images/sickfrednew.gif.)

their state health department through a variety of state and local disease reporting systems, which range from paper-based reporting to secure, Internet-based systems [10]. Nearly all category A agents and most category B agents are included among the Nationally Notifiable Infectious Diseases [12].

State and local health departments have the principal responsibility of protecting the public's health and take the lead in conducting disease surveillance and organizing public health response efforts [10]. Generally, local health departments are responsible for conducting initial investigations into reports of infectious diseases. Such investigations might be launched by reporting to 24-hour telephone systems, such as Chicago's 311 system that is intended to receive calls regarding urgent public health issues originating in Chicago or involving Chicago residents [13]. Information obtained from health care providers or other sources is shared with the state health department, typically through completion of paper or electronic disease report forms or a telephone call when an urgent consultation is needed. State health departments are responsible for collecting statewide surveillance information, coordinating disease investigations especially when they involve more than one local health departments' jurisdiction, analyzing disease-specific data, and sharing surveillance data with the CDC and other agencies, such as the US Department of Agriculture and Food and Drug Administration. Case definitions for reportable diseases that are nationally notifiable are determined by the Council of State and Territorial Epidemiologists and can be found on the Internet (http://www.cste.org/position%20statements/

searchbyyear2005.asp). State health departments may play a more immediate role in the investigation of bioterrorism agents, such as category A agents, because of the lack of familiarity with such investigations by local health departments outside of large urban centers.

Federal agencies collect and analyze surveillance data gathered from the states [10]. For example, CDC analyzes reports it receives from state health departments on cases of notifiable infectious diseases. Reports submitted by the states are used by CDC to monitor national health trends, formulate and implement prevention strategies, and evaluate state and federal disease prevention efforts [10]. The US Department of Agriculture collects surveillance data on the presence of specific confirmed clinical diseases in livestock, poultry, and aquaculture species from participating state veterinarians. Often in cooperation with CDC, the Food and Drug Administration analyzes state data on foodborne disease outbreaks and uses this information to trace back food items to their origin and investigate potential sources of contamination [10]. All of these surveillance-based intergovernmental relationships can play an important role in responding to a bioterrorism event, such as intentional contamination of the food supply at the farm or retail level.

Criteria for bioterrorism surveillance

A surveillance system for a bioterrorism agent should strike a balance between simplicity, flexibility, data quality, acceptability, sensitivity, positive predictive value, representativeness, timeliness, and stability [14]. Although it is not possible to have 100% on each attribute, it is important to decide which attributes are essential to a particular surveillance system because surveillance systems vary in methods, scope, purpose, and objectives. Attributes that are important to one system might be less important to another. Timeliness, high sensitivity and specificity, and periodic analysis of the surveillance system to inform public health decision-making are priorities when designing a system for bioterrorism surveillance [15].

Timeliness reflects the delay between any two or more steps in a surveillance system, such as between the date of disease onset and the date of report [16]. Surveillance for bioterrorism-related illness is dependent on a system that promptly collects, analyzes, and reports data to public health officials because the effectiveness of an intervention following a bioterrorism attack has been strongly linked to the promptness of detection [15]. Many local health departments, however, do not have adequate resources to manage, analyze, and interpret large surveillance datasets. Electronic surveillance is still being implemented nationally and does not necessarily replace the need for person-to-person immediate sharing of information by telephone. Reporting of nonspecific indicators of illness, such as school and work absenteeism, calls to nurse help-lines, and over-the-counter pharmacy sales, may provide earlier indication of a bioterrorism event compared with hospital discharge data or coroners' reports [15].

The sensitivity of a surveillance system refers to the completeness of case reporting and the system's ability to detect outbreaks [16]. Surveillance systems used to detect bioterrorism agents that do not have adequate sensitivity may fail to detect cases of bioterrorism-related illness, potentially resulting in significant delays in the triggered actions, such as antimicrobial prophylaxis or immunization with consequent increases in morbidity and mortality [15]. Predictive value positive (PVP) is defined as the proportion of persons identified as case-patients who actually have the condition being monitored. A surveillance system with low PVP results in frequent false-positive case reports, with subsequent costly or time-consuming actions by clinicians and public health officials on cases that in fact do not exist [16]. Other potential problems resulting from a surveillance system with low PVP are desensitization on the part of public health officials or the public to reports of suspect events [15] or masking of a true outbreak because of a continually high level of false-positive reports [16].

Recognizing deliberate release of a biologic agent

Of the major bioterrorism agents, all are naturally occurring except for smallpox (which was eradicated). Any confirmed case of smallpox in the world indicates an intentional attack, or at the very least, an accidental release of the smallpox virus [17]. For the other bioterrorism agents, however, a confirmed case might actually represent naturally occurring disease, such as tularemia caused by handling an infected rabbit or bubonic plague following bites of infectious rodent fleas. In addition, travelers may acquire infection in an endemic area and become ill in another area where the illness is not endemic, as happened for a couple from New Mexico who developed fever and inguinal adenopathy while in New York City in 2002. They were subsequently diagnosed with bubonic plague and likely were infected from rodent fleas on their New Mexico property [18]. Given the severity of illness caused by bioterrorism agents and the potential for widespread social disruption resulting from a bioterrorism outbreak, however, every report of an infection with a bioterrorism agent requires a rapid public health response.

Determining when a reported case most likely represents a deliberate release of a biologic agent (prompting an intensive investigation and full-scale response) and when a reported case most likely represents naturally occurring disease can be a difficult task. Certain epidemiologic features, however, help to distinguish a deliberate release of biologic agents from naturally occurring illness caused by these agents [19,20].

Suddeness

A single aerosol release of a bioterrorism agent could result in the sudden appearance of multiple cases over a few hours or days, whereas naturally occurring disease more frequently results in cases presenting over several days, weeks, or months, because of the sporadic nature of exposure (an exception to this pattern occurs if there is continued deliberate release of a bioterrorism agent).

Severity of disease or unusual clinical presentation

Persons planning deliberate release of a bioterrorism agent may alter the organism to increase its virulence, resulting in greater-than-expected morbidity or mortality among victims. Additionally, an organism not usually transmitted by an aerosol route might be manipulated to allow for aerosol release, thereby increasing severity of disease among victims or causing a disproportionate frequency of pulmonary manifestations. For example, $<20\%$ of plague cases in the United States present with the pneumonic form of the disease [21], so if most cases during an outbreak present with pneumonic plague, deliberate release of aerosolized *Yersinia pestis* should be highly suspected.

Large number of cases

A large number of cases can represent a deliberate attack on a population center or large public gathering. For example, 13 cases of plague are reported on average in the United States each year [21]. Even as few as 10 cases diagnosed in a short period, such as 1 week, is suspicious for a bioterrorism event.

Unusual geographic, temporal, or demographic clustering

Any unusual pattern may indicate deliberate release of a biologic agent. Examples include many cases occurring among residents of a single town or among attendees of a public gathering; geographic clustering of cases consistent with meteorologic conditions; and an unusual age distribution for common diseases, such as an increase in a chickenpox-like illness among adults that might be smallpox. Similarly, Ebola hemorrhagic fever occurring in the United States where it is not endemic is suspicious for bioterrorism. Importation of nonendemic hemorrhagic fever viruses occasionally occurs, however, such as when Lassa fever was diagnosed in an Illinois resident in 1989 [22] and in a New Jersey resident in 2004 [23]. In both instances, the patients had recently traveled to West Africa. Therefore, a travel history is an important early part of any possible bioterrorism investigation.

Bioterrorism surveillance is most effective when health care providers recognize the presenting signs and symptoms of illness caused by bioterrorism agents and promptly report suspicious cases to the local public health authority. Additionally, quality surveillance data are needed for naturally occurring bioterrorism agents to aid in the determination of when bioterrorism is likely enough to warrant investigation of deliberate release [9]. High-quality surveillance is timely, complete, examined often, and results are disseminated to the stakeholders of the system.

Syndromic surveillance

Improving preparedness for possible bioterrorist attacks has prompted increased interest in the timeliness of infectious disease surveillance. Specifically, surveillance systems that can reduce the amount of time from infection with a pathogen to detection of illness or an outbreak caused by the pathogen is highly desirable [24]. Surveillance for clinical syndromes consistent with infection with a bioterrorism agent rather than traditional surveillance for specific diagnoses can result in more rapid detection of a bioterrorist attack, allowing for a more rapid public health response and possibly a consequent reduction in morbidity and mortality after an attack. Surveillance based on detection of a set of predetermined clinical signs or symptoms is referred to as "syndromic surveillance." CDC defines syndromic surveillance as surveillance that uses health-related data that precede diagnosis and signal a sufficient probability of a case or an outbreak to warrant further public health response [25].

Syndromic surveillance systems have been in use for years for nonbioterrorism infectious disease surveillance. An example of this is CDC's Influenza Sentinel Providers Surveillance Network, in which approximately 1000 health care providers in the United States report weekly the total number of patients seen and the total number with influenza-like illness. Influenza-like illness is defined as the clinical syndrome of temperature $>100^{\circ}$F plus either a cough or sore throat. The percentage of influenza-like illness calculated from these weekly reports is then compared with a national baseline percentage to estimate the onset of increased influenza activity in the United States [26]. Other examples of syndromic surveillance for non–bioterrorism-related conditions include surveillance for acute flaccid paralysis as part of the Polio Eradication Initiative [27] and active surveillance for hepatitis and febrile exanthem syndromes along the United States–Mexico border conducted by the Border Infectious Disease Surveillance Project [28].

The anthrax bioterrorist attacks of 2001 stimulated increased research in and funding of syndromic surveillance systems for detection of bioterrorism agents [29]. A syndromic surveillance system to detect a possible bioterrorist attack in the New York City area was begun almost immediately after the attacks on the World Trade Center on September 11, 2001. The New York City Department of Health and Mental Hygiene collaborated with epidemiologists from CDC to initiate an emergency department–based syndromic surveillance system for syndromes consistent with exposure to a bioterrorism agent (respiratory, rash, gastrointestinal, neurologic, and sepsis), and within 2 days of the attacks the system was operational in 15 emergency departments across the city. Health care providers indicated on a form which syndrome best represented the patient's primary diagnosis, and epidemiologists entered the data onsite at the emergency departments. Daily data analysis over the 30-day surveillance period generated a total of 91 alarms for the five syndromes of bioterrorism interest, of which 7%

were attributed to errors in coding or data entry. Investigations of the remainder did not reveal any diagnoses suggestive of a natural outbreak or bioterrorist attack [30].

In addition to the threat of bioterrorist attacks, syndromic surveillance systems have proliferated because of the increased availability of electronic data sources [31]. Many systems make use of existing electronic resources, a practice that potentially increases efficiency and reduces cost, and many systems integrate data from multiple sources. The following are selected examples of prominent systems that make use of multiple electronic data sources.

BioSense

BioSense is a CDC Internet-based syndromic surveillance application in operation in the United States since November 2003 for the early detection of intentional and natural infectious disease outbreaks. BioSense receives data electronically from four sources. The Department of Veterans Affairs and Department of Defense provide *International Classification of Diseases, Ninth Revision, Clinical Modification* (ICD-9-CM) diagnoses and current procedural terminology–coded medical procedures for ambulatory-care visits to their facilities. Certain retail pharmacies provide sales information on select over-the-counter medications. Laboratory Corporation of America provides information on laboratory tests ordered. CDC analysts examine the data daily and certain public health officials can access reports in a timely fashion [32].

Electronic Surveillance System for the Early Notification of Community-based Epidemics

The Electronic Surveillance System for the Early Notification of Community-based Epidemics (ESSENCE) is a syndromic surveillance system operated by the Department of Defense that automatically collects ICD-9 codes for patient visits at participating military treatment facilities and analyzes the frequency and distribution of seven syndrome types: (1) respiratory; (2) gastrointestinal; (3) fever; (4) neurologic; (5) dermatologic (infectious disease); (6) dermatologic (hemorrhagic); and (7) coma or sudden death [31].

Real-time Outbreak and Disease Surveillance

Researchers at the Real-time Outbreak and Disease Surveillance (RODS) Laboratory, a collaboration of the University of Pittsburgh and Carnegie Mellon University, have created software that can collect and analyze many types of clinical data, such as chief complaints or laboratory tests ordered. In 2002, the Utah Department of Health used the software for infectious disease monitoring during the Winter Olympics Games [33].

Syndromic surveillance has several distinct advantages over traditional disease-based surveillance. Most notable is the potential for syndromic surveillance to operate in a timely fashion enabling rapid recognition of an outbreak. In addition, syndromic surveillance systems generally are automated, do not rely on physician reporting, and have the potential to detect nonbioterrorism infectious diseases.

Certain limitations of syndromic surveillance systems for the detection of bioterrorism agents have become apparent, however, as public health practitioners gain experience with these systems. Some limitations relate to the design of the surveillance system, such as deciding which clinical signs or symptoms to include in the syndrome definition or which data source to use. The United States National Capitol Region Emergency Department syndromic surveillance system uses chief complaint to classify patients into one of eight syndromes. A study of this system concluded that there would be substantial differences in the assignment of the sepsis and neurologic syndromes if discharge diagnosis were used instead [34]. Another frequent challenge for syndromic surveillance systems is the lack of historical data for establishing the expected baseline rate of the syndrome of interest [31].

The choice of statistical methods and determination of the alert threshold is also critical, because too low a threshold has the potential for creating false alarms, each one necessitating expenditure of public health resources for an investigation. False alarms also result from mistakes in data translation, such as data being sent multiple times, or mistakes in diagnosis coding (eg, congestive heart failure has been coded as Crimean Congo hemorrhagic fever) [32]. Such mistakes require time on the part of data managers to resolve.

One of the greatest limitations of syndromic surveillance systems for the detection of bioterrorism agents is inherent in their design. These systems cannot detect outbreaks consisting of small numbers of cases. Even the active syndromic surveillance in emergency departments in New York City after the September 11 attacks did not detect the outbreak of anthrax that occurred in mid-October, because it could not detect cases of cutaneous anthrax diagnosed in non–emergency department settings. Six of the seven New York City patients diagnosed with cutaneous anthrax did not seek care in an emergency department, and the system was operational only in emergency departments [30]. The surveillance system did demonstrate value after the single case of inhalational anthrax was diagnosed, because the system did not detect an increase in emergency department visits for respiratory illnesses. This allowed public health officials to reassure the public that no evidence existed of an inhalational anthrax outbreak [31].

Syndromic surveillance systems can be too geographically focused, resulting in too little surveillance data. An investigation of the ICD-9 coding at a single hospital in Chicago during a large outbreak of West Nile Virus in 2002 showed that a simple syndromic surveillance system based on ICD-9 coding data would not have detected the emergence of West Nile Virus in Chicago. Specifically, had such a system been in place, the counts of ICD-9 codes corresponding to encephalitis and other related neurologic diagnoses would not have significantly differed from counts recorded during the previous 6 years at that hospital [35]. It is possible, however, that such surveillance conducted at the level of the city or region would have resulted in detection of the outbreak. Evaluation of bioterrorism surveillance is greatly needed to make decisions about which methods to use and how to respond to results [15].

Syndromic surveillance is not meant to replace traditional disease-based reporting; instead, it should augment the reporting of unusual or suspicious illness by informed health care providers and laboratorians. As a surveillance technique it continues to evolve, and investigations of its potential to detect an outbreak of a bioterrorism agent are ongoing. A challenge that remains is to adequately fund and staff local and state health departments to perform quality surveillance of infectious diseases, which can then be supplemented with high-quality (but not high-cost) syndromic surveillance systems that do not overly sacrifice specificity of outbreak verification.

References

[1] Rotz LD, Khan AS, Lillibridge SR, et al. Public health assessment of potential biological terrorism agents. Emerg Infect Dis 2002;8:225–30.

[2] Centers for Disease Control and Prevention. Biological and chemical terrorism: state plan for preparedness and response. MMWR Morb Mortal Wkly Rep 2000;49:1–14.

[3] US Army Medical Research Institute of Infectious Diseases. USAMRID's medical management of biological casualties handbook. 5th edition. Frederick, (MD): The Institute; 2004. Available at: http://www.usamriid.army.mil/education/bluebook.htm. Accessed October 11, 2005.

[4] Chang M, Glynn MK, Groseclose SL. Endemic, notifiable bioterrorism-related diseases, United States, 1992–1999. Emerg Infect Dis 2003;9:556–64.

[5] Christie AB. Infectious diseases: epidemiology and clinical practice. 4th edition. New York: Churchill Livingstone; 1987.

[6] Henderson DA, Inglesby TV, Bartlett JG, et al. Smallpox as a biological weapon: medical and public health management. JAMA 1999;281:2127–37.

[7] Sepkowitz KA. Occupationally acquired infections in health care workers. Ann Intern Med 1996;125:917–28.

[8] Mandell GL, Bennett JE, Dolin R, editors. Principles and practice of infectious diseases. 6th edition. Philadelphia: Elsevier Churchill Livingstone; 2005.

[9] Heymann DL, editor. Control of communicable diseases manual. 18th edition. Washington: American Public Health Association; 2004.

[10] United States Government Accountability Office. Emerging infectious diseases: review of state and federal disease surveillance efforts. Report to the Chairman, Permanent Subcommittee on Investigations, Committee on Governmental Affairs, US Senate. Washington, DC: US Government Accountability Office; 2004. p. 8–18.

[11] Koo D, Caldwell B. The role of providers and health plans in infectious disease surveillance. Effect Clin Prac 1999;2:247–52.

[12] Centers for Disease Control and Prevention. Nationally notifiable infectious diseases, United States, 2005. Available at: http://www.cdc.gov/epo/dphsi/phs/infdis2005.htm. Accessed October 11, 2005.

[13] The Chicago Department of Public Health. Reporting urgent public health issues. Available at: http://egov.cityofchicago.org.

[14] Centers for Disease Control and Prevention. Updated guidelines for evaluating public health surveillance systems. MMWR Morb Mort Wkly Rpt 2001;50:1–31.
[15] Bravata DM, McDonald KM, Smith WM, et al. Systematic review: surveillance systems for early detection of bioterrorism-related diseases. Ann Intern Med 2004;140:910–22.
[16] Teutch SM, Churchill RE, editors. Principles and practice of public health surveillance. New York: Oxford University Press; 2000.
[17] Masci JR, Bass E. Bioterrorism: a guide for hospital preparedness. Boca Raton (FL): CRC Press; 2005.
[18] Centers for Disease Control and Prevention. Imported plague — New York City, 2002. MMWR Morb Mortal Wkly Rep 2002;52:725–8.
[19] World Health Organization. Public health response to biological and chemical weapons: WHO guidance. 2nd edition. Geneva: WHO Press; 2004.
[20] Centers for Disease Control and Prevention. Recognition of illness associated with the intentional release of a biologic agent. MMWR Morb Mortal Wkly Rep 2001;50:893–7.
[21] Centers for Disease Control and Prevention. Prevention of plague: recommendations of the Advisory Committee on Immunization Practices (ACIP). MMWR Morb Mortal Wkly Rep 1996;45(No. RR-14):1–4.
[22] Holmes GP, McCormick JB, Trock SC, et al. Lassa fever in the United States. N Engl J Med 1990;323:1120–3.
[23] Centers for Disease Control and Prevention. Imported Lassa fever — New Jersey, 2004. MMWR Morb Mortal Wkly Rep 2004;53:894–7.
[24] Buehler JW, Berkelman RL, Hartley DM, et al. Syndromic surveillance and bioterrorism-related epidemics. Emerg Infect Dis 2003;9:1197–204.
[25] Centers for Disease Control and Prevention. Syndromic surveillance: an applied approach to outbreak detection. Available at: http://www.cdc.gov/epo/dphsi/syndromic.htm. Accessed November 18, 2005.
[26] Centers for Disease Control and Prevention. Flu activity. Available at: http://www.cdc.gov/flu/weekly/fluactivity.htm. Accessed November 18, 2005.
[27] Centers for Disease Control and Prevention. Acute flaccid paralysis surveillance systems for the expansion to other diseases, 2003–2004. MMWR Morb Mortal Wkly Rep 2004;53: 1113–6.
[28] Weinberg M, Waterman S, Alvarez Lucas C, et al. The US-Mexico border infectious disease surveillance project: establishing bi-national border surveillance. Emerg Infect Dis 2003;9: 97–102.
[29] Reingold A. If syndromic surveillance is the answer, what is the question? Biosecur Bioterr 2003;1:77–81.
[30] Centers for Disease Control and Prevention. Syndromic surveillance for bioterrorism following the attacks on the World Trade Center—New York City, 2001. MMWR Morb Mortal Wkly Rep 2002;51(Special Issue):13–5.
[31] Rotz LD, Hughes JM. Advances in detecting and responding to threats from bioterrorism and emerging infectious disease. Nat Med 2004;10:S130–6.
[32] Sokolow LZ, Grady N, Rolka H, et al. Deciphering data anomalies in BioSense. Morb Mortal Wkly Rep 2005;54:133–9.
[33] RODS Laboratory. Available at: http://rods.health.pitt.edu. Accessed November 18, 2005.
[34] Begier EM, Sockwell D, Branch LM, et al. The national capitol region's emergency department syndromic surveillance system: do chief complaint and discharge diagnosis yield different results? Emerg Infect Dis 2003;9:393–6.
[35] Weber SG, Pitrak D. Accuracy of a local surveillance system for early detection of emerging infectious disease [letter]. JAMA 2003;290:596–8.

ELSEVIER
SAUNDERS

Infect Dis Clin N Am
20 (2006) 227–251

INFECTIOUS
DISEASE CLINICS
OF NORTH AMERICA

Anthrax: From Antiquity and Obscurity to a Front-Runner in Bioterrorism

Demetrios N. Kyriacou, MD, PhD, DTM&H[a], Alys Adamski, BS[b], Nancy Khardori, MD, PhD[b,*]

[a]*Department of Emergency Medicine and Department of Preventive Medicine, Northwestern University Feinberg School of Medicine, 259 East Erie Street, Suite 100, Chicago, IL 60611, USA*

[b]*Division of Infectious Diseases, Department of Internal Medicine, Southern Illinois University School of Medicine, PO Box 19636, Springfield, IL 62794-9636, USA*

Anthrax infection is caused by *Bacillus anthracis,* a large gram-positive, rod-shaped bacterium found in soil around the world. Under adverse environmental conditions, anthrax bacteria form endospores (Fig. 1) that are resistant to drying, radiation, and disinfectants. Although anthrax is usually a disease of grazing animals, human contact with animal products, such as hides, hairs, and wool, that are contaminated with anthrax endospores can result in clinical infection with cutaneous, inhalational, gastrointestinal, and neurologic manifestations [1–3]. Although highly pathogenic and extremely virulent, there is no human-to-human transmission of *B anthracis.* The cutaneous form of anthrax is most common, but the noncutaneous manifestations of anthrax infection are significantly more severe. Inhalational anthrax is the most concerning because of its rapid progression to respiratory distress, septicemic shock, and death. Despite its high virulence, only 18 cases of inhalational anthrax were documented in the United States during the twentieth century, with most of those cases resulting in death [4].

A more ominous means of human anthrax infection is through the intentional spread of aerosolized anthrax particles in the form of biologic warfare and terrorism [5–7]. In October and November 2001, 22 individuals in the United States were infected with aerosolized anthrax endospores with 11 subsequently developing inhalational anthrax and 11 developing cutaneous anthrax [8–18]. All 11 patients with inhalational anthrax required hospitalization and intensive therapy, and 5 of these patients ultimately died.

* Corresponding author.
E-mail address: nkhardori@siumed.edu (N. Khardori).

0891-5520/06/$ - see front matter
doi:10.1016/j.idc.2006.03.009

id.theclinics.com

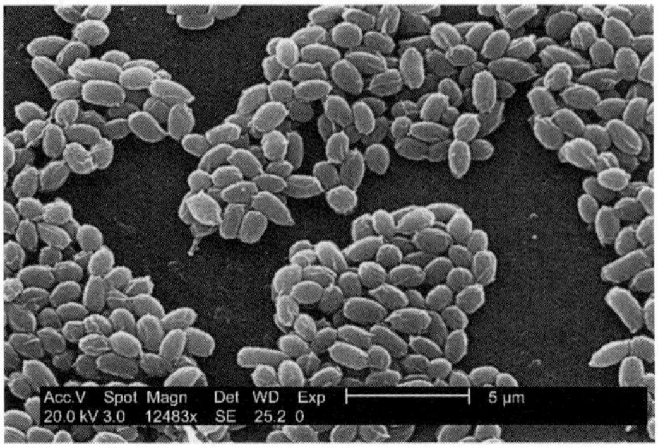

Fig. 1. Scanning electron microscopy of *B anthracis* endospores. (*From* Centers for Disease Control and Prevention, Atlanta, GA. Available at: http://www.cdc.gov.)

Although cutaneous anthrax is easily recognized, the clinical manifestations of inhalational anthrax include a brief but nonspecific prodrome of fever, cough, and chest discomfort that also characterizes many other types of acute respiratory infections [2,3]. Because rapid diagnostic tests for inhalational anthrax are not widely available [19], victims may not be clinically recognized until the onset of respiratory distress and shock.

Although a large-scale bioterrorist anthrax attack has yet to be perpetrated in the United States, previous studies have modeled the potential morbidity and mortality that would be sustained by such an attack (Table 1) [20–22]. These studies have estimated that possibly hundreds of thousands would be infected and die. In addition, the effect of early detection of a bioterrorist anthrax attack has been modeled. It has been estimated that the number of deaths double if it takes 4.8 days to detect an attack instead of 2 days after dissemination of the anthrax endospores [22]. Because the first evidence of a bioterrorist attack likely would be the presentation of victims seeking medical treatment for inhalational anthrax, limiting the effects of such an attack would require the rapid and accurate recognition of the earliest victims seeking medical treatment [3–7].

Table 1
Summary of morbidity and mortality estimates resulting from a large-scale bioterrorist anthrax attack

Source	Simulated population	Amount released (kg)	Estimated morbidity	Estimated mortality
World Health Organization (1970) [20]	Urban population of 5 million	50	250,000	100,000
U S Congressional Office of Technology (1993) [21]	Washington, DC	100	Not estimated	130,000–3,000,000
Anthrax Working Group (Wein et al, 2003) [22]	Urban and rural population of 11.5 million	1	1,490,000	123,400

In response to this potential threat, the Centers for Disease Control and Prevention (CDC) and the Center for Civilian Biodefense Strategies have issued guidelines for the evaluation of individuals with possible inhalational anthrax [23–27]. These guidelines recommend the use of common clinical characteristics to discriminate inhalational anthrax from other acute respiratory illnesses, but are limited by the use of patient-specific information from only 11 cases of bioterrorism-related inhalational anthrax. Subsequently, an evaluation of these guidelines showed that their use would have resulted in the detection of only 1 of the 11 bioterrorism-related cases of 2001 [28]. This article presents a brief history of anthrax, discusses different clinical presentations of anthrax, reviews the clinical characteristics that can be used to recognize inhalational anthrax victims, discusses current diagnostic and treatment modalities, and provides an overview of emerging and investigational therapies and vaccines.

History of anthrax

Anthrax is well described in antiquity and has a crucial place in the development of bacteriology and medical science [29]. The term *anthrax* is derived from the Greek word *anthrakis,* which means "coal" and describes the black eschar lesions that are characteristic of cutaneous anthrax (Fig. 2). In 1872, Koch developed methods to cultivate *B anthracis* and show its growth into long filaments on microscopic slides [30]. He also found that dried spores could remain viable for years, explaining how anthrax recurred in pastures long unused for grazing. Under favorable environmental conditions, the endospores would develop into rod-shaped vegetative bacilli. Although Koch's findings were only fully accepted after the development of a successful anthrax vaccine by Pasteur in 1882, his work with anthrax established his famous postulates [29,31].

In the nineteenth century, anthrax caused several epidemics in the United Kingdom and the United States through the importation, handling, and

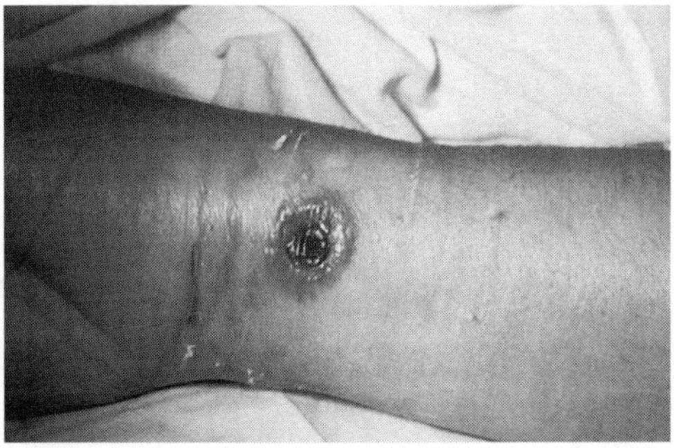

Fig. 2. Cutaneous anthrax infection with characteristic black eschar. (*From* Centers for Disease Control and Prevention, Atlanta, GA. Available at: http://www.cdc.gov.)

processing of wool and other animal products [32–34]. Although classically described as "wool-sorter's disease," individuals typically infected also included workers that cleaned, combed, and dyed wool and other animal hairs. After Koch's and Pasteur's great discoveries of the late 1800s, efforts aimed at protecting these workers led to the rapid development of hygienic measures that significantly reduced the incidence of cutaneous and inhalational anthrax. These measures included washing the wool, burning waste, banning animal grazing on infected pastures, and vaccination of grazing animals. Also during this period, the first bacteriologic and pathologic observations led to theories accounting for the unique pathogenesis of inhalational anthrax [35].

Despite these interventions, including federal regulations to limit the importation of infected materials, several cases still occurred in the United States. During 1916–1919, 126 cases of anthrax were documented in Massachusetts [36]. Of these cases, 23 patients (18.3%) died; there were no gastrointestinal cases and only 3 inhalational cases (all fatal). The remaining cases were cutaneous and treated with surgical excision of the lesions or the newly developed anthrax serum. Information regarding the treatment is available for 113 cutaneous cases. Of the 98 cases treated with anthrax serum, only 13 patients (13.3%) had died. In comparison, of the 15 treated with excision of the skin lesion, 4 patients (26.7%) had died. Although this study was not a formal randomized clinical trial, it provided important evidence regarding the efficacy of a relatively new treatment for a disease that was often disfiguring and frequently life-threatening. Lucchesi's [37] report of the serum treatment of 19 cases of anthrax further confirmed the efficacy of this therapeutic mode.

Although the incidence of new cutaneous anthrax cases in mill workers continued throughout the first half of the twentieth century, the occurrence of inhalational anthrax was becoming exceedingly rare with only uncommon cases reported in the medical literature [38–41]. In 1955, Gold [42] described 117 cases of anthrax. Only one case was inhalational anthrax; the remaining cases had only cutaneous manifestations. In 1957, an outbreak of five cases of inhalational anthrax and four cases of cutaneous anthrax occurred among employees of an industrial goat hair textile mill in Manchester, New Hampshire. Despite extensive therapy and the administration of antibiotics to four of the five patients, only one survived [43,44].

In April 1979, about 1 mg of aerosolized *B anthracis* was released unintentionally from a biologic weapons production facility in Sverdlovsk, Russia [45]. Before the anthrax attacks of 2001 that were perpetrated through the US Postal Service, the Sverdlovsk incident resulted in the only documented cases of inhalational anthrax from weaponized *B anthracis*. Despite an extensive effort to control the outbreak of anthrax with the distribution of antibiotics and vaccinations, approximately 80 individuals developed inhalational anthrax and ultimately died [46]. Although clinical information concerning the Sverdlovsk victims has never been made available, microscopic and macroscopic pathologic investigations of several fatal victims revealed the characteristic mediastinal inflammation, hemorrhage, and lymphadenitis associated with inhalational anthrax [47,48]. These findings suggest few pathophysiologic differences between naturally occurring and bioterrorism-related inhalational anthrax cases. In addition, a comparison of pathologic characteristics among 36 cases of naturally occurring inhalational anthrax from 1880–1976 and 11 cases of bioterrorism-related inhalational anthrax from 2001 found few differences between these two groups [4].

Microbiology and genetics

Bacteria in the genus *Bacillus* are aerobic, spore-forming, nonmotile, gram-positive bacilli. The size of *B anthracis* spores is approximately 1 μm. They grow readily at 37°C with a nonhemolytic "curled hair" colony morphology and "jointed bamboo-rod" cellular appearance [5,49]. Spores germinate readily in nutrient-rich environments, such as blood or tissues, of animals or human hosts. The vegetative forms of *B anthracis* are nonflagellated and large (1–8 μm in length and 1–1.5 μm in breadth). They grow readily on sheep blood agar under aerobic or facultative anaerobic conditions. After overnight growth at 35°C, isolated colonies are 2 to 5 mm in diameter, white or gray-white, tenacious, flat with a "medusa head" appearance (Fig. 3). *B anthracis* is lysed by γ-phage and under natural conditions is susceptible to penicillin. Commercially available API test strips and fluorescent antibody staining can be used for species identification. The CDC guidelines provide details on preliminary testing and transfer to referral public health laboratories for confirmation [50]. Polymerase chain reaction (PCR) and γ-phage lysis are used as confirmatory tests. The polypeptide capsule of *B anthracis* consists of poly-D-glutamic acid and can be visualized by India ink staining. Clinical samples (eg, pus or tissue specimens) from

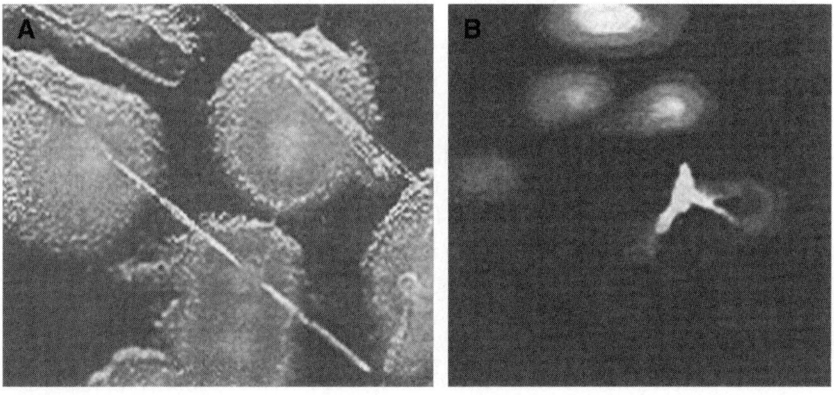

Fig. 3. (*A*) *B anthracis,* colony on sheep blood agar. (*B*) "Sticky" consistency of *B anthracis* colony on SBA. (*From* Centers for Disease Control and Prevention, Atlanta, GA. Available at: http://www.cdc.gov.)

patients suspected to have anthrax should be stained by Gram stain to look for gram-positive bacilli. Polychrome methylene blue can be used to stain the polypeptide capsule [51]. The rapidly multiplying vegetative forms of *B anthracis* form spores only after local nutrients are exhausted, such as when infected body fluids dry.

The Northern Arizona University laboratory has used amplified fragment length polymorphism to study 1200 strains identified around the world over the years. *B anthracis* is a highly monomorphic species with 99% nucleotide sequence identity among different isolates [52]. Multilocus variable number tandem repeat analysis markers are currently the most accurate strain-typing tool and have been used on half of the 1200 known strains of *B anthracis*. They provide a highly precise method for genetic fingerprinting and take the Northern Arizona University laboratory about 12 hours to analyze an anthrax sample. Variable number tandem repeat analysis of the Florida, New York, and Washington, DC, isolates recovered from the 2001 letter attacks suggested that they were all from the same source, a strain originally isolated from a dead cow in Texas in 1981. This strain, designated Ames, has been used in the US Defensive Biological Weapons Program and has been provided to other research laboratories in the United States and Europe. The Institute for Genomic Research in Rockville, Maryland, has completed genome sequencing of a *B anthracis* Ames isolate (the Porton isolate) that lacks the virulence plasmids. The sequences from the Porton chromosome and the previously sequenced *B anthracis* plasmids were aligned to the 2001 Florida isolate. Comparison of the two genomes revealed four high-quality single nucleotide polymorphisms between the two chromosomes and seven differences among different preparations of the reference genome. These markers were found to divide the samples into distinct families when tested on a collection of *B anthracis* isolates. Such genome-based analysis of microbial agents provides a powerful new tool for microbial forensics and for the investigation of natural and intentional infectious disease outbreaks [52].

Virulence factors and pathogenesis

The two unique factors in the fully virulent strains of *B anthracis* are (1) a poly-D-glutamic acid capsule that inhibits phagocytosis and (2) a tripartite toxin [53]. The capsule is produced by virulent strains of *B anthracis* in vivo and under anaerobic conditions on enriched media supplemented with carbon dioxide. The plasmid pXO2 encodes the capsule [54]. In 1955, the injection of sterile plasma from infected guinea pigs was shown to result in local edema and death in a guinea pig model. The three-component toxin is coded by the plasmid pXO1 and consists of edema factor, protective antigen, and lethal factor [55]. The sequencing and organization of both plasmids already have been analyzed [56–58]. Protective antigen, named for its role in inducing protective immunity, binds to cell surface receptors to initiate an uptake system used by edema factor and lethal factor to gain intracellular access. Protective antigen also inhibits phagocytosis of *B anthracis*. The cellular receptor for protective antigen, the anthrax toxin receptor, was identified recently [59]. It is a type 1 membrane protein with an extracellular von Willebrand factor A domain that binds directly to Protective antigen. A soluble version of this domain can protect cells from the toxin activity. The edema factor is a calmodulin-dependent adenylate cyclase leading to increased levels of intracellular cAMP and dysregulation of water and ions, including calcium. Such dysregulation leads to edema in a manner perhaps analogous to the loss of water into the intestinal lumen caused by cholera toxin. Edema factor also inhibits phagocytosis of *B anthracis*. The structure of edema factor shown in 2002 by x-ray crystallography showed it to be activated only after binding to calmodulin and undergoing a conformational change [60]. The lethal factor is a zinc-dependent metallopeptidase that by cleaving members of the mitogen-activated protein kinase leads to the inhibition of one or more signaling pathways. The crystal structure of lethal factor comprises four domains. Domain 1 binds to the protective antigen in the formation lethal toxin [61].

Edema toxin (edema factor plus protective antigen) and lethal toxin (lethal factor plus protective antigen) resemble the A-B enzyme binding structures characteristic of many well-studied bacterial toxins. The lethal toxin was shown to impair the function of dendritic cells severely resulting in a profound impairment of antigen-specific T and B cell immunity [62]. Earlier, lethal toxin had been shown to suppress proinflammatory cytokine production in macrophages [63]. Suppression was seen at very low levels and involves inhibition of transcription of cytokine mRNA.

The pathogenesis of fatal anthrax is not completely known, but is thought to be caused by the tripartite anthrax toxin. The binding of protective antigen to its cellular receptor (anthrax toxin receptor) results in its cleavage into 20-kd and 63-kd portions by a cellular protease. A heptamer is formed by seven copies of the 63-kd protective antigen, and the doughnut-shaped complex binds to the anthrax toxin receptor. Next, lethal factor or edema factor (maximum of three copies) or a combination of both binds to the existing protective antigen heptamer. The complex enters the intracellular endosome. The low pH of the endosome allows the lethal factor and edema factor to cross into the cytosol [64]. In the cytosol, the lethal factor and edema factor trigger the toxin effects, including immune system evasion and cell damage. Sellman and colleagues [65] showed that a mutant protective antigen molecule was able to form a part of the doughnut similar to native protective antigen, but could not disrupt the membrane pore, preventing the escape of edema factor and lethal factor. The pathogenic effects of anthrax toxin have been attributed to macrophage-mediated cytokine release (tumor necrosis factor-α and interleukin-1), toxin-induced lysis of infected macrophages, and sepsis syndrome resulting in death [66]. More recent work in a murine model showed that lethal toxin kills through cytokine-independent mechanisms [67,68]. The death in these mice followed striking tissue hypoxia and liver necrosis. The exact mechanism for this damage remains to be defined.

Recognizing inhalational anthrax victims

After the bioterrorist anthrax attacks of 2001, physicians were called on to provide frontline early recognition and reporting of bioterrorism-related anthrax cases [5]. Because the cutaneous manifestations of anthrax are relatively distinct and rarely fatal, most emphasis has been placed on the recognition of inhalational anthrax victims. CDC directors stated that, "For this frontline surveillance system to function at its best, all clinicians, regardless of their specialty, must have enough basic information about the clinical manifestations of infections caused by the select agents of bioterrorism to raise their suspicion when they see a patient with a compatible illness" [6]. In response to this challenge, several investigators have identified specific individual and sets of clinical predictors that discriminate inhalational anthrax from other infectious diseases to recognize more rapidly and accurately the earliest victims of a bioterrorist anthrax attack.

A study compared patient-specific information regarding clinical characteristics from 47 historical inhalational anthrax cases reported in the medical literature with 376 controls of community-acquired pneumonia or influenza-like illness [4]. Several clinical characteristics were seen more frequently in individuals with inhalational anthrax than in either the community-acquired pneumonia controls or the influenza-like illness controls. In particular, nausea, vomiting, pallor/cyanosis, diaphoresis, altered mental status, heart rate greater than 110 beats/min, temperature greater than 100.9°F, and increased hematocrit all seemed to predict inhalational anthrax. Chest radiographs (when used to detect mediastinal widening or pleural effusion) provide the greatest overall single test accuracy for inhalational anthrax (Fig. 4). This finding was 100% sensitive (95% confidence interval 84.6–100) for inhalational anthrax and 71.8% specific (95% confidence interval 64.8–78.1) compared with community-acquired pneumonia and 95.6% specific (95% confidence interval 90–98.5) compared with influenza-like illness. These radiographic findings also correlate with the thoracic pathologic findings of the historical inhalational anthrax cases that were autopsied.

By introducing the clinical predictors of inhalational anthrax into decision rules, investigators have been able to improve on the recognition of victims in the clinical setting. Kuehnert and colleagues [69] developed clinical scoring systems to discriminate inhalational anthrax from influenza-like illness with a sensitivity of 100% and specificity of 96.1%, and community-acquired pneumonia with a sensitivity of 81.8% and specificity of 81.2%. Hupert developed a screening protocol for presumptive cases of inhalational anthrax by comparing the distribution of presenting symptoms and signs of historical cases of inhalational anthrax and patients with viral respiratory

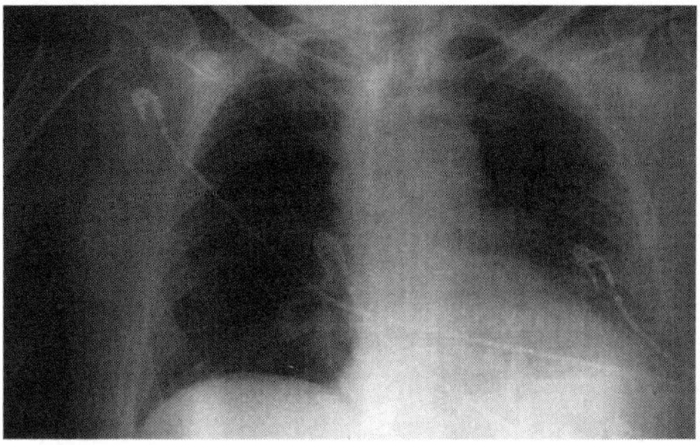

Fig. 4. Chest radiograph of patient with inhalational anthrax showing mediastinal widening and left pleural effusion. (*From* Centers for Disease Control and Prevention, Atlanta, GA. Available at: http://www.cdc.gov.)

tract infections, but did not stipulate measures of sensitivity and specificity. The algorithm developed by Hupert and coworkers [70] was based on comparing symptoms and signs of inhalational anthrax and viral respiratory tract infections, but not community-acquired pneumonia. Consequently, this algorithm could be used only for distinguishing inhalational anthrax from viral respiratory tract illnesses. Howell and associates [71] developed a scoring system of symptoms and signs to discriminate inhalational anthrax from a group of emergency department patients with a sensitivity of 100% and a specificity of 99.8%. The scoring method presented by Howell and associates [71] was based on comparing symptoms and signs of only two cases of inhalational anthrax with a group of emergency department patients that included "all known symptoms and clinical presentations of acute pulmonary anthrax."

Despite differences in methodologies and comparison groups, the four above-reviewed studies found several clinical characteristics of inhalational anthrax in common, including nausea, vomiting, elevated hematocrit, and altered mental status. These clinical features suggest a more systemic nature of inhalational anthrax that is not confined to the respiratory system. It is also likely that mild forms of inhalational anthrax do not exist. A study of workers from the mail distribution centers that sustained the October and November 2001 anthrax attacks found that mild forms of inhalational anthrax did not occur. The authors concluded that surveillance for moderate or severe illness was adequate to identify all inhalational anthrax cases from these attacks [72].

Because all of the studies were based on retrospectively collected information, they have several limitations. Measurements of the predictor variables were from historical reports of the cases and medical records of the controls and are inherently subject to potential bias resulting from missing values. In addition, the clinical characteristics of inhalational anthrax may be subtle, or even absent, early in the disease. In one bioterrorism-related case, mediastinal widening and pleural effusion were missed initially in the emergency department chest radiograph evaluation and were identified only with retrospective review [73]. In another bioterrorism-related case, only a subtle density in the right subhilar region was present in the initial emergency department chest radiograph. Pleural effusion was identified in a subsequent emergency department chest radiograph the following day [74]. Although the clinical predictors may aid in the recognition of inhalational anthrax cases with well-developed symptoms and signs, they may not help identify very early prodromal cases. This also precludes using clinical predictors for identifying inhalational anthrax in individuals with suspected exposure who have yet to develop symptoms or signs.

Knowledge of the clinical predictors of inhalational anthrax can have important implications for the rapid clinical identification of victims in case of a bioterrorism anthrax attack. First, without prior knowledge of a bioterrorist anthrax attack, improving physicians' ability to recognize potential inhalational anthrax victims in clinical settings could enhance surveillance methods to detect an attack rapidly and accurately and save thousands of lives [75]. The CDC describes outbreak detection as the overriding purpose of surveillance for terrorism preparedness [76]. Even with this stated goal, bioterrorism surveillance systems do not have standard case definitions for syndromes, and most systems do not report sensitivities and specificities of their case definitions for detecting bioterrorism-related victims [77]. Systems that are not sensitive would fail to identify cases and detect an attack, whereas systems that are not specific would report cases falsely and trigger needless outbreak investigations and subsequent unnecessary public health responses [78,79].

Implementation of any clinical method of detecting individuals with inhalational anthrax is problematic because of the extremely rare occurrence of this disease. Given this extremely low pretest probability of inhalational anthrax, the post-test probability of inhalational anthrax in an individual patient presenting with respiratory complaints also would be very low. Nevertheless, information regarding clinical characteristics that help discriminate possible inhalational anthrax victims from more common acute respiratory illnesses still would be helpful to frontline physicians responsible for identifying patients with potential bioterrorism-related diseases. The chest radiograph finding of widened mediastinum in a patient can be caused by many different pathologic processes. The combination of widened mediastinum in a patient with fever, vomiting, or altered mental status would narrow the list of potential causes significantly. A small cluster of these types of patients within a limited time period would suggest an outbreak of only a few potential diseases, including inhalational anthrax. The rapid diagnosis of inhalational anthrax can be hastened further by using adjunct diagnostic tests that are currently being developed, including a rapid anthrax test approved by the Food and Drug Administration (FDA) [80–85].

Other clinical manifestations of anthrax

Cutaneous anthrax

"Malignant pustule" or cutaneous anthrax is the most common naturally occurring form of human disease. An estimated 2000 cases are reported worldwide every year [86]. In the United States, 224 cases of cutaneous anthrax were reported in 1944–1994 [87]. One case was reported in 2000. As a consequence of anthrax attacks of 2001, 11 confirmed or probable cases of cutaneous anthrax occurred in the United States. Natural cutaneous anthrax occurs after an exposure to anthrax-infected animals or infected materials and follows the deposition of the spores into the skin. The lesions are commonly on exposed areas of the body, such as arms, hands, neck, and face. Existing cuts or abrasions increase susceptibility to cutaneous anthrax. In the only published case of cutaneous anthrax resulting from the 2001 US attacks, the patient did not have any visible cuts or abrasions at or around the site of the lesions. The mean incubation period was 5 days (range 1–10 days) based on estimated date of exposure to contaminated mail [5]. After germination, the anthrax spores release toxin and lead to localized edema. Edema is followed by a pruritic macule and papule, which then enlarges to become a round ulcer by the second day. The ulcer (malignant pustule) is surrounded by 1- to 3-mm vesicles with clear or serosanguineous fluid that shows gram-positive bacilli on staining. A painless, depressed, black eschar associated with extensive local edema follows. The eschar dries, loosens, and falls off in the next 1 to 2 weeks. Lymphangitis and painful lymphadenitis can be associated with the local lesion.

Infectious causes in the differential diagnosis of cutaneous anthrax include plague, tularemia, scrub typhus, rickettsial spotted fevers, rat bite fever, and ecthyma gangrenosum. Various forms of noninfectious skin lesions, such as vasculitis and arachnid bites, can resemble the eschar caused by anthrax. Excellent resources on clinical diagnosis of cutaneous anthrax are now available [88,89]. Antibiotic therapy of cutaneous anthrax decreases edema and the likelihood of systemic spread, but does not change the course of the skin lesion. The mortality rate in untreated cases has been reported to be 20%, but with antibiotic treatment deaths caused by cutaneous anthrax are rare.

Gastrointestinal anthrax

Outbreaks of gastrointestinal anthrax continue to be reported from Asia and Africa. No culture-proven cases of gastrointestinal anthrax were reported from the United States in the twentieth century. More than 100 cases of the intestinal form of anthrax were reported from the Bekka Valley of Lebanon in 1960–1974 [90]. Two more recent events in which anthrax may have caused intestinal disease were reported in the United States [91,92]. In August 2000, five members of a Minnesota family ate meat from a cow that was found later to be infected with *B anthracis.*

The meat had been cooked well. Two family members developed a self-limited gastrointestinal illness within 48 hours after consumption of the meat. Antibiotic prophylaxis with ciprofloxacin and anthrax vaccine was given to all family members even though the symptoms had resolved. Possible gastrointestinal involvement was reported in one of the patients who died from the 2001 anthrax attack. The patient had nausea and abdominal symptoms, and CT scan showed findings consistent with necrotizing enteritis. At autopsy, 2500 mL of hemorrhagic ascitic fluid with necrotizing infection and gram-positive bacilli in the ileum were seen. Gastrointestinal anthrax occurs from ingestion of insufficiently cooked meat from infected animals [5]. Direct gastrointestinal instillation of *B anthracis* spores has not able to induce experimental infection in primates [93]. The germination of spores may not occur because of the rapid transit time in the gastrointestinal tract. It is more likely that most cases result from the ingestion of large numbers of vegetative forms present in poorly cooked meat from infected animals.

The risks through direct contamination of food and water are largely unknown. The clinical forms of gastrointestinal anthrax are (1) oropharyngeal form with oral or esophageal ulcers and regional lymphadenopathy, edema, and septicemia [94] and (2) intestinal anthrax, the more common form, which presents as primary lesions predominantly in the terminal ileum or cecum [48]. The initial nonspecific abdominal symptoms progress rapidly to bloody diarrhea, acute abdomen, and sepsis syndrome. Massive ascites can occur. Late stage of the disease is similar to the systemic disease or sepsis syndrome secondary to cutaneous or inhalational anthrax [5]. Thick yellow ascites, segmental bowel edema, and mesenteric lymphadenopathy, particularly in the ileocecal area, are seen at surgery. The mortality rate from gastrointestinal anthrax is high owing to difficulty in early diagnosis. Based on the experience from the Lebanese outbreak, intestinal anthrax should be treated with medical therapy, including intravenous antibiotics initially. Wide surgical resection of the involved areas of bowel extending into apparently uninvolved tissue should be performed if a quick response is not seen. The overall estimated mortality rate of intestinal anthrax is 28% to 60% [91].

Hemorrhagic meningoencephalitis

Neurologic complications can be associated with any of the three forms of primary anthrax infections [95,96]. Meningoencephalitis should be considered as the fourth type of initial clinical presentation and should prompt a search for inhalational anthrax and potential bioterrorism [97]. The autopsy reports from accidental cases of inhalational anthrax in Sverdlovsk revealed hemorrhagic meningitis in 50% of patients. The first recognized case in the US 2001 anthrax attack was the Florida patient who presented with hemorrhagic meningitis [9]. The historical case-fatality rate is 95% even after treatment. Other neurologic complications include cerebral edema, parenchymal brain hemorrhages, vasculitis, and subarachnoid hemorrhage.

Microbiologic diagnosis

The first suspicion of an anthrax illness must lead to immediate notification of the local hospital epidemiologist, local or state health department, and local or state public health laboratory. Microbiologic detection of organisms resembling *B anthracis* may lead to initial detection of an outbreak. In advanced infections, the bacilli may be visible on Gram stain of unspun peripheral blood (Fig. 5). The most useful routine diagnostic test is the standard blood culture (Fig. 6). It is important to obtain blood cultures before the initiation of antibiotics. The blood cultures usually grow at 6 to 24 hours and may be negative after only one or two doses of antibiotics. It takes about 24 hours to identify a *Bacillus* species from a blood culture. Isolation of *Bacillus* species in the United States from blood culture most often represents growth of *Bacillus cereus*. If the diagnosis of anthrax is entertained, biochemical testing and colony morphology provide a preliminary identification. After preliminary identification, the isolate should be sent promptly to a level B or level C laboratory in the Laboratory Response Network for bioterrorism [98]. Currently, 81 clinical laboratories in the Laboratory Response Network have diagnostic capabilities for bioterrorism pathogens. Confirmatory tests include immunohistochemical staining, enzyme-linked immunosorbent assay for protective antigen, γ-phage lysis, and PCR assay. The Mayo-Roche Rapid Anthrax Test, a rapid-cycle real-time PCR, is now commercially available [80]. Uhl and colleagues [99] reported the detection of DNA from vaccinia virus, herpes simplex virus, varicella-zoster virus, and *B anthracis* by light cycle PCR after autoclaving the specimens and eliminating infectivity. Specific qualified laboratories without biosafety level 4 facilities may be able to offer such tests for immediate diagnosis. PCR to amplify specific virulence plasmid markers in *B anthracis* may become available soon [2]. Because of the pathogenesis of inhalational anthrax, respiratory secretions are unlikely to reveal the organism by Gram stain and culture. Gram stain of the sputum revealed *B anthracis* in only one patient from the 2001 US inhalational anthrax cases. A Gram stain and culture of the vesicular fluid from skin lesions should be obtained. If the patient is already on antibiotics or Gram stain of the fluid is negative, punch biopsy of the skin should be sent to an appropriate laboratory for immunohistochemical staining or PCR assays. Blood cultures from patients with cutaneous anthrax should be obtained before starting antibiotics. The presence of gram-positive bacilli in the cerebrospinal fluid in a patient with a compatible clinical illness should make anthrax a serious consideration. This is how the index case of inhalational anthrax in the 2001 anthrax attacks was diagnosed [9]. Autopsy findings of thoracic necrotizing hemorrhagic

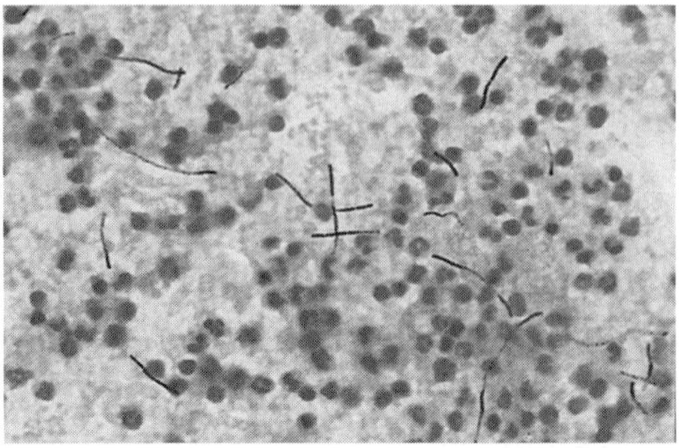

Fig. 5. Gram stain of peripheral blood buffy coat from a patient with inhalational anthrax. (*From* Borio L, Frank D, Mani V, et al. Death due to inhalational anthrax. In: Henderson, Inglesby, Toole, editors. Bioterrorism: guidelines for medical and public health management. Chicago: AMA Press; 2002; with permission.)

lymphadenitis and mediastinitis or hemorrhagic meningitis in a case with unexplained death should strongly favor the diagnosis of anthrax.

Current therapies and postexposure prophylaxis

Current antibiotic management guidelines were developed by the CDC shortly after recognition of the bioterrorist anthrax attacks in October 2001 [24]. These guidelines were based on antimicrobial susceptibility patterns that were determined for the 11 *B anthracis* isolates from the victims of the intentional exposures in Florida, New York City, and Washington, DC. All of these isolates were susceptible to penicillin, amoxicillin, ciprofloxacin, doxycycline, chloramphenicol, clindamycin, tetracycline, rifampin, clarithromycin, and vancomycin. The isolates also are susceptible to

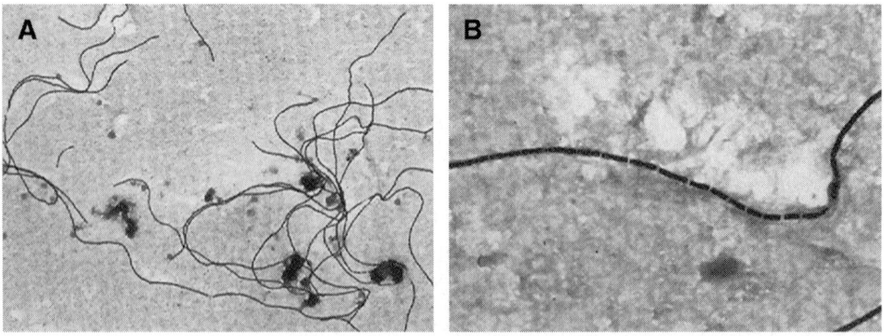

Fig. 6. (*A*, *B*) Gram stain of blood culture media from a patient with inhalational anthrax. (*From* Borio L, Frank D, Mani V, et al. Death due to inhalational anthrax. In: Henderson, Inglesby, Toole, editors. Bioterrorism: guidelines for medical and public health management. Chicago: AMA Press; 2002; with permission.)

imipenem and likely to be susceptible to meropenem. The isolates showed intermediate susceptibility to ceftriaxone and erythromycin. In addition, studies at the CDC showed the presence of a cephalosporinase and other β-lactamases in the isolates.

Based on laboratory and animal studies, the CDC recommends that ciprofloxacin or doxycycline should be used for initial intravenous therapy until susceptibility results become established. They also recommend at least two antimicrobial agents because of the significant mortality associated with inhalational anthrax. Despite these recommendations, the specific effectiveness of ciprofloxacin and doxycycline, compared with other antibiotics in humans, has not been studied sufficiently because of the lack of clinical trials and small numbers of naturally occurring cases of inhalational anthrax.

A review of 82 cases of inhalational anthrax found that the median time from symptom onset to the initiation of antibiotics for all cases in the review was 4.7 days [100]. Victims who had received antibiotic therapy in 4.7 days or sooner had a 40% mortality rate. If antibiotic therapy was initiated after 4.7 days, the mortality rate was 75%. These findings emphasize that the most crucial aspect of medical care of inhalational anthrax victims is the rapid initiation of any potentially effective antibiotic therapy. The review also suggested that patients who received multidrug antibiotic therapy and pleural fluid drainage had higher rates of survival. Nevertheless, even with modern supportive therapies, patients who progressed to the fulminant phase of inhalational anthrax had a mortality rate of 97%, regardless of the treatment they received.

Although data are limited, combination antimicrobial therapy seems a prudent therapeutic approach to life-threatening anthrax. This approach may be particularly useful for central nervous system involvement because of the poor penetration of many antibiotics. Ciprofloxacin in combination with chloramphenicol, rifampin, or penicillin is recommended for anthrax meningitis [5]. The addition of clindamycin for any form of anthrax also has been recommended based on the theoretical benefit of diminishing bacterial toxin production [101].

In the contained casualty setting, initial intravenous antibiotic therapy (ciprofloxacin or doxycycline) followed by oral therapy with the same agents is recommended. In a mass causality setting, intravenous therapy or combination therapy may not be feasible. Under these circumstances, oral therapy with ciprofloxacin or doxycycline is recommended for adults for therapy and postexposure prophylaxis. Ciprofloxacin, doxycycline, and amoxicillin are recommended for children and pregnant women. There are no FDA-approved antibiotic regimens for post–anthrax exposure chemoprophylaxis. Antibiotic therapy or prophylaxis should be continued for at least 60 days after exposure because of the possibility of delayed germination of spores. Cutaneous anthrax should be treated for 60 days after exposure because of presumed concomitant inhalational exposure in the setting of a potential bioterrorism event.

Emerging and investigational therapies

Passive immunotherapy with plasma from vaccinated horses was the only available treatment for anthrax in the preantibiotic era and is still used in Russia and China [102]. There are no data on its efficacy in humans. In animal studies, antibody therapy for anthrax was shown to be effective only when given before infection. The CDC and other federal agencies have been discussing the potential use of plasma from military personnel vaccinated against anthrax to provide preformed antibodies against the anthrax toxin. Such "antitoxin" therapy would be used as an adjunct to antibiotics, especially in patients not responding to antibiotics alone. The US Army Medical Research Institute of Infectious Diseases in collaboration with the CDC and the National Institutes of Health is conducting animal experiments on efficacy and dosing. The United States currently has a small plasma supply collected from military personnel. The second larger batch from vaccinated volunteers would add modestly to these supplies, some of which would be needed for animal studies. Selected antibodies from an *Escherichia coli* expression system were shown to bind to protective antigen with high affinity [103]. The antibody (IH) with the highest affinity for protective antigen prevented anthrax toxin from binding to its receptor and protected rats against a lethal challenge with the anthrax toxin. Iverson and Georgiou (unpublished data, as cited in [103]) reported a monoclonal antibody against anthrax toxin with 50-fold improved affinity for anthrax toxin compared with the original fragments. The monoclonal antibody protected rats from a lethal challenge with anthrax toxin.

A drug based on mutant protective antigen has the potential of being useful in the treatment of anthrax. Rats survived injection of lethal factor plus mutant protective antigen [65]. A peptide isolated from a phage display library was shown to bind weakly to the heptameric cell-binding subunit of anthrax toxin, but prevented the interaction between cell-binding and enzymatic moieties [104]. A polyvalent molecule of this non-natural peptide prevented assembly of the toxin complex in vitro and blocked the effects of the toxin in an animal model. The characterization of the crystal structure of lethal factor and edema factor and the cellular receptor for protective antigen is expected to help identify drugs that interfere with the binding and the activity of anthrax toxin [59–61]. The phage lysin γ (PlyG lysin) isolated from the γ phage of *B anthracis* was shown specifically to kill vegetative cells and germinating spores of *B anthracis* and other members of the *B anthracis* "cluster" in vitro and in vivo [105]. The lytic specificity of PlyG lysine rapidly identified *B anthracis*.

Human vaccination

The current human anthrax vaccine in the United Kingdom and the United States consists of alum precipitated cell-free filtrate with protective antigen from an avirulent noncapsulated strain [5,106]. The US vaccine,

AVA, is adsorbed onto aluminum hydroxide. Licensed in 1970, AVA currently is manufactured by BioPort Corporation (Lansing, MI) and is given in a series of six inoculations over 18 months. Numerous animal studies have shown efficacy of pre-exposure vaccination with AVA [107,108]. A predecessor vaccine to AVA showed 92.5% efficacy against human cutaneous anthrax in a placebo-controlled trial in 1950 [109]. The efficacy of AVA in inhalational anthrax has been studied in monkeys [110]. After exposure to 8 LD_{50} of *B anthracis* spores, 9 of 10 control animals and 8 of 10 vaccinated animals died. All nine animals receiving doxycycline for 30 days plus vaccine at baseline and 2 weeks after exposure survived even after being rechallenged. The US Department of Defense initiated the compulsory anthrax vaccine immunization program for 2.4 million military personnel in 1997 [106]. A report from the Institute of Medicine concluded that AVA is effective against inhalational anthrax and in combination with appropriate antibiotic therapy may prevent the development of disease after exposure [111]. The report also concluded that AVA has acceptable safety. *Mycoplasma* contamination of AVA administered to military personnel thought to be associated with Persian Gulf syndrome was ruled out [112].

The civilian use of AVA in the United States currently is limited to individuals at high risk of exposure to contaminated materials or environments, including personnel working with environmental specimens and workers performing confirmatory testing for *B anthracis* in the US Laboratory Response Network, workers making repeated entries to known spore-contaminated areas, and others in whom repeated exposure to aerosolized spores may occur [97]. AVA was given under investigational new drug procedures as an adjunct to the 60-day postexposure antibiotic prophylaxis during the 2001 anthrax attacks [5]. The US Department of Health and Human Services recommended three options for individuals at risk for inhalation anthrax [113]: (1) antimicrobial prophylaxis for 60 days accompanied by monitoring for illness and adverse events, (2) 40 more days of antimicrobial prophylaxis (intended to provide protection against the possibility that anthrax spores may cause illness 100 days after exposure) accompanied by monitoring for illness and adverse reactions, or (3) 40 more days of antimicrobial prophylaxis plus three doses of AVA administered over 4 weeks. Because the vaccine is not approved by the FDA for postexposure prophylaxis, it was administered with informed consent.

Anthrax vaccines in development

A vaccine containing recombinant Protective antigen produced by non–spore-forming *B anthracis* protects rhesus monkeys against inhalational anthrax [114]. Fewer injections of this vaccine might be needed to elicit an effective immune response, and the vaccine might have fewer side effects than AVA. The recombinant anthrax vaccine currently is being developed under a fast-track program. Avant Immunotherapeutics (Needham, MA) is developing a rapidly acting oral one-dose anthrax vaccine made from protective antigen-producing attenuated *Vibrio cholerae*. A critical level of vaccine-induced IgG antibody against the protective antigen of *B anthracis* is known to confer protective immunity. The role of IgG antibody against the poly γ-D-glutamic acid (γ_DPGA) capsule in protective immunity was studied. Schneerson and colleagues [115] compared the nonimmunogenic γ_DPGA or corresponding synthetic peptides bound to BSA, recombinant *B anthracis* Protective antigen (*r*PA), or recombinant *Pseudomonas aeruginosa* exotoxin A (*r*EPA) for their immunogenicity. The anti-γ_DPGA antibodies induced opsonophagocytic killing of capsulated toxin-negative *B anthracis*. The γ_DPGA-*r*PA conjugates induced antibodies against Protective antigen and γ_DPGA. A dually active anthrax vaccine such as the one used in these studies confers simultaneous protection against the replicating bacilli and the toxin [116]. The conjugation of capsular γ_DPGA to Protective antigen converted the weakly immunogenic PGA to a potent immunogen and synergistically enhanced the humeral response to Protective antigen. The concept of dually active anthrax vaccine introduces a novel vaccine design with the potential of wide application against infectious diseases, including those related to bioterrorism.

Infection control and decontamination

Standard barrier precautions are recommended for all hospitalized patients. In addition, contact isolation precautions should be used for patients with draining cutaneous anthrax lesions [51]. Dressings removed from the draining lesions should be disposed of as biohazardous waste. Health care workers, household contacts, or other contacts who are determined to have been exposed to aerosol or surface contamination should receive post-exposure prophylaxis [5]. When a diagnosis of anthrax is suspected, the hospital epidemiologist, the hospital microbiology laboratory, and the state health department should be notified immediately. Appropriate specimen handling in the laboratory involves biosafety level 2 conditions and referral to the nearest facility in the Laboratory Response Network under appropriate handling and shipping conditions. Individuals coming in direct contact with a substance alleged to be containing *B anthracis* should wash the exposed skin and clothing thoroughly with soap and water. For environmental surfaces contaminated with infected body fluids, a disinfectant such as hypochlorite, used for standard hospital infection control, is adequate. Human and animal remains should be handled under protocols to prevent further transmission of the disease. Cremation should be recommended in preference to burial [5]. Embalming of bodies should be considered a special risk. All autopsy-related instruments and materials should be incinerated or autoclaved.

The spores of *B anthracis* may not be eliminated by the usual decontamination procedures. The sporicidal activity of various agents is determined by contact time, temperature, concentration, pH, and relative humidity [117]. The US Environmental Protection Agency recommends the use of sodium hypochlorite as a sporicidal agent under an emergency exemption because it needs to be used under specified conditions [118]. For effective sporicidal activity, common household bleach must be diluted with water to increase the free available chlorine and acetic acid added to change the pH of the solution to 7. Fumigation with formaldehyde vapor has been used in the past to decontaminate textile mills. The *B anthracis* spores were greatly reduced immediately after treatment and were undetectable after 6 months of fumigation. The deliberate spore contamination at Gruinard Island, Scotland, occurred during British military testing of explosives. Spores remained viable for 36 years after the experiments. Gruinard Island was declared anthrax-free after decontaminating it in stages between 1979 and 1987. Materials used for decontamination included 280 tons of formaldehyde and 2000 tons of seawater. The carcinogenic properties of formaldehyde are reduced by using ammonium bicarbonate after fumigation. Gamma radiation was used in the 1960s and 1970s for disinfection of bailed goat hair contaminated with *B anthracis* spores [117]. Based on a study by Horne and associates [119], 2 megarads of gamma radiation kill most resistant spores and include a margin of safety. This was the method used to decontaminate all mail from contaminated US Postal Service facilities in 2001.

The greatest risk to humans from an aerosol occurs from primary aerosolization, when *B anthracis* spores first are made airborne. There is evidence to suggest that after an outdoor aerosol release, the threat would be similar to individuals indoors and outdoors [49]. Kournikakis and coworkers [120] showed that even "low-tech" delivery systems, such as the opening of envelopes containing spores in dry powder form, can deliver high concentrations of spores rapidly to people in the vicinity. During the 2001 attacks, infection occurred even in individuals who handled or processed unopened letters in Washington, DC [5]. These cases showed that *B anthracis* spores of "weapons grade" quality are able to leak out of the edges or the pores of envelopes. The only explanation for two fatal inhalational anthrax cases in New York and Connecticut during the 2001 attacks was inhalation of small numbers of spores present in cross-contaminated mail. The risk from secondary aerosolization (resuspension of spore into the air) is uncertain and would be expected to depend on many variables. The question of illnesses from secondary aerosolization in the Sverdlovsk experience has been debated. The epidemic curve is typical, however, for a common source with virtually all confirmed cases having occurred within the area of the plume on the day of the accident. The risk from secondary aerosolization of *B anthracis* spores was assessed by the US Environmental Protection Agency in the office of Senator Daschle in the Hart Building in Washington, DC. The experiments showed that routine activity could cause significant resuspension *B anthracis* spores [121]. These findings do not allow conclusions about the risk of occupants developing anthrax infection under these conditions. They do have important implications for addressing decontamination, respiratory protection, and reuse of contaminated buildings. The methods used to decontaminate or sterilize laboratory or food industry settings perhaps can be used to decontaminate buildings. Multiple technologies may be needed to decontaminate buildings and their contents. Decontamination of sections of the Hart Senate Office Building in Washington, DC, after the opening of a letter laden with *B anthracis* was estimated to cost $23 million.

Summary

The earliest known writings about anthrax are from Egypt and Mesopotamia and date back to 5000 BC. The Book of Exodus in the Bible describes the Fifth plague killing the Egyptians' cattle and the Sixth plague, which may have been outbreaks of anthrax in humans. The early literature of Hindus, Romans, and Greeks contains descriptions of anthrax. Anthrax became the first human infectious disease with specific microbial etiology when *B anthracis* was used to fulfill Koch's postulate in 1877. The attenuated anthrax spore vaccine was first tested by Pasteur in 1881. In the early 1900s, improved industrial and animal husbandry hygiene and decreased use of potentially contaminated imported animal products caused a steady and significant decline in the number of cases in the developed world. This decline was aided further by the Sterne animal vaccine from the spore suspension by an avirulent nonencapsulated strain in 1939. This is the currently used animal vaccine. Anthrax in its natural form became an obscure disease in many parts of the world.

Because of the ease with which *B anthracis* could be cultivated, it gained notoriety during World War I and World War II as a biologic weapon and was included in the offensive biologic weapons programs of Germany, Great Britain, the United States, and the USSR. Accidental release of anthrax spores from a biologic weapons facility in Sverdlovsk, Russia, caused the first documented outbreak from weapons grade *B anthracis*. The new age doomsday cult Aum Shinrikyo in Japan (1995) attempted to use anthrax spores along with other microbial agents to cause mass casualties, but all attempts failed. Larry Wayne Harris, a microbiologist in the United States, threatened to release "military grade anthrax" in Las Vegas, Nevada. He had obtained the veterinary vaccine strains of anthrax and was arrested when he openly talked about the use of biologic agents. The sensational media coverage of this event may have had the unintended effect of popularizing anthrax as a potential tool for terrorists. The first wave of anthrax hoaxes in the United States followed the report of this event. New legislation came into effect to ensure legitimate medical and scientific purposes for possession and transfer of biologic agents.

The use of the US Postal Service to disseminate *B anthracis* intentionally in 2001 brought into focus the diversity of biologic threats. It also provided impetus and funding for research on microbial forensics, newer treatment modalities, and improved vaccines for anthrax. The scientific knowledge that has been gained using *B anthracis* potentially has a much wider application to infectious disease in general. To quote Albert Einstein: "In the middle of difficulty lies opportunity."

References

[1] Wilkinson L. Anthrax. In: Kiple K, editor. The Cambridge world history of human disease. New York: Cambridge University Press; 1993. p. 582.
[2] Dixon TC, Meselson M, Guillemin J, et al. Anthrax. N Engl J Med 1999;341:815–26.
[3] Swartz MH. Recognition and management of anthrax—an update. N Engl J Med 2001; 345:1621–6.
[4] Kyriacou DN, Stein AC, Yarnold PR, et al. Clinical predictors of bioterrorism-related inhalational anthrax. Lancet 2004;364:449–52.
[5] Inglesby TV, O'Toole T, Henderson DA, et al. Anthrax as a biological weapon, 2002. JAMA 2002;287:2236–52.
[6] Cieslak TJ, Eitzen EM. Clinical and epidemiologic principles of anthrax. Emer Infect Dis 1991;5:552–5.
[7] Brachman PS. Bioterrorism: an update with a focus on anthrax. Am J Epidemiol 2002;155: 981–7.
[8] Jernigan JA, Stephens DS, Asford DA, et al. Bioterrorism-related inhalational anthrax: the first 10 cases reported in the United States. Emerg Infect Dis 2001;7:933–44.
[9] Bush LM, Abrams BH, Beall A, et al. Index case of fatal inhalational anthrax due to bioterrorism in the United States. N Engl J Med 2001;345:1607–10.
[10] Traeger MS, Wiersma ST, Rosenstein NE, et al. First case of bioterrorism-related inhalational anthrax in the United States, Palm Beach County, Florida, 2001. Emerg Infect Dis 2002;8:1029–34.
[11] Mayer TA, Bersoff-Match S, Murphy C, et al. Clinical presentation of inhalational anthrax following bioterrorism exposure: report of 2 surviving patients. JAMA 2001;286:2549–53.
[12] Dewan PK, Fry AM, Laserson K, et al. Inhalational anthrax outbreak among postal workers, Washington, D.C., 2001. Emerg Infect Dis 2002;8:1066–72.
[13] Borio L, Frank D, Mani V, et al. Death due to bioterrorism-related inhalational anthrax: report of 2 patients. JAMA 2002;286:2554–9.
[14] Greene CM, Reefhuis J, Tan C, et al. Epidemiologic investigations of bioterrorism-related anthrax, New Jersey, 2001. Emerg Infect Dis 2002;8:1048–55.
[15] Mina B, Dym JP, Kuepper F, et al. Fatal inhalational anthrax with unknown source of exposure in a 61-year-old woman in New York City. JAMA 2002;287:858–62.
[16] Krol CM, Uszynski M, Dillon EH, et al. Dynamic CT features of inhalational anthrax infection. AJR Am J Roentgenol 2002;178:1063–6.
[17] Gill JR, Melinek J. Inhalational anthrax: gross autopsy findings. Arch Pathol Lab Med 2002;126:993–4.
[18] Barakat LA, Quentzel HL, Jernigan JA, et al. Fatal inhalational anthrax in a 94-year-old Connecticut woman. JAMA 2002;287:863–8.
[19] Enserink M. Biodefense hampered by inadequate tests. Science 2001;294:1266–7.
[20] World Health Organization. Health aspects of chemical and biological weapons: report of a WHO group of consultants. Geneva: World Health Organization; 1970.
[21] Office of Technology Assessment, US Congress. Proliferation of weapons of mass destruction. Publication OTA-ISC-559. Washington, DC: US Government Printing Office; 1993. Available at: www.wws.princeton.edu/ota/disk1/1993/9341_n.html.
[22] Wein LM, Craft DL, Kaplan EH. Emergency response to an anthrax attack. Proc Natl Acad Sci U S A 2003;100:4346–51.

[23] Centers for Disease Control and Prevention. Update: investigation of anthrax associated with intentional exposure and interim public health guidelines, October 2001. MMWR Morb Mortal Wkly Rep 2001;50:889–93.
[24] Centers for Disease Control and Prevention. Update: investigation of bioterrorism-related anthrax and interim guidelines for exposure management and antimicrobial therapy, October 2001. MMWR Morb Mortal Wkly Rep 2001;50:909–19.
[25] Centers for Disease Control and Prevention. Update: investigation of bioterrorism-related anthrax and interim guidelines for clinical evaluation of persons with possible anthrax. MMWR Morb Mortal Wkly Rep 2001;50:941–8.
[26] Centers for Disease Control and Prevention. Investigation of bioterrorism-related anthrax and adverse events from antimicrobial prophylaxis. MMWR Morb Mortal Wkly Rep 2001; 50:973–6.
[27] Centers for Disease Control and Prevention. Notice to readers: considerations for distinguishing influenza-like illness from inhalational anthrax. MMWR Morb Mortal Wkly Rep 2001;50:984–6.
[28] Mayer TA, Morrison A, Bersoff-Matcha S, et al. Inhalational anthrax due to bioterrorism: would current centers for the Disease Control and Prevention have identified the 11 patients with inhalational anthrax from October through November 2001? Clin Infect Dis 2003;36: 1275–83.
[29] Sternbach G. The history of anthrax. J Emerg Med 2003;24:463–7.
[30] Munch R. Robert Koch. Microbes Infect 2003;5:69–74.
[31] Weiss R. Robert Koch: the grandfather of cloning? Cell 2005;123:539–42.
[32] Tenth Annual Report of the Local Government Board, 1880–81. Supplement containing the report of the Medical Officer. London: Her Majesty's Stationery Office; 1881.
[33] Bell JH. Anthrax. In: Allbutt TC, editor. A system of medicine, vol. 2. New York: MacMillan; 1901. p. 525–52.
[34] Macher A. Industry-related outbreak of human anthrax, Massachusetts, 1868. Emerg Infect Dis 2002;8:1182.
[35] Albrink WS. Pathogenesis of inhalational anthrax. Bacteriol Rev 1961;25:268–73.
[36] Osborn SH. Anthrax problem in Massachusetts. Am J Public Health 1920;10:657–65.
[37] Lucchesi PF. Serum treatment of 19 cases of anthrax including one of external, internal, and bacteremic type. Am J Med Sci 1932;133:795–802.
[38] Case records of the Massachusetts General Hospital, case #14032: an acute infection with bloody fluid in the right pleural space. N Engl J Med 1928;198:148–53.
[39] Brooksher WR, Briggs JA. Pulmonary anthrax: report of a case. JAMA 1920;74:323–4.
[40] Bell HH. Pulmonary anthrax, with report of case. J Missouri State Med Assoc 1924;21: 407–8.
[41] Cowdery JS. Primary pulmonary anthrax with septicemia. Arch Pathol 1947;43:396–9.
[42] Gold H. Anthrax: a report of one hundred seventeen cases. Arch Intern Med 1955;96: 387–96.
[43] Plotkin SA, Brachman PS, Utell M, et al. An epidemic of inhalation anthrax, the first in the twentieth century: I. clinical features. Am J Med 1960;29:992–1001.
[44] Brachman PS, Plotkin SA, Bumford FH, et al. An epidemic of inhalation anthrax: the first in the twentieth century: II. epidemiology. Am J Hyg 1960;72:6–23.
[45] Meselson M, Guillemin J, Hugh-Jones M, et al. The Sverdlovsk anthrax outbreak of 1979. Science 1994;266:1202–8.
[46] Brookmeyer R, Blades N. The statistical analysis of truncated data: application to the Sverlovsk anthrax outbreak. Biostatistics 2001;2:233–47.
[47] Grinberg LM, Abramova FA, Yampolskaya OV, et al. Quantitative pathology of inhalational anthrax: I. quantitative microscopic findings. Mod Pathol 2001;14:482–95.
[48] Abramova FA, Grinberg LM, Yampolskaya OV, et al. Pathology of inhalational anthrax in 42 cases from the Sverdlovsk outbreak of 1979. Proc Natl Acad Sci U S A 1993;90: 2291–4.

[49] Inglesby TV, Henderson DA, Bartlett JG, et al. Anthrax as a biological weapon: medical and public health management. JAMA 1999;281:1735–45.

[50] CDC Laboratory Response Network (LRN). Level A laboratory procedures for identification of *Bacillus anthracis*. 2003; p. 1–18. Available at: www.bt.cdc.gov/agent/anthrax/LevelAProtocol./anthraxlabprotocol.pdf.

[51] Lew D. *Bacillus anthracis* (anthrax). In: Mandell GL, Bennett JE, Dolin R, editors. Mandell, Douglas, and Bennett's principles and practice of infectious diseases. Philadelphia: Churchill Livingstone; 2000. p. 2215–20.

[52] Read TD, Salzberg SL, Pop M, et al. Comparative genome sequencing for discovery of novel polymorphism in *Bacillus anthracis*. Science 2002;296:2028–33.

[53] Farrar WE. Anthrax: virulence and vaccines. Ann Intern Med 1994;121:379–80.

[54] Green BD, Battisti L, Koeler TM, et al. Demonstration of a capsule plasmid in *Bacillus anthracis*. Infect Immun 1985;49:291–7.

[55] Mikesell P, Ivins BE, Ristroph JD, et al. Evidence for plasmid-mediated toxin production in *Bacillus anthracis*. Infect Immun 1983;39:371–6.

[56] Beauregard KE, Collier RJ, Swanson JA. Proteolytic activation of receptor-bound anthrax antigen on macrophages promotes its internalization. Cell Microbiol 2000;2:251–8.

[57] Okinaka RT, Cloud K, Hampton O, et al. Sequence and organization of pX01, the large *Bacillus anthracis* plasmid harboring the anthrax toxin genes. J Bacteriol 1999; 181:6509–15.

[58] Okinaka RT, Cloud K, Hampton O, et al. Sequence, assembly and analysis of pX01 and pX02. J Appl Microbiol 1999;87:261–2.

[59] Bradley KA, Mogridge J, Mourez M, et al. Identification of the cellular receptor for anthrax toxin. Nature 2001;414:225–9.

[60] Drum CL, Yan SZ, Bard J, et al. Structural basis for the activation of anthrax adenylyl cyclase exotoxin by calmodulin. Nature 2002;415:396–402.

[61] Pannifer AD, Wong TY, Schwarzenbacher R, et al. Crystal structure of the anthrax lethal factor. Nature 2001;414:229–30.

[62] Agrawal A, Lingappa J, Leppla SH, et al. Impairment of dendritic cells and adaptive immunity by anthrax lethal toxin. Nature 2003;424:329–33.

[63] Erwin J, DaSilva LM, Bavar S, et al. Macrophage-derived cell lines do not express proinflammatory cytokines after exposure to *Bacillus anthracis* lethal toxin. Infect Immun 2001; 2:1175–7.

[64] Young JA, Collier RJ. Attacking anthrax. Sci Am 2002;286:48–59.

[65] Sellman BR, Mourez M, Collier RJ. This time it was real—knowledge of anthrax put to the test. Science 2001;292:695–7.

[66] Hanna PC, Acosta D, Collier RJ. On the role of macrophages in anthrax. Proc Natl Acad Sci U S A 1993;90:10198–201.

[67] Moayeri M, Haines D, Young HA, et al. *Bacillus anthracis* lethal toxin induces TNF-α-independent hypoxia-mediated toxicity in mice. J Clin Invest 2003;112:670–82.

[68] Prince AS. The host response to anthrax lethal toxin: unexpected observations. J Clin Invest 2003;112:656–8.

[69] Kuehnert MJ, Doyle TJ, Hill HA, et al. Clinical features that discriminate inhalational anthrax from other acute respiratory illnesses. Clin Infect Dis 2003;36:328–36.

[70] Hupert N, Bearman GML, Mushlin AI, et al. Accuracy of screening for inhalational anthrax after a bioterrorist attack. Ann Intern Med 2003;139:337–45.

[71] Howell JM, Mayer TA, Handflin D, et al. Screening for inhalational anthrax due to bioterrorism: evaluating proposed screening protocols. Clin Infect Dis 2004;39:1842–7.

[72] Baggett HC, Rhodes JC, Fridkin SK, et al. No evidence of a mild form of inhalational *Bacillus anthracis* infection during a bioterrorism-related inhalational anthrax outbreak in Washington, D.C. in 2001. Clin Infect Dis 2005;41:991–7.

[73] Barakat LA, Quentzel HL, Jernigan JA, et al. Fatal inhalational anthrax in a 94-year-old Connecticut woman. JAMA 2002;287:863–8.

[74] Borio L, Frank D, Mani V, et al. Death due to bioterrorism-related inhalational anthrax: report of 2 patients. JAMA 2002;286:2554–9.
[75] Bravata DM, Sundaram V, McDonald KM, et al. Evaluating detection and diagnostic decision support systems for bioterrorism response. Emerg Infect Dis 2004;10:100–8.
[76] Bravata DM, McDonald KM, Smith WM, et al. Systematic review: surveillance systems for the early detection of bioterrorism-related diseases. Ann Intern Med 2004;140: 910–22.
[77] Bravata DM, Sundaram V, McDonald KM, et al. Evaluating detection and diagnostic decision support systems for bioterrorism response. Emerg Infect Dis 2004;10:100–8.
[78] Dworkin MS, Ma X, Golash RG. Fear of bioterrorism and implications for public health preparedness. Emerg Infect Dis 2003;9:503–5.
[79] Blank S, Moskin LC, Zucker JR. An ounce of prevention is a ton of work: antibiotic prophylaxis for anthrax, New York City, 2001. Emerg Infect Dis 2003;9:615–22.
[80] De BK, Bragg SL, Sanden GN, et al. Two-component direct fluorescent-antibody assay for rapid identification of *Bacillus anthracis*. Emerg Infect Dis 2002;8:1060–5.
[81] Uhl JR, Bell CA, Sloan LM, et al. Application of rapid-cycle real-time polymerase chain reaction for the detection of microbial pathogens: the Mayo-Roache rapid anthrax test. Mayo Clin Proc 2002;77:673–80.
[82] Succhi CT, Whitney AM, Mayer LW, et al. Sequencing the 16S rRNA gene: a rapid tool for identification of *Bacillus anthracis*. Emerg Infect Dis 2002;8:1117–23.
[83] Quinn CP, Semenova VA, Elie CM, et al. Specific, sensitive, and quantitative enzyme-linked immunosorbent assay for human immunoglobulin G antibodies to anthrax toxin protective antigen. Emerg Infect Dis 2002;8:1103–10.
[84] Fasanella A, Losito S, Adone R, et al. PCR assay to detect *Bacillus anthracis* spores in heat-treated specimens. J Clin Microbiol 2003;41:896–9.
[85] Stephenson J. Rapid anthrax test approved. JAMA 2004;294:30.
[86] Brachman P, Friedlander A. Anthrax. In: Plotkin S, Orenstein W, editors. Vaccines. Philadelphia: WB Saunders; 1999. p. 629–37.
[87] Centers for Disease Control and Prevention. Summary of notifiable diseases, 1945–1994. MMWR Morb Mortal Wkly Rep 1994;43:70–8.
[88] American Academy of Dermatology. Anthrax. Available at: www.aad.org/BioInfo/anthrax.html. Accessed 2003.
[89] The Universidad Peruana Cayetano Heredia Gorgas course in clinical tropical medicine. Available at: http//info.dom.edu/gorgas/anthrax/html. Accessed 2003.
[90] Kanafani ZA, Ghossain A, Sharara AI, et al. Endemic gastrointestinal anthrax in 1960's Lebanon: clinical manifestations and surgical findings. Emerg Infect Dis 2003;9:520–5.
[91] Centers for Disease Control and Prevention. Human ingestion of *Bacillus anthracis*-contaminated meat—Minnesota. MMWR Morb Mortal Wkly Rep 2000;49:813–6.
[92] Borio L, Frank D, Mani V, et al. Death due to bioterrorism-related inhalational anthrax: report of 2 patients. JAMA 2001;286:2554–9.
[93] Lincoln R, Hodges D, Klein F, et al. Role of the lymphatics in the pathogenesis of anthrax. J Infect Dis 1965;15:481–94.
[94] Sirisanthana T, Navachareon N, Tharavichitkul P, et al. An outbreak of oral-pharyngeal anthrax. Am J Trop Med Hyg 1984;33:144–50.
[95] Meyer MA. Neurological complications of anthrax: a review of the literature. Arch Neurol 2003;60:483–8.
[96] Lanska DJ. Anthrax meningoencephalitis. Neurology 2002;59:327–34.
[97] Lucey D. *Bacillus anthracis* (anthrax). In: Mandell GL, Bennett JE, Dolin R, editors. Mandell, Douglas, and Bennett's principles and practice of infectious diseases. Philadelphia: Churchill Livingstone; 2000. p. 2485–91.
[98] Centers for Disease Control and Prevention. 2002. Available at: http://www.bt.cdc.gov/LabIssues/index.asp.

[99] Uhl JR, Bell CA, Sloan LM, et al. Application of rapid-cycle real-time polymerase chain reaction for the detection of microbial pathogens: the Mayo-Roche rapid anthrax test. Mayo Clinic Proc 2002;77:673–80.
[100] Holty JEC, Bravata D, Liu H, et al. Systematic review: a century of inhalational anthrax cases for 1900 to 2005. Ann Intern Med 2006;144:270–80.
[101] Stevens DL, Gibbons AE, Bergstron R, et al. The Eagle effect revisited. J Infect Dis 1988; 158:23–8.
[102] Enserink M. 'Borrowed immunity' may save future victims. Science 2002;295:777.
[103] Maynard JA, Maassan CB, Leppla SH, et al. Protection against anthrax toxin by recombinant antibody fragments correlates with antigen affinity. Nat Biotechnol 2002;20:597–601.
[104] Mourez M, Kane RS, Mogridge J, et al. Designing a polyvalent inhibitor of anthrax toxin. Nat Biotechnol 2001;19:958–61.
[105] Schuch R, Nelson D, Fischetti VA. A bacteriolytic agent that detects and kills *B. anthracis*. Nature 2002;418:884–8.
[106] Jefferson T. Bioterrorism and compulsory vaccination. BMJ 2004;329:524–5.
[107] Ivins BE, Fellows P, Pitt ML, et al. Efficacy of standardized human anthrax vaccine against *Bacillus anthracis* aerosol spore challenge in rhesus monkeys. Salisbury Med Bull 1996;87: 125–6.
[108] Fellows P, Linscott M, Ivins B, et al. Efficacy of a human anthrax vaccine in guinea pigs, rabbits, and rhesus macaques against challenge by *Bacillus anthracis* isolates of diverse geographical origin. Vaccine 2001;20:635.
[109] Brachman PS, Gold H, Plotkins SA, et al. Field evaluation of human anthrax vaccine. Am J Public Health 1962;52:632–45.
[110] Friedlander AM, Welkos SL, Pitt ML, et al. Post exposure prophylaxis against experimental inhalation anthrax. J Infect Dis 1993;167:1239–42.
[111] Committee to Assess the Safety and Efficacy of the Anthrax Vaccine, Medical Follow-Up Agency. The anthrax vaccine: is it safe? Does it work? Washington, DC: Institute of Medicine, National Academy Press; 2002. Available at:. http://www.iom.edu/iom/iomhome.nsf/WFiles/Anthrax-8-pager1FINAL/$file/Anthrax-8-pager1FINAL.pdf/.
[112] Hart MK, Del Giudice RA, Korch GW Jr. Absence of mycoplasma contamination in the anthrax vaccine. Emerg Infect Dis 2002;8:94–6.
[113] Centers for Disease Prevention and Control. Additional options for preventive treatment for person exposed to inhalational anthrax. MMWR Morb Mortal Wkly Rep 2001;50: 11–42.
[114] Friedlander AM. New anthrax vaccine gets a green light. Science 2002;296:639–40.
[115] Schneerson R, Kubler-Kielb J, Liu TY, et al. Poly (γ-D-glutamic acid) protein conjugates induce IgG antibodies in mice to the capsule of *Bacillus anthracis*: a potential addition to the anthrax vaccine. Proc Natl Acad Sci U S A 2003;100:8945–50.
[116] Rhie GE, Roehrl MH, Mourez M, et al. A dually active anthrax vaccine that confers protection against both bacilli and toxins. Proc Natl Acad Sci U S A 2003;100:10925–30.
[117] Spotts-Whitney EA, Beatty ME, Taylor TH, et al. Inactivation of *Bacillus anthracis* spores. Emerg Infect Dis 2003;9:623–7.
[118] US Environmental Protection Agency. Pesticides: topical and chemical fact sheets [cited 2003 March 31]. 2003. Available at: http://www.epa.gov/pesticides/factsheets/chemicals/bleachfactsheet.htm#bkmrk7.
[119] Horne T, Turner G, Willis A. Inactivation of spores of *Bacillus anthracis* by G-radiation. Nature 1959;4659:475–6.
[120] Kournikakis B, Armour SJ, Boulet CA, et al. Risk assessment of anthrax threat letters. Defense Research Establishment Suffield; 2001. Available at: http://www.dres.dnd.ca/Meetings/FirstResponders/tr01-048annex.pdf.
[121] Weis CP, Intrepido AJ, Miller AK, et al. Secondary aerosolization of viable *Bacillus anthracis* spores in a contaminated US Senate office. JAMA 2002;288:2853–8.

ELSEVIER
SAUNDERS

Infect Dis Clin N Am
20 (2006) 253–272

INFECTIOUS
DISEASE CLINICS
OF NORTH AMERICA

Impact of Plague on Human History

Cheston B. Cunha[a], Burke A. Cunha, MD[b,c,*]

[a]*Pennsylvania State University College of Medicine, Hershey, PA 17033, USA*
[b]*Infectious Disease Division, Winthrop-University Hospital, Mineola, NY 11501, USA*
[c]*State University of New York School of Medicine, Stony Brook, NY, USA*

There is little doubt that plague has existed since ancient times. The oldest written description of plague is of the epidemic in 1320 BC that occurred among the Philistines. Plague was first mentioned in the Book of Samuel in the Old Testament and was described as "the great dying" and "the great pestilence." Victims were described as having "boils," and an association with rodents (ie, mice) was noted. Since the Philistine plague, there have been many descriptions of plagues through the ages. Some of these epidemics may have been due to plague, but other pestilences may not have been plague related. Without specific paleopathologic evidence from ancient remains of plague victims, the likely cause of the plague epidemics in ancient times rests heavily on the interpretation/translation descriptions in ancient texts. Translation problems are complicated further by the difference in medical terminology used by the ancients compared with today's medical descriptive terms. Observers writing about ancient plagues varied in their descriptive ability and their use of medical terms [1,2].

Contemporary notions about ancient plagues have been derived from translations by classical scholars on the one hand and infectious disease physicians on the other hand. Classical scholars are familiar with the nuances of language, but lack the appreciation of the significance of descriptive medical terms. Infectious disease clinicians are often unfamiliar with the variations and nuances of terms used in ancient texts (ie, *buboes* could be translated as "ulcers," "sores," or "boils"). Until paleopathologic proof from ancient remains is available, clinicians are left with different possible explanations causing ancient plagues based on different observers writing in different

* Corresponding author. Infectious Disease Division, Winthrop-University Hospital, 222 Station Plaza North, Suite 432 Mineola, NY 11501, USA.

doi:10.1016/j.idc.2006.03.001

languages, subject to interpretational difficulties by contemporary classical scholars and infectious disease physicians [3–5].

Plague bacillus

The causative agent of plague (ie, the plague bacillus) was first identified simultaneously by two individuals, Yersin and Kiasato. In the 1890s, plague epidemics were occurring in China, and the Japanese government sent Kiasato, who had studied with Koch in Berlin, to China to determine the cause of the epidemic there. The French government sent Yersin to Hanoi in French Indochina for the same reason. Apparently, Kiasato was the first to make the observation that the "plague bacillus" was responsible for the plague, but he published his findings in Japanese and English. Apparently, Yersin published his observations on the plague bacillus in French in a rapid publication journal, assuring that his report would be published first. The plague bacillus subsequently was named *Pasteurella pestis*. Yersin suspected insect vectors (ie, flies) as the primary vector in plague. Ogata, a Japanese investigator, theorized the tropical rat flea was the vector of plague. Later in the same year, Simond, a French navy physician also working in Indochina, identified the tropical rat flea, *Xenopsylla cheopis*, as the vector of plague. Later in 1898, he determined that rats were the reservoir. He also showed that fleas from dead rats transmitted *P pestis* to other animals. In 1970, in honor of Yersin's first publication, *P pestis* was renamed *Yersinia pestis* [6–9].

Clinical manifestations of plague

Plague caused by *Y pestis* most often presents as bubonic plague and less commonly as pneumonic plague or septicemic plague. Bubonic or septicemic plague may be complicated by secondary hematogenously spread plague pneumonia. Primary plague pneumonia, also known as "demic plague," occurs from direct inhalation of the plague bacillus and is highly contagious and lethal. Transmission may occur within 2 to 6 ft of aerosolization from a patient with primary plague pneumonia. Bubonic plague may be complicated rarely by secondary plague pneumonia.

Pestis minor is the term used for mild localized lymphadenitis resulting from plague. Spontaneous recovery is the rule. The clinical manifestations of plague are well recognized, but approximately 5% of patients in endemic plague areas have serologic evidence of previous exposure or subclinical plague. In endemic areas, during outbreaks, approximately 50% of individuals in the outbreak area have serologic evidence of plague exposure. Spontaneous rupture and drainage of lymph nodes with plague lymphadenitis mark the end of illness and the beginning of recovery. Pestis minor occurs as part of the spectrum of disease in an epidemic ranging from subclinical plague to pestis minor to the clinically recognizable variants of plague (ie, bubonic, pneumonic, and septicemic plague) [10–12].

Bubonic plague

Bubonic plague was known as the "Black Death." This term may have been derived from the local hemorrhage accompanying necrosis in suppurative lymphadenitis of bubonic plague or from the purplish black appearance of the entire body resulting from disseminated intravascular coagulation complicating bubonic or septicemic plague. The incubation period of bubonic plague is 3 to 6 days (range 10 hours–10 days) after an infected rodent flea bite. *Y pestis* is carried via the lymph system to regional lymph nodes, resulting in initially painless lymphadenopathy with the sudden onset of fever and chills. The fever is accompanied by malaise, weakness, and prominent headache. Suppurative lymphadenitis is the pathologic lesion in bubonic plague and may involve any of the lymph node chains (in descending order of frequencythe nodes most frequently involved are femoral nodes > inguinal nodes > cervical nodes > axillary nodes > epitrochlear nodes, popliteal nodes, and periaortic nodes). The suppurative lymphadenitis of bubonic plague is exquisitely tender, and even light touch results in intense discomfort. Necrosis follows lymphadenitis, and the suppurative nodes drain with a serosanguineous discharge. Neurologic features are characteristic of plague and caused by the neurotoxins of *Y pestis*. Neurologic abnormalities include delirium, stupor, and sleeplessness. Weakness, vertigo, a staggering gait, and slurred speech are common. Insomnia and loss of memory are common long-term sequelae in survivors. Bacterial superinfection may complicate suppurative lymphadenitis [10–12].

In addition to generalized suppurative lymphadenitis, involvement of the spleen, and to a lesser extent the liver, is common. Gastrointestinal symptoms, including nausea and vomiting and abdominal pain, are most common in patients with septicemic plague. Plague meningitis may occur from hematogenous dissemination to the central nervous system, complicating bubonic plague. Secondary plague pneumonia may occur after bubonic or septicemic plague. The kidneys are not usually involved with bubonic plague [11–13].

Plague meningitis is a recognized complication of bubonic plague and usually occurs 10 to 17 days with untreated bubonic plague. Axillary lymphadenitis correlates with the development of plague meningitis (ie, approximately one third of patients with axillary lymphadenitis develop plague meningitis, but plague meningitis may occur in the absence of lymphadenitis). The clinical presentation of plague meningitis is indistinguishable from other causes of acute bacterial meningitis [10–13].

Septicemic plague

Septicemic plague is also known as "pestis siderans." Although approximately 25% of patients with bubonic plague are bacteremic, the hallmark of septicemic plague is high-grade *Y pestis* bacteremia in all patients. Symptoms are nonspecific and usually include gastrointestinal symptoms, and death ensues rapidly. As with pneumonic plague, septicemic plague victims have no buboes because overwhelming infection and death occur before suppurative lymphadenitis can occur. Septicemic plague may be complicated by secondary hematogenously spread plague pneumonia. Patients with secondary plague pneumonia have respiratory symptoms and a thick mucopurulent sputum that distinguishes secondary hematogenous plague pneumonia from primary inhalation pneumonia [10–13].

Pneumonic plague

During the incubation period (24–60 hours), patients present with a dry, unproductive cough and shortness of breath. The sputum is thin, watery, and blood tinged. The onset and severity of primary inhalation plague pneumonia is related to inoculum size.

Cause of ancient plagues

Because laboratory tests were unavailable to the ancients, a clear analysis of their findings rests on careful interpretation of their clinical description compared with current understanding of infectious diseases. Given the vagaries and variability of translation, it is possible to arrive at a presumptive clinical explanation for most of the ancient plagues. Knowledge of the varied clinical manifestations of plague may account for some of the variability in the descriptions from antiquity. It is also possible, but unlikely, that bubonic plague has changed its clinical manifestations over the centuries, which may account for differences, frequency, severity, and location of plague epidemics. The history of human plague is closely related to endemic zoonotic plague in rodents. Plague epidemics occur when rodent plague comes into contact with humans. Endemic plague foci were established centuries ago from a confluence of Eurasian and North African disease pools. Plague was spread along trade routes by humans and rodents introducing plague into new areas, which subsequently became endemic foci for plague. The potential for pandemic plague remains a constant threat waiting for a disruption in the equilibrium between zoonotic and human plague precipitated by famine, wars, or a breakdown in general sanitation [1,6–9].

By comparing the clinical features of bubonic, pneumonic, and septicemic plague as exist now, one can attempt to determine the causes of the major plagues of antiquity. The plague of Athens, the Antonine plague, and the plague of Justinian are the classic examples of well-described ancient plagues thought to be due to bubonic plague. The likelihood that plague was the cause of each of these plagues may be determined by a clinical analysis of clinical manifestations of plague compared with the original descriptions written by authors who were physically present, who survived, and whose writings have survived through the ages (Table 1) [1,6,8–13].

Table 1
Clinical presentations of plague

Clinical features	Bubonic[a] plague	Pneumonic plague	Septicemic[a] plague
Symptoms			
Fever/chills	+++	+	+
Malaise/anorexia	+	+	+
Slurred speech/memory loss	++	−	−
Lethargy/delirium/stupor	+++	−	−
Weakness	++	−	−
Ataxia/vertigo	+	−	−
Insomnia	+++	−	−
Dry cough	−	−	
Shortness of breath	−	+	−
Nausea/vomiting/diarrhea	++	−	−
Abdominal pain	+++	−	+
Signs			
Cervical adenitis	+++	−	−
Suppurative lymphadenitis	+++	−	−
Hemorrhagic mediastinitis	−	+	−
Tracheobronchitis	−	++	−
Multilobar pneumonia	−	+++	−
Pleural effusion	−	++	−
Cyanosis (late)	+	−	+
Splenomegaly	+	−	−
Petechiae	++	−	−

[a] Secondary plague pneumonia (hematogenous) may complicate bubonic or septicemia plague. Sepsis precedes secondary plague pneumonia by 1–2 days and is characterized by sudden onset of chest pain with hemoptysis and thick mucopurulent sputum.

Data from Refs. [1,10–13].

Three great plagues of antiquity

Plague of Athens (430–426 BC)

Historical background

Athens and Sparta represented two of the most powerful and influential civilizations on mainland Greece in the ancient world. The two powers cooperated during the great Persian wars to fend off successfully the much larger forces of Darius I in 490 BC and his son Xerxes in 479 BC, who sought to dominate the Greek mainland. The victory of the Greeks over Persia left Athens with the most powerful fleet in the Aegean and the Spartans with a formidable reputation in land warfare. Immediately after their victory over Xerxes, in part because many of the Greek states feared the return of the Persian armies, most city-states joined with the Athenians to form the Delian League. This alliance, based on naval dominance and trade, played a crucial role in the liberation of Greek colonies in Asia Minor from the Persian Empire in the years after the League's formation. The states not in the Delian League banded together under Sparta's leadership to form the Peloponnesian League, which retained most of the land-based power on the Peloponnese. By the 460s, the threat from Persia having lessened, Sparta became increasingly nervous and suspicious concerning the actions of the Delian League, and in 460 BC open hostilities erupted between Athens and Sparta. While the peace treaty of 446 BC temporarily put a stop to fighting, in 431 BC, the Peloponnesian War between Athens and Sparta began. The Spartans, because their strength relied on land-based forces, wished to ensure that the war would be decided via ground engagement. Led by Pericles, the Athenians wished to use their naval superiority to their advantage and engage primarily in battles that would require naval assets to win. The Peloponnesian League sought to destroy the Athenian Empire and not vice versa. Athens, it would seem, had only to survive to claim a victory, whereas the Spartans and their allies would have to conquer Athens itself. Pericles proposed that the Athenians surrender their territory in Attica and move the entire population into the city of Athens itself, protected by the great Themistoclean walls. These walls not only guarded the city proper, but also a walled corridor connecting it with the harbor of Piraeus, 9 km from Athens. With control of the seas and guarded access to its port, it seemed Athens would be impregnable for the Spartans. Several events occurred after the outset of war, however, that eventually resulted in the defeat of Athens in 404 BC.

The most important factor leading to the Athenian defeat was the great plague of Athens, described precisely by Thucydides. A plague descended on the city of Athens in the summer of 430 BC wreaking havoc on the Athenian population. Although not a physician, Thucydides was an astute observer and was careful to use medical vocabulary developed by Hippocrates in use at the time. Thucydides himself contracted and survived the plague and wrote an accurate and meticulous account of the disease [1,2,14].

Thucydides' description of the plague of Athens[1]

"It first began, so it is said, in *Ethiopia above Egypt*, and then descended into Egypt and Libya and into most of the King's land. Suddenly falling upon Athens, and first attacked the population at Piraeus, so that they themselves said that the Peloponnesians had thrown poison into their wells: for there were, as yet, no cisterns there. But afterwards it came to the upper city as well, and from that time the deaths became much greater. Therefore, anyone, either physician or layman, might by his own opinion, speak on its origins and the causes that produced so great a departure from normal conditions; but I shall talk about its course, and explain the symptoms, by which it could be recognized in the future, having knowledge of it beforehand. For I myself was ill and saw others suffer from it."

"That year, as agreed by all, had been unprecedentedly disease-free in respect to other sicknesses; but if anyone suffered with anything before, all

[1] Translation with italics added by C.B. Cunha.

separated into this. In other cases, there was no apparent cause, but suddenly, healthy men were seized first *with mighty heats in the head,* and *redness, and inflamed eyes,* and the inside, both the *throat and tongue, immediately became blood-red* and *emitted an atypical, foul breath.*"

"After which came *sneezing and hoarseness*, and in not much time the pain descended into the chest, and produced a *severe cough*; and *when it fixed in the stomach, it upset it,* and *vomiting of bile* of every kind named by physicians ensued, accompanied by *great suffering*; and in most cases *nonproductive retching* followed, giving way to *violent spasms,* which sometimes abated soon after, in others, long after."

"Externally, the body was *not very hot to the touch,* and was not pale, *but reddish, livid, and flowering with small blisters and wounds.* But *internally was lit such a heat that the patients could not bare garments or fine cloths being laid on them, nor be anything but naked, and would have liked best to hurl themselves into cold water,* as in fact, many of those neglected did, throwing themselves into cisterns, tormented by unquenchable thirst. And it was the same whether they drank much or little."

"Also, they were ceaselessly tormented by the *inability to rest or sleep*. And the body, while the disease flourished, did not whither, but withstood the ravages of the disease; so *that when they died, as most did, on the seventh or ninth day from the burning heat, they still had some strength.* But if they escaped this, *the disease descended into the bowels, creating a great ulceration,* and at the same time, *accompanied by acute diarrhea,* and many later *died from exhaustion* because of this. *For the disease starting from above in the head, where it first settled, then throughout the whole body,* and if one survived the worst, *it left its mark on the extremities. For it fell upon the genitals, and the tips of the hands and the feet, and many escaped, being deprived of these, some also lost their eyes.* Others again were taken with a *complete loss of memory* after recovery, and they failed to know either themselves or friends" [15].

Infectious disease aspects

Ever since Thucydides first described the plague, physicians from every era have attempted to determine the precise cause of the plague of Athens. The limitations inherent in translation of the original Greek prevents a definitive explanation based on Thucydides' description. Possible infectious diseases responsible for the plague of Athens are bubonic plague, typhoid fever, smallpox, measles, and epidemic typhus. All of these infectious diseases were present in the ancient world and have some of the clinical features described by Thucydides.

The word *plague* in ancient descriptions meant pestilence in general, rather than a specific disease entity (ie, bubonic plague). Thucydides' description of the buboes is critical in the diagnosis of bubonic plague if his words φλυκταινα μικραιζ and ελκσζ are taken to represent the characteristic buboes of bubonic plague and not nonspecifically sores or blisters. There is also lack of evidence of black rats in Athens at the time, which would be important in suggesting the plague was bubonic plague. By analyzing the clinical features described by Thucydides, the great plague of Athens may have been caused by bubonic plague, but measles has more clinical features in common with Thucydides' description. In the plague of Athens, plague pneumonia could explain the absence of buboes in Thucydides' careful clinical descriptions (Table 2) [15–17].

Historical importance

The plague reduced the population of Athens by approximately 25%. The plague killed Pericles, leaving Athens without one of its greatest statesmen. Athens' ultimate defeat in the Peloponnesian War ultimately was determined by the plague. Their Spartan adversaries were comparably untouched by the disease. The great plague of Athens effectively altered the outcome of the Peloponnesian War and had a profound impact on subsequent Hellenistic and Western history [1,8–10,14].

Antonine plague (166–270 AD)

Historical background

By the second century AD, the Roman Empire stretched from Arabia in the east to Hispania in the west and from Britannia in the north to Aegyptus

Table 2
Differential diagnostic features of the Athenian plague

Clinical description by Thucydides	Time of occurrence	Bubonic plague	Typhoid fever	Smallpox	Measles	Epidemic typhus
Rapid onset	Early	+	−	+	+	+
Fever	Early	+	+	+	+	
Red eyes	Early	−	−	+	+	+
Runny nose and sneezing	Early	+	−	−	+	+
Red throat and hoarseness	Early	−	−	−	+	+
Foul breath	Early	−	−	−	+	+
Retching and convulsions	Middle	−	−	−	−	+
Livid red rash	Middle	−	−	+	+	+
Blisters and sores	Middle	+	−	+	−	+
Sensation of intense internal heat	Middle	−	−	+	+	+
Sleeplessness	Late	+	−	−	+	−
Diarrhea	Late	−	+	+	−	+
Gangrene of the body or extremities	Late	−	−	+	−	+
Loss of sight	Late	−	−	+	−	+
Loss of memory	Late	−	−	−	−	+
Death by exhaustion	Late	−	−	−	+	+

Data from Refs. [1,5,10,16,17].

in the south, encompassing most of the known world. No detailed description exists for the Antonine plague, in contrast to the earlier plague of Athens. All that remains are some notes made by Galen, an allusion to the epidemic by the emperor Marcus Aurelius in his writings, two references by Lucian, and some other, minor text references. Apparently, the Antonine plague originated in the Middle East and was brought to Europe by Roman troops returning home after the Parthian War. Spreading through the Roman Empire, the Antonine Plague lasted until 270 AD and took the lives of millions of Romans, including Marcus Aurelius. Although exact numbers of deaths are unknown, Cassius Dio suggested that at one point during the Antonine plague more than 2000 people a day were dying from plague in Rome itself [1,2,8,9].

Galen's description of the Antonine plague[2]

Exanthem. "On the ninth day a certain young man was *covered over his whole body with an exanthem,* as was the case with almost all who survived. Drying drugs were applied to his body. *On the twelfth day he was able to rise from bed.*"

"On those who would survive who had diarrhea, *a black exanthem* appeared on the whole body. *It was ulcerated in most cases and totally dry.* The blackness was due to a remnant of blood that had putrefied in the fever blisters, like some ash which nature had deposited on the skin. 'Of some of these which had become *ulcerated, that part of the surface called the scab fell away and then the remaining part nearby was healthy and after one or two days became scarred over.* In those places where it was not ulcerated, *the exanthem was rough and scabby and fell away like some husk* and hence all became healthy.'"

"In many cases where there was *no bloody colliquescences* (diarrhea), the entire body was covered by a black exanthem 'and sometimes a sort of scale fell off, when the exanthem had dried and dissipated, little by little, over a period of many days after the crisis.'"

Fever. "Those afflicted with plague *appear neither warm, nor burning to those who touch them, although they are raging with fever inside,* just as Thucydides describes."

"Galen calls the plague a *fever plague.*"

Bowels. "*Black excrement* was a symptom of those who had the disease, whether they survived or perished of it. Colliquescence (diarrhea) was first auburn, then yellowish red, later black, like fecal matter of blood."

"Colliquescence of evacuation was an inseparable symptom of the plague."

[2] Italics added by C.B. Cunha.

"In many who survived, black stools appeared, mostly on the ninth day or even the seventh or eleventh day. Many differences occurred. Some had stools that were nearly black; some had neither pains in their excretions, nor were their excretions foul smelling. Very many stood in the middle. If the stool was not black, the exanthem always appeared. *All those who excreted very black stool died.*"

Vomiting. "Occurred in some cases."

Stomach upset. "Occurred in all cases."

Fetid breath. "Occurred."

Cough-catarrh. "On the ninth day a young man had a *slight cough.* On the tenth day the *cough became stronger and with it he brought up scabs.*"

"After having catarrh for many days, first with a cough *he brought up a little bright, fresh blood,* and afterwards even part of the membrane which lines the artery and rises through the larynx to the pharynx and mouth."

Internal ulcerations and inflammation. "On the tenth day a young man coughed and brought up a scab, which was an indication of an ulcerated area in the windpipe in the region of the trachea near the jugular vein. *No ulcers were present in the mouth or throat* (there was no problem of ingesting food). *The larynx was infected, and the man's voice was damaged.*"

Duration of the disease. "The crisis appeared on the ninth to twelfth day. *On the third day after the ninth the young man was able to rise from his bed*" [18].

Infectious disease aspects

Although the description of the Antonine plague is not as thorough as Thucydides' description of the plague of Athens, Galen characterizes the plague as a rash extending over the entire body rather than as buboes in the groin and axilla. Galen's description of the exanthem that was pustular and later became blackened could represent buboes or the pustular stage of smallpox. Galen's description of the blackened pustules indicates that the Antonine plague could be bubonic plague or possibly smallpox (Table 3) [1,8–10,19].

Historical importance

The Antonine plague was a crucial factor in the decline and fall of the Roman Empire. With deaths from the plague and renewed offensives by the Germanic tribes on the northern borders of Rome, the Empire could not maintain an adequate army. The plague affected all levels of Roman life. The social order was disrupted, and Romans all across the Empire became panicked and believed their gods had abandoned them. The Antonine plague finally subsided a century after it began and contributed to Rome's eventual fall [1,2,9,20,21].

Table 3
Differential diagnostic features of the Antonine plague

Clinical description by Galen	Time of occurrence	Bubonic plague	Typhoid fever	Measles	Epidemic typhus	Smallpox
Rapid onset	Early	+	−	+	+	+
Slight fever	Early	+	+	+	+	+
Foul breath	Middle	−	−	+	+	+
Livid red rash	Middle	−	−	+	+	+
Blisters and sores	Middle	−	−	−	+	+
Sensation of intense internal heat	Middle	−	−	+	+	+
Sleeplessness	Late	+	−	+	−	−
Diarrhea	Late	−	+	−	+	+
Ulcers of the trachea/larynx	Late	−	−	−	−	+
Red throat and hoarseness	Late	−	−	+	+	+
Death by hemorrhage	Late	−	−	−	−	+

Data from Refs. [1,5,8–10,18,19].

Justinian plague (542–590 AD)

Historical background

By the end of the fourth century, Rome had withdrawn from some of its western territories, but the Empire was able to maintain its new borders and developed a relatively secure boundary with the Germanic tribes to the north and east. In the eastern Roman Empire, Justinian began his campaign in the western Roman Empire in 532 AD, retaking much of North Africa, Carthage, Sicily, parts of Hispania, and much of the Italian peninsula. By 540 AD, Germanic resistance was collapsing, and Justinian hoped to attack Gaul and possibly Britain. It seemed as though the reign of Justinian would re-establish the glory of the Roman Empire. All that changed when the Justinian plague struck in 542 AD. The Justinian plague probably originated in Africa to Constantinople. The enclosed city of Constantinople, similar to Athens during the Peloponnesian War, was ideal for the spread of a contagious infectious disease in a closed population.

There are several descriptions of the Justinian plague by John of Ephesus, Evagrius Scholasticus, and Procopius. Although all provide descriptions of the Justinian plague, Procopius' account is considered to be the most accurate description of the plague. Procopius was one of Emperor Justinian's principal archivists. When the plague arrived in Constantinople where Procopius was, he chronicled the plague epidemic firsthand [2,6–9].

Procopius' description of the Justinian plague[3]

"During this time there was a plague, by which all men were almost completely destroyed..."

[3] Translation with italics added by C.B. Cunha.

"... For it did not come in a part of the world nor to certain men, nor did it confine itself to any season of the year, so that from such circumstances it might be possible to find explanations of a cause, but it encompassed the entire world, and destroyed the lives of all men, though differing from one another in the most marked degree, respecting neither sex nor age."

"For just as men differ with regard to places in which they live, or in the law of their daily life, or in natural bent, or in active pursuits, or in whatever else man differs from man, in the case of this disease alone the difference availed naught. And it attacked some in the summer season, others in the winter, and still others at the other times of the year. Now let each one express his own judgment concerning the matter, both sophist and astrologer, but as for me, I shall proceed to tell where this disease originated and the manner in which it destroyed men."

"*It came from the Egyptians who live in Pelusium.* And it split, and in one direction came toward Alexandria and the rest of Egypt, and in the other it came to Palestine bordering Egypt, and from there spread everywhere, always moving forward and going whenever time favored it. For it seemed to move by a set arrangement and delayed in each land for a certain time, casting its blight slightingly upon none, but spreading in either direction right out to the ends of the world, as if fearing lest some corner of the earth might escape it. For it left neither island nor cave nor mountain ridge which had human inhabitants; and if it had passed by any land, either not affecting the men there or touching them in indifferent fashion, still at a later time it came back; then those who lived near this land, whom formerly it had afflicted most sorely, it did not touch at all, but it did not retire from the place in question until it had given up its just and proper toll of dead, so as to correspond exactly to the number destroyed at the earlier time among those who lived nearby. And this disease always *started on the coast and from there moved to the interior.*"

"And in the second year it reached Byzantium in the midst of spring, where I happened to be staying at the time. And it came thusly. The spirits of divine beings in human form of every kind were seen by many people, and those who encountered them thought that they were struck by the man they had met in this or that part of the body, as it havened, and immediately upon seeing this apparition they were seized also by the disease."

"Now at first those who met these creatures tried to turn them aside by uttering the holiest of names and exorcising them in other ways as well as each one could, but they accomplished absolutely nothing, for even in the sanctuaries where the most of them fled for refuge they were dying constantly. But later on they were unwilling even to give heed to their friends when they called to them, and they shut themselves up in their rooms and pretended that they did not hear, although their doors were being beaten down, fearing that he who was calling was one of those demons. But in the case of some, the pestilence did not come in this way, but they saw a vision in a dream and seemed to suffer the very same thing at the hands of the creature who stood over them, or else to hear a voice prophesizing that they were written down in the number of those who were to die. But with most it happened that they were seized by the disease without being made aware of what would come by a waking vision or a dream. And they were taken as follows.

"They had a *sudden fever,* some when they awoke from sleeping, others while walking around, and still others while otherwise busy, without any respect for what they were doing. And the body showed no change in its original color, neither was it as hot as expected when attacked by the fever, nor did any inflammation occur, but the fever was of such a lethargic kind from its onset until the evening that it would not grant any suspicion of danger either to the sick themselves of a physician. Therefore, it was natural for none of those who had contracted the disease expected to die because of it. But in some cases on the same day, in others on the day following, and in the rest not many days later, a *bubonic swelling developed, there in the groin of body, which is below the abdomen, but also in the armpit, and also behind the ear and at different places along the thighs*. Up to this point, then, everything went in about the same way with all who had taken the disease."

"But from then on very marked differences developed; and I am unable to say whether the cause of this diversity of symptoms was to be found in the difference in bodies, or in the fact that it followed the wish of Him who brought the disease into the world. For there ensued for some a deep *coma,* with others a *violent delirium,* and in either case they suffered the characteristic symptoms of the disease. For those who were under the spell of the coma forgot all those who were familiar to them and seemed to lie sleeping constantly. And if anyone cared for them, they would eat without waking, but some also were neglected, and these would die directly through lack of sustenance. But those who were seized with delirium suffered from *insomnia* and were victims of a *distorted imagination*; for they suspected that men were coming upon them to destroy them, and they would become excited and rush off in flight, crying out at the top of their voices."

"And those who were attending them were in a state of constant exhaustion and had a most difficult time of it throughout. For this reason everybody pitied them no less than the sufferers, not because they were threatened by the pestilence in going near it, *for neither physicians nor other persons were found to contract this malady through contact with the sick or with the dead,* for many who were constantly engaged either in burying or in attending those in no way connected with them held out in the performance of this service beyond all expectation, while with many others the disease came on without warning and they died straightway; but they pitied them because of the great hardships which they were undergoing. For when the patients fell from their beds and lay rolling upon the floor, they kept putting them back in place, and when they were struggling to rush headlong out of their houses, they would force them back by shoving and pulling against them. And when water chanced to be near, they wished to fall into it, not so much because of a desire for drink, for the most of them rushed into the sea, but the cause was to be found chiefly in the diseased state of their minds."

"*They had also great difficulty in the matter of eating,* for they could not easily take food. And many perished through lack of any man to care for them, for they were either overcome by hunger, or threw themselves down from a height. And in those cases where neither coma nor delirium came on, the bubonic swelling became mortified and the sufferer, no longer able to endure the pain, died. And one would suppose that in all cases the same thing would have been true, but since they were not at all in their senses, some were quite unable to feel the pain; for owing to the troubled condition of their minds they lost all sense of feeling."

"In some cases death came immediately, in others, after many days; and with some the body broke out with *black pustules* about as large as a lentil and these did not survive even one day, but all succumbed immediately. With many also a *vomiting of blood* ensued without visible cause and straightway brought death. Moreover I am able to declare this, that the most illustrious physicians predicted that many would die, who unexpectedly escaped entirely from suffering shortly afterwards, and that they declared that many would be saved, who were destined to be carried off almost immediately. So it was that in this disease there was no cause that came within the province of human reasoning; for in all cases the issue tended to be something unaccountable."

"Now in those cases where the swelling rose to an unusual size and a discharge of pus had set in, it came about that they escaped from the disease and survived, for clearly the acute condition of the carbuncle had found relief in this direction, and this proved to be in general an indication of returning health; but in cases where the swelling preserved its former appearance there ensued those troubles which I have just mentioned. And with some of them it came about that the thigh was withered, in which case, though the swelling was there, it did not develop the least suppuration. With others who survived the tongue did not remain unaffected, and they lived on either lisping or speaking incoherently and with difficulty" [22].

Infectious disease aspects

The most critical signs described by Procopius were bubonic swellings (υσερσν βσυβων) in the groin and axilla. Even without other symptoms, the well-described buboes indicate bubonic plague. Bubonic plague was certainly the cause of the Justinian plague (Table 4) [1,8,23].

Historical importance

The effects of the Justinian plague were disastrous for the Roman Empire. Procopius and others estimated that more than a third of the Roman Empire's population was eliminated by this plague at the end of the sixth century. Procopius described much of the infected surviving population of the Roman Empire as suffering from debilitating and crippling effects

Table 4
Differential diagnostic features of the Justinian plague

Clinical description by Procopius	Time of appearance	Typhoid fever	Measles	Epidemic typhus	Smallpox	Bubonic plague
Rapid onset	Early	−	+	+	+	+
Slight fever	Early	+	+	+	+	+
Coma	Middle	−	−	−	−	+
Buboes	Middle	−	−	−	−	+
Delirium	Middle	−	−	+	−	−
Vomiting blood	Middle	−	−	−	−	+
Sleeplessness	Middle	−	+	−	−	+
Diarrhea	Middle	+	−	+	−	−
Red throat and hoarseness	Middle	−	+	+	+	+
Death by hemorrhage	Late	−	−	−	+	−
Disease leaves many survivors crippled	Late	−	−	−	−	+

Data from Refs. [1,5,10,22–24].

of the plague. The plague so weakened the Roman Empire that not long after the plague had passed, Roman borders were overrun by Huns, Goths, Moors, and other "barbarians." The plague so weakened the eastern Roman Empire (Byzantium) that it survived only until its eventual fall [1,2,6,8,24].

Plague pandemics through the ages

Beginning with the plague of Justinian (ie, the first plague pandemic), two other plague pandemics have occurred up to the present time. The three plague pandemics in history have had a major effect on human populations and the course of history itself. The first plague pandemic (plague of Justinian) precipitated the collapse of the eastern Roman Empire. The plague-induced weakness of the eastern Roman Empire permitted barbarian invasions to occur, resulting in the end of Byzantium. The second pandemic resulted in the "great plague" or the Black Death, which decimated the population of Europe in the Middle Ages. Details of the Black Death in Europe are well documented and need no re-review here. In the modern era, the third plague endemic occurred beginning in China in the 1890s. Asia, particularly China, had long been a focus of endemic plague. Plague had moved from east to west during the second plague pandemic via overland trade routes, which resulted in the introduction of the plague into Europe. In the 1890s, plague was spread from China via ships. Ships engaging in trade, taking goods from China to other continents, introduced plague into North and Latin America, Japan, Australia, the Philippines, and southern Africa, establishing endemic plague in these areas (Table 5) [1,10,11,25].

Table 5
Plague pandemics

Plague pandemic	Year	Location	Vector	Historical significance
Plague of Athens	430–426 BC	Athens	Unknown. No antecedent rat deaths described	Decimated military/civilian population of Athens. Pericles died of plague. Spartans victorious over Athens. End of Greece's Golden Age. Western civilization changed forever. Cause: Possibly plague versus measles
Antonine plague	166–270 AD	Pelusium, Egypt, to Roman Empire, (Mediterranean Europe/Asia Minor)	Unknown. No antecedent rat deaths described	Decisively weakened the Roman army resulting in subsequent Barbarian invasions and eventual fall of the Western Roman Empire. Cause: Probably plague versus smallpox
Justinian Plague (1st pandemic)	542–590 AD	Africa to Byzantium	Unknown. No antecedent rat deaths described	Reduced population of Roman Empire by one third resulting in subsequent Barbarian invasions and final collapse of the eastern Roman Empire (Byzantium). Cause: Definitely bubonic plague
"Black Death" of Europe (2nd pandemic)	Early 1300s–late 1600s	Began in China and spread via caravan trade routes to the Middle East. Reached Messina in 1347 and ravaged Europe for centuries	Rats	Decimated European population by one third to one half, Mortality varied by location from 25–70%
Modern era (3rd pandemic)	1894–early 1900s	Began in China and spread via ships to ports worldwide	Rats, rodents	Plague introduced in North America, Latin America, Australia, Philippines, Japan, and Southern Africa resulting in the establishment of endemic plague in the Americas and Africa

Data from Refs. [1,4,7–10,14,15,20,25].

There is no infectious disease in history that has had a more profound effect on world history and has resulted in so many victims. Plague has killed more than wars, famines, and other pestilences combined. The Black Death, the second plague endemic, reduced Europe's population in the Middle Ages from one third to one half. Plague epidemics continue to the present whenever the equilibrium between rodents and humans is altered in favor of the plague vectors [8,9]. Outbreaks and epidemics of pneumonic plague without bubonic plague remain unexplained (Table 6) [26–28]. Because of the lethality of plague as an infectious disease, the concept of using plague as a weapon has occurred to many, and it has been used as a biological weapon in history.

Plague biological warfare in history

In ancient civilizations, the virulence and potential lethality of plague was appreciated. The use of plague as a biological weapon in warfare was limited by its lethality on the attacker and potential victims. Without fully appreciating the epidemiology of human plague, ancient attempts to use plague as a weapon were limited. Undoubtedly there were many attempts to use plague-infected humans or animals as weapons, but no record of the failed attempts is available. Many individuals trying to use plague-infected carcasses as weapons were infected themselves, and biowarfare attempts had counterproductive effects limiting more widespread use of plague as a weapon.

Two applications of plague in biological warfare were in the siege of Caffa in 1346 AD and in World War II in China. The siege of Caffa in the Crimea occurred in 1346. Tartars used plague-infected corpses against the Genoese. The Genoese fled to Sicily and later returned to their home city of Genoa and brought the plague with them. The plague spread from Sicily throughout Europe and initiated the great Plague of 1348 [7,29]. The most recent and best-documented use of plague in biological warfare was during World War II. The Japanese had biological warfare capability; they used aircraft to drop rice contaminated with infected fleas on several Chinese cities. Apparently thousands became infected with plague, and there were

Table 6
Selected plague epidemics/outbreaks

Year	Location	Clinical presentations	Vector	Effects
1910–1911	Manchuria	Pneumonic plague. No cases of bubonic plague	Marmots	43,942 plague deaths (100% mortality)
1924	Los Angeles	Pneumonic plague. No cases of bubonic plague	Rats	30 plague deaths (100% mortality)
1994	India	876 cases of bubonic plague	Rats	54 plague deaths
1995–1996	Madagascar	Bubonic plague endemic in Madagascar since 1898	Rats, shrews	60 plague deaths

Data from Refs. [1,4,26–28].

Table 7
Plague biological warfare

Years	Location	Attackers/defenders	Methods	Effects
300 BC–1100 AD	Ancient Greco-Roma-Persian world	Greeks, Romans, local enemies	Plague-infected corpses catapulted[a] into walled fortifications	Possible local spread of plague/unknown effects
1346 AD	Caffa (Crimea)	Tartars/Genoese	Plague-infected corpses catapulted[a] into walled fortifications	Effect of plague decisive. Defenders return to Sicily with plague. Subsequent spread of plague from Sicily to Europe beginning the Great Plague of 1348
1710 AD	Keval	Russians/Swedes	Plague-infected corpses catapulted[a] into walled fortifications	Possible local spread of plague/unknown effects
1915	St. Petersburg	Germans/Russians	Ground delivered—plague-contaminated food/objects	Unproven allegations/unknown effects
1940–1942	Chuhsien/Chinese cities	Japanese/Chinese	Air delivered—rice contaminated with infected fleas	Thousands infected with bubonic plague; ~700 plague-related deaths

[a] Catapults were incapable of hurling corpses over walls. Trebouchets were used to catapult corpses over walls (a trebouchet could hurl 300 lb 300 yards).
Data from Refs. [1,2,4,29,30,33–35].

approximately 700 plague-related deaths (Table 7) [3–35]. Using biological warfare is a double-edged sword, posing problems for the attackers and the defenders as the history of plague when used as a weapon illustrates. With increasingly sophisticated facilities to produce biological weapons and improved means to deliver them, the potential for biological warfare using plague and other agents remains an ever-present threat [36,37].

References

[1] Kiple KF. The Cambridge world history of human diseases. New York: Cambridge University Press; 1993.
[2] Murray O. The Oxford history of the classical world. Oxford: Oxford University Press; 1997.
[3] Allbutt TC. Greek medicine in Rome. London: Macmillan & Co; 1921.
[4] Titball RW, Leary SEC. Plague. Br Med Bull 1998;54:625–33.
[5] Scarborough J. Roman medicine. Ithaca (NY): Cornell University Press; 1969.
[6] Brothwell D, Sandison AT. Diseases in antiquity. Springfield: Charles C Thomas; 1967.
[7] Bollet AJ. Plagues and poxes. New York: Demos Publications; 1987.
[8] Cartwright FF. Disease and history. New York: Dorset Press; 1991.
[9] McNeill WH. Plagues and peoples. New York: Anchor Books; 1976.
[10] Christie AB. Infectious diseases: epidemiology and clinical practice. 4th edition. New York: Churchill Livingstone; 1987.
[11] Cleri DJ, Ricketti AJ, Panesar M, et al. Plague (*Yersinia pestis*): Part I. Infect Dis Pract 2004; 28:259–65.
[12] Cleri DJ, Ricketti AJ, Panesar M, et al. Plague (*Yersinia pestis*): Part II. Infect Dis Pract 2004;28:271–5.
[13] Adamovicz JL, Worsham PL. Plague. In: Swearengen JR, editor. Biodefense: research methodology and animal models. Boca Raton (FL): CRC Press; 2006. p. 107–35.
[14] Soupios MA. Impact of the plague in Ancient Greece. Infect Dis Clin N Am 2004;18:45–51.
[15] Thucydides. The Peloponnesian War. New York: Cambridge University Press; 1989.
[16] Cunha BA. The cause of the plague of Athens: plague, typhus, smallpox, or measles? Infect Dis Clin N Am 2004;18:29–43.
[17] Shrewsbury JFD. The plague of Athens. Bull Hist Med 1950;24:1–25.
[18] Galen. Methodus Medendi. Cambridge: Harvard University Press; 1984.
[19] Littman RJ, Littman ML. Galen and the Antonine plague. Am J Philol 1973;94:243–55.
[20] Fears JR. The Plague under Marcus Aurelius and the decline and fall of the Roman Empire. Infect Dis Clin N Am 2004;20:65–77.
[21] Gilliam JF. The Plague under Marcus Aurelius. Am J Philol 1961;30:225–51.
[22] Procopius. Histories of the wars. Cambridge: Harvard University Press; 1981.
[23] Bratton TL. The identity of the plague of Justinian. Trans Stud Coll Physicians Phila 1981;3: 113–24.
[24] Allen P. The Justinian plague. Revue internationale des etudes Byzantines 1979;49–58.
[25] Gottfried RS. The Black Death: natural and human disaster in medieval Europe. New York: The Free Press; 1987.
[26] Chernin E. Richard Pearson Strong and the Manchurian epidemic of pneumonic plague, 1910–1911. J Hist Med Allied Sci 1989;44:296–319.
[27] Viseltear AJ. The pneumonic plague epidemic of 1924 in Los Angeles. Yale J Biol Med 1974; 1:40–54.
[28] Kamat V. Resurgence of malaria in Bombay (Mumbai) in the 1990s: a historical perspective. Parasitologia 2000;42:135–48.
[29] Derbes VJ. De Mussis and the Great Plague of 1348. JAMA 1966;196:179–82.
[30] Khardori N, Kanchanapoom T. Overview of biological terrorism: potential agents and preparedness. Clin Microbiol Newsl 2005;27:1–8.

[31] Poupard J, Miller L. History of biological warfare: catapults to capsomeres. Ann N Y Acad Sci 1992;666:9–20.

[32] Christopher GW, Cieslak TJ, Pavlin JA, et al. Biological warfare: a historical perspective. JAMA 1997;278:412–7.

[33] Eitzen EM Jr, Takafuji ET. Historical overview of biological warfare. In: Geissler E, van Courtland Moon JE, editors. Biological and toxin weapons: research, development and use from the Middle Ages to 1945. Stockholm International Peace Research Institute. Oxford: Oxford University Press; 1999. p. 415–23.

[34] Carus WS. Working paper: bioterrorism and biocrimes. The illicit use of biological agents in the 20th century. Washington, DC: Center for Counterproliferation Research, National Defense University; 1999. p. 13–26.

[35] Geissler E, van Courtland Moon JE, editors. Biological and toxin weapons: research, development and use from the Middle Ages to 1945. Stockholm International Peace Research Institute. Oxford: Oxford University Press; 1999.

[36] Tucker JB. Historical trends related to bioterrorism: an empirical analysis. Emerg Infect Dis 1999;5:498–504.

[37] Beeching NJ, Dance DA, Miller AR, et al. Biological warfare and bioterrorism. BMJ 2002; 324:336–9.

ELSEVIER
SAUNDERS

Infect Dis Clin N Am
20 (2006) 273–287

INFECTIOUS
DISEASE CLINICS
OF NORTH AMERICA

Plague: Disease, Management, and Recognition of Act of Terrorism

Janak Koirala, MD, MPH

Division of Infectious Diseases, Department of Internal Medicine, Southern Illinois University School of Medicine, 751 North Rutledge, Room 1100, Springfield, IL 62702, USA

Plague is an ancient disease caused by *Yersinia pestis*, a member of Enterobacteriaceae family. Plague is maintained in nature as a zoonosis among wild rodents and fleas. Humans acquire it most often through infected flea-bites. Many outbreaks of plague have been described since the beginning of the history of mankind. Plague has caused numerous epidemics and three recorded pandemics, including Justinian plague, Black Death, and the modern plague pandemic that began a little over a century ago in China [1–3].

Natural foci and global epidemiology

The natural foci of plague exist in Asia, Africa, North America, South America, and South-East Europe (Fig. 1). The World Health Organization (WHO) reported 80,613 cases of plague from 38 countries between 1954 and 1997, including 6587 plague-related deaths. The largest proportion (58%) of these cases was from Asia and it included epidemics in India and Vietnam [4,5]. A WHO analysis of plague distribution by continent showed that a few countries in each continent have most of the disease burden (Box 1). For example, during 1982 to 1997, Madagascar and Tanzania accounted for 62.5% of the total plague cases in Africa, Brazil and Peru accounted for 83% of the total cases in the Americas, and Myanmar and Vietnam for 78.5% of the cases reported in Asia [5]. Seven countries reported plague virtually every year over the latter half of the twentieth century: (1) Brazil, (2) Democratic Republic of Congo, (3) Madagascar, (4) Myanmar, (5) Peru, (6) United States, and (7) Vietnam [4].

The Centers for Disease Control and Prevention (CDC) recorded 390 cases of plague in the United States over a 50-year period between 1947

E-mail address: jkoirala@siumed.edu

0891-5520/06/$ - see front matter
doi:10.1016/j.idc.2006.02.004

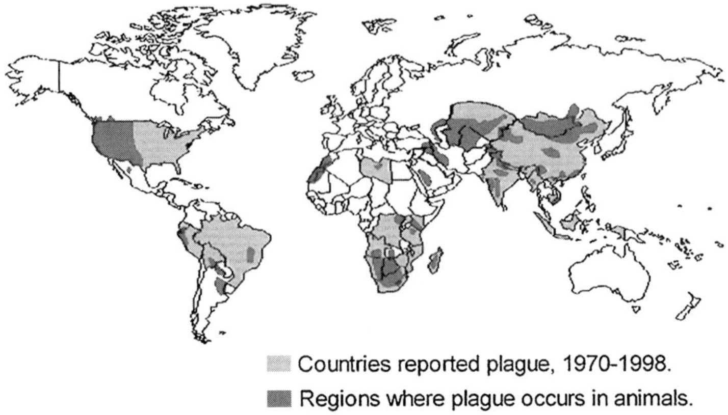

Fig. 1. Global distribution of plague, 1970 to 1998. (*From* the Centers for Disease Control and Prevention. Available at: http://www.cdc.gov/ncidod/dvbid/plague/world98.htm.)

and 1996. These mostly included cases of bubonic plague (84%) followed by septicemic (13%) and pneumonic plague (2%). The natural foci of plague in North America occur in 15 western states of the United States, and its bordering regions including southwestern Canada and northern Mexico. The natural foci of plague in South America exist in Argentina, Bolivia, Brazil, Ecuador, Peru, and Venezuela.

In its natural cycle, *Y pestis* survives between rodents and fleas. Rat fleas, such as *Xenopsylla cheopis*, serve as the vector and maintain the zoonotic form of plague by transmission of *Y pestis* among the wild rats, squirrels, prairie dogs, voles, chipmunks, rabbits, and other small mammals [5,6]. Human cases of plague are relatively sparse in natural foci. Most of the isolated cases occur among people who come in contact with wild rodents in the course of their work, hunting, or camping. Larger epidemics and pandemics have occurred when *Y pestis* invaded the domestic rodents (*Rattus species*).

Rodent-to-human transmission generally occurs by fleabites. Less common modes of transmission include direct contact or handling infected materials. Human-to-human transmission can occur through direct contact with infected materials from patients with plague, respiratory exposure to patients with pneumonic plague, or through human flea after biting patients with septicemic plague [6]. Twenty-three cases of cat-associated human plague were reported from eight western states in the United States between 1977 and 1998 [7].

Bacteriology and evolutionary genomics

Yersinia pestis is a member of the Enterobacteriaceae family. It is a gram-negative coccobacillus measuring 0.75 × 1.5 μm, and is nonmotile and nonspore forming. It has a bipolar appearance on staining, which is also

Box 1. Global distribution of plague during 1980 to 1997

Africa

Human plague was reported from 13 countries: Angola, Botswana, Democratic Republic of Congo, Kenya, Libya, Madagascar, Malawi, Mozambique, South Africa, Uganda, Republic of Tanzania, Zambia, and Zimbabwe.
Total cases: 19,349 (66.8% of the world total)
Total deaths: 1781 (75.8% of the world total)
Yearly average: 1073 cases and 99 deaths
Mean case-fatality rate: 9.2%

Americas

Human plague was reported from five countries: Bolivia, Brazil, Ecuador, Peru, and the United States.
Total cases: 3137 (10.8% of the world total)
Total deaths: 194 (8.3% of the world total)
Yearly average: 175 cases and 11 deaths
Mean case-fatality rate: 6.2%

Asia

Human plague was reported from seven countries: China, India, Kazakhstan, Lao People's Democratic Republic, Mongolia, Myanmar, and Vietnam.
Total cases: 6501 (22.4% of the world total)
Total deaths: 374 (15.9% of the world total)
Yearly average: 361 cases and 21 deaths
Mean case-fatality rate: 5.8%

described as a "safety pin appearance." *Y pestis* grows on sheep blood agar forming gray-white, translucent colonies, and has a "fried egg" appearance after 48 to 72 hours of incubation. They form small, nonlactose-fermenting colonies on MacConkey or eosin methylene blue agar. *Y pestis* grows in clumps in general nutrient-rich broths, such as brain-heart infusion, and gives a "flocculant" or "stalactite" appearance. Although under controlled conditions *Y pestis* has been shown to be viable for few to several hours on environmental surfaces (eg, steel, polythene, or glass), they have low resistance to environmental factors, such as sunlight, high temperatures, and desiccation. Ordinary disinfectants, such as Lysol and chlorine-containing preparations, kill *Y pestis* within 1 to 10 minutes [6,8].

Yersinia pestis has been classified into three biovars (*Antiqua*, *Mediaevalis*, and *Orientalis*) according to their ability to reduce nitrate and use glycerol. Biovar *Mediaevalis* is negative for nitrate reduction and positive for glycerol use, biovar *Orientalis* is positive for nitrate reduction and negative for glycerol use, and biovar *Antiqua* is positive for both characteristics. Each biovar corresponds to one of the three pandemics of plague [6,9]. Biovar *Antiqua* is thought to be the cause of Justinian plague, or the first pandemic. It is prevalent in Central Asia, Southeastern Russia, and Africa. Biovar *Mediaevalis* is believed to be the cause of Black Death, the second pandemic. It is currently prevalent in the Caspian Sea region. Biovar *Orientalis* is the cause of the modern plague, the third pandemic, and it is still circulating in Asia and the Western hemisphere.

The complete genomes of two virulent strains of *Y pestis*, *Orientalis* (CO92) and *Mediaevalis* (KIM), have been sequenced [10–12]. These works have provided important data for genomic research in general. Transmissibility of *Y pestis* by fleabite is believed to be a recent evolutionary adaptation that distinguishes it from *Y pseudotuberculosis* and other enteric bacteria [13]. The phylogenetic analyses suggest that *Y pestis* evolved from *Y pseudotuberculosis* about 1500 to 20,000 years ago, most likely shortly before the first known pandemic of human plague [9]. In addition, genomic analysis of a nonvirulent strain of *Y pestis* (strain 91,001 isolated from *Microtus brandti* in Inner Mongolia) has provided further insights into the evolution. The comparison of genomes of these three strains suggests that the ancestral *Y pestis* strain was probably virulent only to rodents. Some strains probably obtained genes by horizontal transfer of genetic materials and were able to jump species barriers leading to human infection [14,15].

The CCR5-Delta32 mutation that confers resistance to entry of HIV into human T-lymphocytes has been speculated to have expanded among whites under a selective pressure from plague or another illness. One of the most widely held theories is that *Y pestis* was unable to affect people with CCR5-Delta32 resulting in their survival, whereas others died from the pandemic. Others have argued against it because they could amplify the CCR5-Delta32 DNA sequence from up to 2900-year-old skeletal remains from central Germany and southern Italy, long before plague epidemics [16]. Animal studies have demonstrated no difference in either bacterial growth or survival time in mice with and without CCR5-Delta32 mutations [17].

Pathogenesis and virulence factors

A plague-infected fleabite leads to the inoculation of thousands of organisms into the human skin. From the skin, *Y pestis* migrates through cutaneous lymphatics to the regional lymph nodes causing regional lymphadenopathy and abscess formation, which are commonly known as "buboes." They resist phagocytosis by neutrophils and macrophages by various mechanisms. The bacteria rapidly replicate as aggregates of extracellular bacteria within necrotic lesions in the lymphoid tissue. Destruction of the lymph nodes is followed by bacteremia, septicemia, and endotoxemia.

Several virulence factors produced by *Y pestis* make it capable of overcoming the host factors and causing a severe form of infection (Table 1)

Table 1
Virulence factors of *Yersinis pestis*

Factors	Effects on the host
F1 antigen	An antiphagocytic factor, elicits humoral responses, used for immunologic diagnostic tests
Yersinia outer proteins	Inhibit phagocytosis, platelet aggregation, and effective inflammatory response
Lipopolysaccharide endotoxin	Cause of classic endotoxic shock, lacks O-antigen
Plasminogen activator	Facilitates systemic spread by degrading fibrin and other extracellular proteins
Hemin storage system	Enhances survival in phagocytes, increases uptake by eukaryocytic cells, a laboratory marker of pigmentation
V and W antigens	Mediate resistance to phagocytosis
Low-calcium-response plasmid	Activates V-antigen under low calcium conditions, activates *Yersinia* outer proteins
Phospholipase D	Allows to survive in the flea gut

[6,18,19]. Antiphagocytic factors, such as *Yersinia* outer proteins (Yops), low-calcium-response V (LcrV), F1, and W antigens protect *Y pestis* from destruction by phagocytosis. F1 (a protein fibrillar capsule) and LcrV antigens elicit protective humoral response against *Y pestis* and are currently the targets for vaccines under development [20–22]. F1 antigen, an antiphagocytic factor encoded in *pFra* plasmid, is also the target for commonly used immunologic diagnostic tests.

A type III secretion system encoded on the 70-kb plasmid functions to export multiple proteins (Yops and LcrV), which act in concert to inhibit phagocytosis and to down-regulate inflammation [23]. Yops are a group of pathogenicity factors consisting of two transporter and six effector proteins. The effector Yops counteract multiple signaling responses initiated by phagocytic receptors, Toll-like receptors, translocator Yops, and additional mechanisms [24]. As a result Yops inhibit phagocytosis, platelet aggregation, and an effective inflammatory response. Similar to the other members of the Enterobacteriaceae family, lipopolysaccharide is a major outer membrane component of *Y pestis*. The lipopolysaccharide of *Y pestis* is rough and lacks an important virulence factor, O-antigen (O-ag), as a consequence of the mutations within the biosynthesis cluster of O-antigen. The advantage of genetic loss of O-antigen in the highly pathogenic *Y pestis* remains unresolved [10,25].

Clinical presentations

Bubonic, septicemic, and pneumonic forms are the three classic presentations of plague. The most common type is bubonic plague, which typically occurs 2 to 6 days after a fleabite or after a direct exposure of skin or mucous membrane to the infected material. A local skin lesion, such as papule, vesicle, pustule, ulcer, or eschar, at the inoculation site may be present in some cases. Bubonic plague is characterized by a sudden onset of illness with headache, shaking chills, fever, and malaise, followed by pain in the affected regional lymph nodes. The regional lymph nodes are enlarged and very tender, hence the name "bubo" (in Greek, "boubon" means groin or swollen groin). Buboes usually become visible after 24 hours, and the size may vary from 1 to 10 cm in diameter. The surrounding skin is warm, erythematous, edematous, and adherent. Rarely, the bubo may become fluctuant and suppurate. Buboes may occur in any regional lymph nodes, such as inguinal, axillary, supraclavicular, cervical, postauricular, epitrochlear, popliteal, and pharyngeal sites. Deeper sites, such as intra-abdominal or intrathoracic lymph nodes, may also be involved. In untreated cases, such complications as secondary septicemia, secondary pneumonia, and meningitis are common. The case fatality rate for bubonic plague is 60% in untreated cases and less than 5% with appropriate antibiotic treatment [5,18,19,26].

Primary pneumonic plague results from the inhalation of droplets containing *Y pestis* after a short incubation period (usually 1–3 days). Pneumonic plague begins with a sudden onset of chills, fever, headache, body aches, weakness, and chest discomfort. Patients develop a productive cough, chest pain, shortness of breath, hypoxia, and hemoptysis. Chest radiograph may show a segmental or lobar involvement in the beginning, which may evolve into bilateral pneumonia, cavitations, pleurisy, and adult respiratory distress syndrome. Primary pneumonic plague is the most fulminant and fatal form of plague, usually resulting in death within 24 hours of the onset of illness [5,26,27].

Septicemic plague can be primary or secondary. Primary septicemic plague is characterized by an overwhelming *Y pestis* bacteremia usually after a cutaneous exposure in the absence of primary lymphadenopathy. It can occur in all age groups, but the elderly are at the greatest risk. Secondary septicemic plague results from spread of bacteria after establishing an identifiable localized infection, such as bubonic or pneumonic plague. The clinical picture is generally indistinguishable from other gram-negative septicemias. The septicemic plague results in sepsis syndrome, disseminated intravascular coagulopathy, multiorgan dysfunction, and adult respiratory distress syndrome, as a result of triggering a widespread immunologic cascade. Gangrene of the fingers and toes or the tip of the nose caused by small vessel thrombosis may appear in advanced stages (black death). *Y pestis* bacteremia may result in other complications, such as pneumonia, meningitis, hepatic or splenic abscesses, endophthalmitis, or generalized lymphadenopathy. Case fatality rate in untreated cases approaches 100% [5,26].

Less commonly, plague may present with pharyngitis as a result of ingestion or inhalation of *Y pestis*. Asymptomatic colonization of the pharynx has also been reported in contacts of pneumonic plague. Patients present with swollen tonsils and inflamed cervical lymph nodes [26]. Plague may rarely present with primary meningitis.

Plague as a biological weapon

Plague has been used as a biological weapon since the fourteenth century. The Tartar army (AD 1346) hurled its plague-infected corpses over the walls of the city during the siege of Caffa. This forced the Genoese defenders to flee, taking the illness with them and spreading to other cities and villages. The Russian army used similar tactics in the eighteenth century in the war against Sweden. During World War II, a secret branch of the Japanese army reportedly developed and dropped plague-infected fleas along with grains over populated areas of China on several occasions, which resulted in small epidemics in at least three cities. The grains were supposed to attract rats, which would help in spreading plague [28]. The United States and the Soviet Union were involved in developing aerosolized *Y pestis* before the 1972 convention on prohibition of biologic and toxin weapons [29].

The global distribution of *Y pestis* along with the ease for its mass production and aerosolized dissemination makes it a highly potential biological weapon. Aerosolization of *Y pestis* can result in primary pneumonic plague with a high fatality rate. It also has a potential for spreading from person to person during an epidemic leading to a large number of secondary cases. According to a WHO estimate, if 50 kg of *Y pestis* were aerosolized and spread over a city of 5 million people, pneumonic plague could occur in as many as 150,000 persons with 36,000 deaths. The plague bacilli would remain viable in the air for an hour and travel up to 10 km downwind. Significant numbers of city inhabitants might attempt to flee the infected area, which can further spread the disease to the people in other towns and cities [29,30].

Expected features of plague in a deliberate attack

The most likely form of plague used as a biological weapon is by aerosolization. Aerosolized *Y pestis* can result in a clinically evident pulmonary infection within 1 to 6 days after exposure. Symptoms, such as fever with cough and dyspnea, can be easily confused with those of other severe respiratory illnesses. This is followed by a rapidly progressive pulmonary disease and secondary septicemia with high case fatality rates. Gastrointestinal symptoms, such as nausea, vomiting, abdominal pain, and diarrhea, may also be present.

If an outbreak of plague occurs in a place that is not epidemiologically known to have enzootic plague or if there has been no prior rodent deaths in the area, an act of bioterrorism should be suspected. It should also be suspected if a diagnosis of plague is made in a person without risk factors, such as contact with rodents or fleas, or recent travel to an enzootic area. Plague outbreak in individuals without a common source of exposure should also raise the index of suspicion.

Application of the newer molecular epidemiologic techniques, such as multiple-locus variable number of tandem repeat analysis (MLVA), combined with epidemiologic information should be helpful to differentiate naturally occurring plague from that occurring from an intentional *Y pestis* release [31].

Laboratory diagnosis

Naturally occurring plague should be suspected based on clinical and epidemiologic features. In contrast, an outbreak of pneumonic plague might occur as a result of deliberate aerosolization without initially obvious environmental factors. When a case of plague is suspected, collection of clinical specimens followed by initiation of appropriate antimicrobial therapy should occur without any delay. Before sending the specimens containing suspected *Y pestis*, the microbiology laboratory should be notified about the possibility of plague because they are required to follow Biological Safety Level-2 (BSL-2) practices. Diagnostic specimens should include blood cultures. In addition, appropriate site-specific samples should be collected for staining and cultures, such as aspirates from suspected buboes, pharyngeal swabs, sputum, or endotracheal wash for suspected plague pharyngitis or pneumonia, and cerebrospinal fluid from those with suspected meningitis [8,26,29,32].

Under the microscope, *Y pestis* appears as a plump, gram-negative coccobacillus, 1 to 2 μm × 0.75 μm, mostly as single cells, or in pairs and short chains in liquid media. Its characteristic bipolar appearance on Wright-Giemsa or Wayson stain can provide a reasonable clue in an appropriate clinical setting. A positive direct fluorescent antibody testing that detects F1 antigen in tissues or body fluids is considered a presumptive evidence of plague [32].

On solid culture media, *Y pestis* grows as gray-white, translucent colonies, usually too small to be seen at 24 hours. *Y pestis* grows well in brain-heart infusion broth, sheep blood agar, or MacConkey agar. Definite identification of *Y pestis* culture is done with specific phage lysis. Automated bacteriologic test systems can misidentify or overlook *Y pestis* if the system is not properly programmed. *Y pestis* has been falsely identified as *Y pseudotuberculosis*, *Shigella*, *Salmonella*, or *Acinetobacter* [8].

When a case of plague is suspected and *Y pestis* is not isolated from cultures, a serologic diagnosis can be useful. The CDC recommends detection of antibodies against F1 antigen by the hemagglutination inhibition test. Using this method, a fourfold or greater change in antibody titer between acute and convalescent phase sera or a single titer of >1:128 is considered confirmatory of plague in a person previously unexposed to the infection or vaccine. A single titer of >1:10 is considered presumptive positive [32].

The WHO collaborative group and Pasteur Institute tested a rapid diagnostic test based on monoclonal antibodies against F1 antigen. This rapid diagnostic test detected presence of *Y pestis* in 41% more clinical specimens than by the bacteriologic methods, and in 31% more specimens than by the F1 ELISA method. The positive and negative predictive values of this rapid diagnostic test were 91% and 87%, respectively, with 100% sensitivity and specificity [33]. An F1 antigen-capture ELISA has also been described, which has 100% sensitivity for specimens from affected lymph nodes in patients with bubonic plague. This test's sensitivities, however, for serum and urine specimens are only 52% and 58%, respectively [34]. Various polymerase chain reaction assays, including multiplex polymerase chain reaction microarray assays for plague, anthrax, and tularemia, are under development [35].

The CDC has recommended a set of diagnostic criteria for a uniform notification and surveillance of plague [32]. Case definitions of suspect, presumptive, and confirmed cases of plague are shown in Box 2.

Management

If a case of plague is suspected, clinical specimens should be promptly obtained from the patient and specific antimicrobial therapy should be started

Box 2. Diagnostic criteria for plague

Suspect plague

- Clinical symptoms compatible with plague (fever and lymphadenopathy) in a person who resides or recently traveled to a plague-endemic area
- Small gram-negative or bipolar-staining coccobacilli on a smear from affected tissues (eg, a bobo, blood, tracheal or lung aspirate)

Presumptive plague

- Immunofluorescense stain (direct fluorescent antibody) positive for *Y pestis* F1 antigen
- A single serum specimen with anti-F1 antigen titer >1:10 by agglutination[a]

Confirmed plague

- A culture isolate lysed by specific bacteriophage for *Y pestis*
- Paired serum specimens (acute and convalescent) demonstrate greater than or equal to fourfold change in anti-F1 antibody titer by agglutination[a]
- A single serum specimen tested by agglutination[a] has a titer of >1:128 and the patient has no known previous plague exposure or vaccination history

[a] *Y pestis* F1 antigen-specific hemagglutination inhibition test.

Modified from Centers for Disease Control and Prevention. CDC case definitions. Atlanta (GA): Centers for Disease Control and Prevention; 2005.

without delay. Patients with suspected pneumonic plague should be managed under respiratory droplet precautions. Supportive care is an important part of the management, which may include immediate fluid resuscitation, vasopressors, hemodynamic monitoring, and respiratory care including ventilator support.

Streptomycin has been the preferred drug for treatment of plague, and should be administered intramuscularly for a total of 10 days, or until 3 days after the temperature returns to normal. Gentamicin is the alternative aminoglycoside used. In less severe cases, oral alternatives, such as tetracyclines and chloramphenicol, can be used. A retrospective data analysis of 75 cases from New Mexico showed similar outcomes in patients who received streptomycin alone, gentamicin alone, or gentamicin in combination with tetracyclines [36]. Chloramphenicol should be used in cases of plague meningitis.

The animal and in vitro studies suggest an equivalent or higher efficacy of ciprofloxacin compared with the aminoglycosides, although there are no clinical data in humans [29,37,38]. In animal studies, ciprofloxacin, ofloxacin, moxifloxacin, and gatifloxacin were shown to have equivalent efficacy [39–41]. Based on these data, the Working Group on Civilian Biodefense has recommended ciprofloxacin as an alternative agent for plague [29].

Although sulfonamides have been used extensively in the management of plague, their use has been associated with relatively higher mortality, increased complications, and slower defervescence of fever compared with other antibiotics used. Rifampin, aztreonam, and β-lactam antibiotics including cephalosporins should not be used to treat plague because they are ineffective. Use of β-lactam antibiotics has been associated with higher mortality rates in humans and mice [36,38]. Multidrug-resistant *Y pestis* has been reported from Madagascar [42]. Some Russian publications have reported ciprofloxacin resistance in virulent laboratory isolates of *Y pestis* [43,44].

Streptomycin or gentamicin can be used to treat plague in children. Gentamicin is preferred in pregnant women because of its safety; easy administration (intravenous or intramuscular); and wider availability of blood concentration monitoring (Table 2).

In a large outbreak or mass casualty situation from pneumonic plague, the Working Group on Civilian Biodefense recommends pre-emptive antibiotic treatment for all persons developing a temperature of 38.5°C or higher, or a new cough. In this setting, oral antibiotics are recommended because the number of people requiring treatment can exhaust local health care resources. Most patients do not need parenteral antibiotics. Preferred oral antibiotics are doxycycline or ciprofloxacin for both children and adults for large-scale outbreaks (Table 3). Alternatively, chloramphenicol can be used. Although the use of chloramphenicol in children less than 2 years old and doxycycline in those less than 8 years old should be avoided, in an outbreak setting the benefit of using these antibiotics outweighs the side effects. Recommended duration of treatment is 10 days [29].

Table 2
Recommended antibiotic treatment for plague

Adults	
Preferred agent	
Streptomycin	30 mg/kg/d (up to 1 g twice daily), IM
Alternative agents	
Gentamicin	5 mg/kg IM or IV once daily, or 2 mg/kg loading dose followed by 1.7 mg/kg every 8 h
Doxycycline	100 mg IV twice daily (or 200 mg once daily)
Chloramphenicol	25 mg/kg IV every 6 h
Ciprofloxacin[a]	400 mg IV or 500 mg oral twice daily
Children	
Preferred agents	
Streptomycin	15 mg/kg IM twice daily (maximum daily dose, 2 g)
Gentamicin	2.5 mg/kg IM or IV every 8 h
Alternative agents	
Doxycycline (for children >8 y)	
weight <45 kg	2.2 mg/kg IV twice daily (maximum daily dose, 200 mg)
weight ≥45 kg	Same as adult
Ciprofloxacin[a]	15 mg/kg IV twice daily (maximum daily dose, 1 g)
Chloramphenicol (>2 y)	25 mg/kg IV every 6 h (maximum daily dose, 4 g)
Pregnancy	
Gentamicin	Same as adult dose
Duration of treatment	10 d or until 2 d after the temperature has returned to normal

[a] Only in vitro and animal data are available to support use of fluoroquinolones in plague.

Prevention and infection control

Prevention of transmission of plague is challenging because *Y pestis* is a highly infectious agent that can be transmitted by multiple routes. Because plague exists as a zoonosis in its natural foci, public education on control of rodents and fleas in human dwellings can be helpful in reducing transmission to humans. These measures include environmental sanitation to remove food sources of rodents, building rodent-proof houses, and use of rodenticides and insecticides around human dwellings. Hunters and travelers to areas known to be the natural foci of plague should use insect repellents, such as DEET, and avoid contact with rodents and other sick or dead animals [5,29,45].

Immunization

Two types of plague vaccines have been available for human use since the early twentieth century: live attenuated and formalin-killed. Their efficacy in preventing bubonic plague has been variable. They do not protect against primary pneumonic plague, nor are they useful in outbreak settings. These vaccines are variably immunogenic and moderately to highly reactogenic. After immunization with these vaccines, it generally takes more than a month to develop a protective immune response [46,47]. Plague vaccines

Table 3
Treatment and postexposure prophylaxis for plague in a mass casualty setting

Preferred agents		
Doxycycline:	Adults	100 mg, po, twice daily
	Children <45 kg	2.2 mg/kg, po, twice daily
Ciprofloxacin:	Adults	500 mg, po, twice daily
	Children	20 mg/kg, po, twice daily
Alternative agent		
Chloramphenicol:	Adults or children	25 mg/kg, po, four times daily
Duration		
Treatment:	10 days	
Postexposure prophylaxis:	7 days	

are not currently available in the United States, because the manufacturing was stopped in 1999. They are available in most other countries. Their use is limited to high-risk groups only, such as laboratory technicians in plague reference and research laboratories or persons studying infected rodent colonies.

The current focus for developing plague vaccines is on two immunogenic proteins: F1 and V [46–48]. Vaccines based on these two purified recombinant antigens, rF1 and rV, have been found to be effective of protecting mice against both the bubonic and pneumonic forms of plague. A recombinant fusion vaccine (rF1V) tested by the United States Army Research Institute of Infectious Diseases has been shown to induce a significant level of protection in nonhuman primates. Both these candidate vaccines were scheduled for human trials in 2005. A novel DNA vaccine expressing a modified V antigen (LcrV) of *Y pestis* has been reported to be highly immunogenic in mice [49].

Antibiotic prophylaxis

Postexposure antibiotic prophylaxis for plague should begin within 6 days from exposure. Preferred antimicrobials are tetracyclines or ciprofloxacin (see Table 3). Alternatively, chloramphenicol or one of the effective sulfonamides (eg, sulfamethoxazole) can bc used. Prophylaxis should be given for 7 days [29].

Pre-exposure antibiotic prophylaxis may be used in persons who must travel to a plague-active area for a short duration under circumstances in which exposure to plague sources (eg, fleas, pneumonic cases) is inevitable.

Infection control

In general, plague requires standard precautions but patients with pneumonic plague, both primary and secondary, require droplet precautions. Pneumonic plague can be transmitted from person to person by respiratory droplets to close contacts within a 2-m distance. Patients with pneumonic plague require respiratory isolation, use of standard surgical masks, and avoidance of close contact. This needs to be followed for the first 48 hours from initiation of antibiotics or until clinical improvement. All suspected and confirmed cases of plague should be reported to the hospital epidemiologist or infection control practitioner, and to the local or state health department. Microbiology laboratory personnel should be alerted about any specimen suspected to have *Y pestis* because they are required to follow Biological Safety Level-2 precautions for general procedures and Biological Safety Level-3 precautions for procedures that can result in aerosol or droplet production. Autopsy procedures likely to cause aerosols (eg, bone sawing) need to be avoided. Persons exposed to *Y pestis* should immediately wash with soap and plenty of water, and promptly begin postexposure antibiotic prophylaxis. Because *Y pestis* is very sensitive to the sunlight and heating, it does not survive very long outside the host. Environmental decontamination is done with a 0.5% hypochlorite solution or a 1:10 dilution of household bleach [29].

Summary

Plague is a zoonosis caused by *Y pestis* that classically presents in one of three clinical forms: (1) bubonic, (2) septicemic, and (3) pneumonic. Aerosolized *Y pestis* is the most likely method used in a bioterrorist attack, which can lead to a rapidly fatal pneumonic plague. Plague should be suspected when the clinical picture is consistent and bipolar staining gram-negative rods are present. Diagnosis is confirmed by direct fluorescent antibody (presumptive); culture; polymerase chain reaction; or serology (paired sera). Preferred antibiotics are streptomycin or gentamicin, whereas tetracyclines, fluoroquinolones, and chloramphenicol are alternatives. Because vaccines are not currently available in the United States, pre-exposure and postexposure chemoprophylaxis should be used. Recent advances in genomic research on *Y pestis* should help in better understanding the epidemiology. and in the development of rapid diagnostic tests and safer and more effective vaccines.

References

[1] Achtman M, Morelli G, Zhu P, et al. Microevolution and history of the plague bacillus, *Yersinia pestis*. Proc Natl Acad Sci U S A 2004;101:17837–42.
[2] Kostis KP. In search of the plague: the Greek peninsula faces the Black Death, 14th to 19th centuries. Dynamis 1998;18:465–78.
[3] Dols MW. The second plague pandemic and its recurrences in the Middle East: 1347–1894. J Econ Soc Hist Orient 1979;22:162–89.
[4] WHO report on global surveillance of epidemic-prone infectious diseases. Geneva: World Health Organization; 2000.

[5] Dennis DT, Gage KL, Gratz N, et al. In: Plague manual: epidemiology, distribution, surveillance and control. Geneva: World Health Organization; 1999. p. 11–171.
[6] Perry RD, Fetherston JD. *Yersinia pestis*-etiologic agent of plague. Clin Microbiol Rev 1997;10(1):35–66.
[7] Gage KL, Dennis DT, Orloski KA, et al. Cases of cat-associated human plague in the Western US, 1977–1998. Clin Infect Dis 2000;30:893–900.
[8] Centers for Disease Control and Prevention. ASM, APHL basic protocols for level A laboratories for the presumptive identification of *Yersinia pestis*. Atlanta: CDC; 2001.
[9] Achtman M, Zurth K, Morelli G, et al. *Yersinia pestis*, the cause of plague, is a recently emerged clone of *Yersinia pseudotuberculosis*. Proc Natl Acad Sci U S A 1999;96:14043–8.
[10] Parkhill J, Wren BW, Thomson NR, et al. Genome sequence of *Yersinia pestis*, the causative agent of plague. Nature 2001;413:523–7.
[11] Deng W, Burland V, Plunkett G, et al. Genome sequence of *Yersinia pestis* KIM. J Bacteriol 2002;184:4601–11.
[12] Drancourt M, Roux V, Dang LV, et al. Genotyping, Orientalis-like *Yersinia pestis*, and plague pandemics. Emerg Infect Dis 2004;9:1585–92.
[13] Hinnebusch BJ. The evolution of flea-borne transmission in *Yersinia pestis*. Curr Issues Mol Biol 2005;7:197–212.
[14] Woolhouse ME, Taylor LH, Haydon DT. Population biology of multihost pathogens. Science 2001;292:1109–12.
[15] Song Y, Tong Z, Wang J, et al. Complete genome sequence of *Yersinia pestis* strain 91001, an isolate avirulent to humans. DNA Res 2004;11(3):179–97.
[16] Hummel S, Schmidt D, Kremeyer B, et al. Detection of the CCR5-Delta32 HIV resistance gene in Bronze Age skeletons. Genes Immun 2005;6:371–4.
[17] Mecsas J, Franklin G, Kuziel WA, et al. Evolutionary genetics: CCR5 mutation and plague protection. Nature 2004;427:606.
[18] McGovern TW, Friedlander A. Plague. In: Zajtchuk R, Bellamy RF, editors. Medical aspects of chemical and biological warfare. Bethesda: Office of the Surgeon General; 1997. p. 479–502.
[19] Dennis D, Meier F. Plague. In: Horsburgh CR, Nelson AM, editors. Pathology of emerging infections. Washington: ASM Press; 1997. p. 21–47.
[20] Philipovskiy AV, Cowan C, Wulff-Strobel CR, et al. Antibody against V antigen prevents Yop-dependent growth of *Yersinia pestis*. Infect Immun 2005;73:1532–42.
[21] Hill J, Copse C, Leary S, et al. Synergistic protection of mice against plague with monoclonal antibodies specific for the F1 and V antigens of *Yersinia pestis*. Infect Immun 2003;71:2234–8.
[22] Anderson GW Jr, Worsham PL, Bolt CR, et al. Protection of mice from fatal bubonic and pneumonic plague by passive immunization with monoclonal antibodies against the F1 protein of *Yersinia pestis*. Am J Trop Med Hyg 1997;56:471–3.
[23] Pujol C, Bliska JB. Turning *Yersinia* pathogenesis outside in: subversion of macrophage function by intracellular yersiniae. Clin Immunol 2005;114:216–26.
[24] Viboud GI, Bliska JB. *Yersinia* outer proteins: role in modulation of host cell signaling responses and pathogenesis. Annu Rev Microbiol 2005;59:69–89.
[25] Kukkonen M, Suomalainen M, Kyllonen P, et al. Lack of O-antigen is essential for plasminogen activation by *Yersinia pestis* and *Salmonella enterica*. Mol Microbiol 2004;51:215–25.
[26] Bossi P, Tegnell A, Baka A, et al. Bichat guidelines for the clinical management of plague and bioterrorism-related plague. Euro Surveill 2004;9:E5–6.
[27] Cleri DJ, Vernaleo JR, Lombardi LJ, et al. Plague pneumonia disease caused by *Yersinia pestis*. Semin Respir Infect 1997;12:12–23.
[28] McGovern TW, Friedlander AM. Plague. In: Sidell FR, Takafuji ET, Franz DR, editors. Textbook of military medicine: medical aspects of chemical and biological warfare. Washington: Borden Institute; 1997.

[29] Inglesby TV, Dennis DT, Henderson DA, et al. Plague as a biological weapon: medical and public health management. Working Group on Civilian Biodefense. JAMA 2000;283: 2281–90.
[30] WHO. Health aspects of chemical and biological weapons. Geneva: WHO; 1970.
[31] Lowell JL, Wagner DM, Atshabar B, et al. Identifying sources of human exposure to plague. J Clin Microbiol 2005;43:650–6.
[32] CDC. Laboratory testing criteria for diagnosis of plague. Available at: http://www.cdc.gov/ncidod/dvbid/plague/lab-test-criteria.htm. Accessed January 13, 2006.
[33] Chanteau S, Rahalison L, Ralafiarisoa L, et al. Development and testing of a rapid diagnostic test for bubonic and pneumonic plague. Lancet 2003;361:211–6.
[34] Chanteau S, Rahalison L, Ratsitorahina M, et al. Early diagnosis of bubonic plague using F1 antigen capture ELISA assay and rapid immunogold dipstick. Int J Med Microbiol 2000; 290:279–83.
[35] Tomioka K, Peredelchuk M, Zhu X, et al. A multiplex polymerase chain reaction microarray assay to detect bioterror pathogens in blood. J Mol Diagn 2005;7:486–94.
[36] Boulanger LL, Ettestad P, Fogarty JD, et al. Gentamicin and tetracyclines for the treatment of human plague: review of 75 cases in new Mexico, 1985–1999. Clin Infect Dis 2004;38: 663–9.
[37] Bonacorsi SP, Scavizzi MR, Guiyoule A, et al. Assessment of a fluoroquinolone, three beta-lactams, two aminoglycosides, and a cycline in treatment of murine *Yersinia pestis* infection. Antimicrob Agents Chemother 1994;38:481–6.
[38] Byrne WR, Welkos SL, Pitt ML, et al. Antibiotic treatment of experimental pneumonic plague in mice. Antimicrob Agents Chemother 1998;42:675–81.
[39] Steward J, Lever MS, Russell P, et al. Efficacy of the latest fluoroquinolones against experimental *Yersinia pestis*. Int J Antimicrob Agents 2004;24:609–12.
[40] Russell P, Eley SM, Green M, et al. Efficacy of doxycycline and ciprofloxacin against experimental *Yersinia pestis* infection. J Antimicrob Chemother 1998;41:301–5.
[41] Russell P, Eley SM, Bell DL, et al. Doxycycline or ciprofloxacin prophylaxis and therapy against experimental *Yersinia pestis* infection in mice. J Antimicrob Chemother 1996;37: 769–74.
[42] Galimand M, Guiyoule A, Gerbaud G, et al. Multidrug resistance in *Yersinia pestis* mediated by a transferable plasmid. N Engl J Med 1997;337:677–80.
[43] Ryzhko IV, Shcherbaniuk AI, Skalyga E, et al. Formation of virulent antigen-modified mutants (Fra-, Fra-Tox-) of plague bacteria resistant to rifampicin and quinolones. Antibiot Khimioter 2003;48:19–23.
[44] Kasatkina IV, Shcherbaniuk AI, Makarovskaia LN, et al. Chromosomal resistance of plague agent to quinolones. Antibiot Khimioter 1991;36:35–7.
[45] Gage KL, Denis DT, Tsai TF. Prevention of plague: recommendations of the Advisory Committee on Immunization Practices (ACIP). MMWR 1996;45:1–15.
[46] Titball RW, Williamson ED. *Yersinia pestis* (plague) vaccines. Expert Opin Biol Ther 2004;4: 965–73.
[47] Jefferson T, Demicheli V, Pratt M. Vaccines for preventing plague. Cochrane Database Syst Rev 2000;2:CD000976.
[48] Williamson ED, Flick-Smith HC, Lebutt C, et al. Human immune response to a plague vaccine comprising recombinant F1 and V antigens. Infect Immun 2005;73:3598–608.
[49] Wang S, Heilman D, Liu F, et al. A DNA vaccine producing LcrV antigen in oligomers is effective in protecting mice from lethal mucosal challenge of plague. Vaccine 2004;22: 3348–57.

ELSEVIER
SAUNDERS

Infect Dis Clin N Am
20 (2006) 289–311

INFECTIOUS
DISEASE CLINICS
OF NORTH AMERICA

Tularemia: Current Epidemiology and Disease Management

Henrik Eliasson, MD[a,*], Tina Broman, DVM, PhD[b], Mats Forsman, PhD[b], Erik Bäck, MD, PhD[a,c]

[a]*Department of Infectious Diseases, Örebro University Hospital, Infektionskliniken, Universitetssjukhuset, SE-70185 Örebro, Sweden*

[b]*Department of NBC Analysis, Swedish Defence Research Agency, FOI, SE-90182 Umeå, Sweden*

[c]*Department of Clinical Medicine, Örebro University, Örebro, Sweden*

Background

Francisella tularensis was first isolated in 1912 by McCoy and Chapin as the causative agent of a disease among ground squirrels in Tulare County, California. McCoy subsequently named the organism *Bacterium tularense* after the area of its first isolation [1]. In the sixteenth century, a disease of lemmings in Norway was described by Ziegler [2]; this is probably the oldest existing documentation of tularemia. Tularemia also was described in Japan in 1818 as a disease in humans that was contracted through contact with hares [3]. In the 1920s, Francis [4,5] reported on isolation of the organism from humans, naming the disease tularemia and the organism *Pasteurella tularensis* because of its resemblance to the plague bacterium. Francis [4,5] also classified the disease according to clinical picture, described insect vectors, and developed the serum agglutination test. In honor of his contributions, the organism, a small, fastidious gram-negative rod, was renamed *Francisella tularensis* [6].

At present, four subspecies of *F tularensis* are recognized [7]: (1) *F tularensis* subsp. *tularensis* (or type A) is the most virulent subtype. It is almost exclusively isolated in North America except for a single report from Europe [8]. Two genetically and geographically distinct subpopulations of this subspecies, AI and AII, have been defined [9]. (2) *F tularensis* subsp. *holarctica*

* Corresponding author.
E-mail address: henrik.eliasson@orebroll.se (H. Eliasson).

doi:10.1016/j.idc.2006.03.002

id.theclinics.com

(or type B) gives rise to a milder infection. It occurs over almost the entire Northern Hemisphere and causes disease in animals and humans. (3) *F tularensis* subsp. *mediasiatica* is a subspecies with low virulence that has been isolated from animals in central parts of Asia. (4) *F tularensis* subsp. *novicida* has been isolated only rarely, and its ability to cause disease in immunocompetent humans is still unclear [10,11].

There are few, if any, zoonotic diseases with an epidemiology as complex as is the case with tularemia. The organism has been found in more than 200 animal species—warm-blooded and cold-blooded vertebrates, invertebrates, and numerous arthropods [12,13]. Transmission to humans can occur by several routes.

Almost 100 years since the first isolation of the pathogen, there is still a limited understanding of the ecology and epidemiology of the organism. In many areas, the intervals between outbreaks span several years or decades, and the reasons for these variations are unknown. Geographically, the disease shows a patchy distribution with certain natural foci. The underlying mechanisms have not been clarified. In recent years, tularemia has emerged in new geographic locations, populations, and settings. Natural factors, such as climate, variations in numbers of suitable hosts and vectors, and level of susceptibility to infection in different host species, undoubtedly influence the local ecology and can be expected to be involved in the emergence of tularemia in new areas. Clinicians still have a poor understanding, however, of the interplay between such factors and of how they govern the spread and persistence of the organism.

Ecology

Two ecologic cycles of tularemia have been described, one mainly terrestrial and one mainly aquatic. Transmission of *F tularensis* subsp. *tularensis* is associated predominantly with rabbits and ticks in comparatively dry environments, whereas *F tularensis* subsp. *holarctica* often is isolated from hares, small rodents, mosquitoes, and ticks in association with streams, ponds, lakes, or rivers [12]. There also is evidence that the subspecies *holarctica* can persist for prolonged periods in watercourses [14], possibly in association with protozoa [15,16]. Water-borne transmission of type B tularemia frequently has been reported [17–25], and in Russia outbreaks of tularemia commonly occur in flooded areas close to large rivers and along shores of lakes [26]. The role of natural waters in the ecology of the organism is not well characterized, however, largely as a result of the fact that the bacterium has been impossible to culture from water samples. Its presence in water and sediments nonetheless has been proven, through inoculation of samples into laboratory animals from which culturable bacteria subsequently have been isolated [17]. Further experimental studies have indicated that the organism reaches higher concentrations in mud or sediments than in the pelagic zone [17].

A large variety of water-associated mammals and other organisms have been suggested to constitute the natural reservoir of the organism or to sustain the temporal persistence in natural waters through a constant seeding of bacteria to aquatic milieus. In Russia, the water vole (*Arvicola terrestris*) has been depicted as a major amplifier of *F tularensis* subsp. *holarctica* [26], whereas the water-living muskrat (*Ondatra zibethicus*) is considered the main source of type B infection in Canada [27]. Contamination of water has been suggested to occur from decomposing *F tularensis*–infected carcasses or through shedding of bacteria via urine from occasional surviving chronic carriers [28]. The relevance of the latter view could be questioned because few rodents survive infection, and because experimental infections have failed to produce conclusive results concerning development of chronic nephritis as a consequence of *F tularensis* infection. Nevertheless, either process would explain contamination of water only during epizootics, but each fails to explain persistence between outbreaks. The latter could be explained, however, by the survival and multiplication of *Francisella* intracellularly in protozoa [16].

Some species of birds have been shown to be susceptible to tularemia [29,30]. Transmission by birds or ticks transported or dropped by birds possibly could explain sporadic cases of tularemia in nonendemic areas, but seems unlikely as a general mode of transmission because tularemia has not been reported to occur along migration routes to the Southern Hemisphere [31].

Arthropods commonly are reported to act as vectors of tularemia, but no consistent evidence exists showing that they would constitute a reservoir for the organism. *F tularensis*–infected ticks have a high mortality rate, and the possibility of transovarial transmission remains dubious [18,32,33]. It is probable, however, that the bacteria can circulate in the tick-animal cycle for several years and promote local persistence. Mosquitoes of certain species in some areas, such as Russia and Sweden, have been shown to carry the organism [34,35], but experimental infections do not indicate that the organism is capable of multiplication in the vector [34]. Several researchers have suggested that mosquitoes transmit the disease mechanically from an infected to a susceptible host during repeated feeding [34]. Others suggest that mosquito larvae could become infected during their development in water [26]. Also, tabanid flies are known to transmit tularemia and have been suggested to become infected while drinking *F tularensis*–contaminated water [34].

Present knowledge suggests that *F tularensis* of the *holarctica* subspecies are adapted to existence in aquatic ecosystems, although the mechanistic features that enable persistence in water remain to be elucidated. Less is known about the natural reservoir of *F tularensis* subsp. *tularensis,* but this subspecies seems to be more dependent on nonaquatic ecologic niches and vector-animal cycles for persistence and transmission. The division of type A strains into two major subpopulations, AI and AII, suggests that different ecologic niches exist among type A strains [9]. The AI subpopulation primarily occurs in the central United States and is spatially correlated with the distribution of the eastern cottontail rabbit (*Sylvilagus floridanus*), the American dog tick

(*Dermacentor variabilis*), and the Lone Star tick (*Amblyomma americanum*). The AII group primarily occurs in the western United States and is associated with the wood tick (*Dermacentor andersoni*), the deerfly (*Chrysops discalis*), and the mountain cottontail rabbit (*Sylvilagus nuttallii*).

In addition to this complexity, several other organisms, based on a high degree of similarity in 16S rRNA gene sequences, have been classified as probable members of Francisellaceae [7]. Such *Francisella*-like organisms have been detected by DNA-based methods in ticks and in soil and water samples [36–38]. The gene sequences obtained from environmental samples indicated that within the family Francisellaceae organisms may exist that are distinct from known species and that potentially represent novel species and genera. These findings indicate that a wide range of closely related *Francisella*-like bacteria exist in the environment, and that the pathogenic subspecies may form just one branch, or possibly even just a clone, within a large group of diverse *Francisella*-like environmental bacteria.

Geographic distribution and epidemiology

Tularemia exists over almost the entire Northern Hemisphere, but with great variation in geographic and temporal occurrence. A single isolate of *F tularensis* subsp. *novicida* has been reported from the Southern Hemisphere [11]. On the American continent, the disease has been reported from the United States, Mexico, and Canada. In the United States, cases have been reported from every state except Hawaii, with most from Arkansas, South Dakota, Missouri, and Oklahoma. A decreasing incidence of tularemia has been noted since the 1930s, possibly as a result of a changing society with fewer people being exposed to vectors and wild animal hosts. In the period between 1990 and 2000, 1368 cases were reported to Centers for Disease Control and Prevention. Of cases in the United States, 80% are thought to be caused by *F t tularensis* [39]. Few scientific reports on tularemia in the United States state the frequency of *F t tularensis* and *F t holarctica* possibly because diagnosis is confirmed mainly by serologic methods that do not enable subspecies specification.

There are two major routes of transmission of tularemia to humans in the United States—through ticks and rabbits. Tick-borne tularemia dominates west of the Mississippi and occurs mainly in the summer. East of the Mississippi, the disease generally has been contracted through direct contact with animals, mainly cotton-tailed rabbits (*Sylvilagus* spp), during the winter hunting season [40]. To date, the winter peak is less prominent, possibly because of a decrease in rabbit hunting [41]. A higher incidence of tularemia has been reported among American Indians/Alaska Natives; this is probably a consequence of a greater exposure to the organism rather than to immunologic differences [40,41].

In 2000 an outbreak comprising 15 cases, of which 11 developed respiratory tularemia, occurred on Martha's Vineyard, Massachusetts [42]. Most of the disease victims were professional landscapers, and a case-control study showed grass mowing and brush-cutting as risk factors for tularemia [42]. In 1995, tularemia was removed from the list of notifiable diseases in the United States. Notifiable status was restored in 2000 because of the increasing focus on possible bioterrorism.

Tularemia has constituted a major health problem in parts of the former Soviet Union, presumably causing more than 100,000 cases during World War II [43]. A vast Russian documentation exists on the disease, and considerable efforts have been made to investigate natural foci of the disease and possible reservoirs. In all probability, the incidence of tularemia could have been even higher, had not large populations been immunized with a live vaccine [43]. Reports of the disease, or at least identification of the organism, also have been published from China, Mongolia, and Iran [44–47]. In Japan, most infections have occurred in the northeastern part of the country, mainly after contact with lagomorphs [48,49]. Tick-borne infection also has been described in Japan [50]. Outbreaks caused by contaminated drinking water have been reported from Turkey [23,51,52].

In Europe, tularemia has been reported from all countries except Iceland, Portugal, and the British Isles. Reports from central and southern Europe mainly indicate transmission through direct contact with animals such as hares and hamsters, but tick-borne infection and transmission through contaminated water and food also has been reported [25,31,53–55]. From Austria and former Czechoslovakia, several reports have been published describing airborne transmission in sugar plants, presumably caused by contaminated aerosols produced during washing of the sugar beets [56]. In recent years, outbreaks of disease through contact with hares have been reported from Spain, and an outbreak associated with crayfish fishing has been reported [24,57]. Whether crayfish are carriers of the organism or the patients simply were infected by contaminated water, through skin lesions, is unclear. Tularemia is a rare disease in Germany and Denmark. In Norway, infection through contaminated water supplies has been reported in a considerable proportion of cases [2]. Probably the highest incidence rates in the world have been reported from certain areas in Sweden and Finland. There is a remarkable variation in number of human cases between different years. Only 27 cases of type B tularemia were reported in Sweden in 2001, whereas 464 cases were reported in 2000, and 698 cases were reported in 2003. In Sweden, most patients are infected by mosquito bites, but transmission by ticks and rain flies (*Hematopota pluvialis*) also occurs [35,58–60]. Some, but not all, outbreaks have been linked to an increase in rodent tularemia [61,62]. In Sweden and Finland, outbreaks, or at least several scattered cases, of respiratory tularemia occasionally occur among farmers during summer [63]. An extraordinary outbreak occurred in northern Sweden in the winter of 1966–1967. Traditionally, farmers in northern Sweden kept hay stored in barns in wetland areas until the ground was frozen, which facilitated transportation. During this particular winter, massive death occurred among voles, leaving large amounts of carcasses and vole feces in the hay. While sorting the hay to get rid of dead voles, more than 600 individuals contracted respiratory tularemia. To the authors' knowledge, this is the largest outbreak of respiratory tularemia ever reported [62].

Tularemia as an emerging disease

A zoonotic disease such as tularemia, with a capacity to infect several species of animals, bears the potential of emergence in new areas. This potential has become evident as tularemia in recent years has emerged or reemerged in several countries [64]. Since the 1990s, tularemia emerged in new areas in central Sweden [59,65]. An example is the county of Örebro, where only a handful of cases were noted during the 1990s, whereas more than 300 cases of type B tularemia, mainly vector-borne, have been reported over 6 years. The underlying causes for the rapid increase in incidence are unknown. In Spain, tularemia was unrecognized until 1996, when 585 cases were reported from a limited region, most of them contracted through contact with hares [24,57]. Hares are frequently imported, for hunting purposes, to Spain from central Europe; this possibly explains the emergence of tularemia in Spain [64]. The risks concerned with international trade and transportation of wild animals also were illustrated during an outbreak of tularemia among wild-caught prairie dogs (*Cynomys ludovicianus*) in Texas. Several animals that had been in contact with the infected prairie dogs had been sold within the United States, but also exported overseas to the Netherlands, Belgium, and the Czech Republic. An isolate of *F t holarctica,* identical to isolates from animals in Texas, could be cultured from one of the prairie dogs in the Czech Republic, and another five animals were polymerase chain reaction (PCR) positive [66,67].

A breakdown of infrastructure, caused by war or natural disaster, may lead to the emergence of tularemia. This was experienced in Kosovo in 2000, where an outbreak was assumed to be caused by food and water contaminated by rodents, the animals appearing in abundance during the postwar era [25]. Similarly, outbreaks of what was called "trench tularemia" occurred in military personnel and civilians in the Soviet Union during World War II. In Turkey, outbreaks of tularemia have been associated with infrastructural breakdown after earthquakes [52].

Routes of transmission

Direct contact with infected animals

In 1925, Ohara [68] in a classic experiment rubbed infected rabbit tissue onto the left hand of his wife, who "courageously volunteered herself". He later removed enlarged lymph nodes from her axilla, from which he was able to culture the bacteria, showing the ability of *F tularensis* to penetrate seemingly intact skin. This route of transmission is an important mode of acquiring tularemia worldwide and occurs mainly among hunters, who become infected during handling of trapped or killed animals such as rodents and lagomorphs [48,53,54,69–71].

Vectors

Several arthropods, insects and ticks, have been implicated in the spread of tularemia. In North America and central Europe, different species of ticks have been shown to harbor *Francisella* [12,72,73]. Tularemia also has been linked to transmission by flies of the family Tabanidae [1,60,74]. This family includes true horseflies (*Tabanus* spp. and *Chrysozona* spp.) and deerflies (*Chrysops* spp.). Mosquitoes also may act as vectors for tularemia and constitute the dominant mode of transmission in Sweden and Finland, where transmission by ticks or deerflies is seen only occasionally [35,59,61]. Vector-borne infection generally leads to the ulceroglandular form of tularemia.

Inhalation

The inhalation route of transmission has been implicated in outbreaks of disease among farmers in Scandinavia and landscapers in the United States, the common factor being harvesting, grass cutting, or similar activities [42,62,63,75]. The inhaled vehicle may consist of aerosolized contaminated water or dust. Other outbreaks through inhalation of the bacteria have been described from sugar plants in central Europe [31,56]. Laboratory staff also is at high risk of infection via the respiratory route [76–78]. This has implications for the handling of diagnostic samples. Infection through inhalation generally leads to the typhoidal or respiratory form of tularemia.

Ingestion

Infection through contaminated water, rarely described in the United States and northern Europe, was considered the cause for the largest suspected outbreaks in the world, during World War II. Water from contaminated wells occasionally causes outbreaks of tularemia in Turkey and southern Europe. An outbreak in a nursing home in Czechoslovakia in the 1970s was caused by contaminated apple juice [19,23,51,52,56]. An outbreak of oropharyngeal tularemia, constituting 262 laboratory-confirmed cases, was reported from Bulgaria [55]. This tularemia outbreak indicated consumption of contaminated food and water as sources for the human infection.

Pathogenesis

Although the bacteria have the ability to penetrate intact skin, it is generally believed that invasion occurs through abrasions of the skin or mucous membranes. The infective dose is extremely low, especially if inhaled, when

10 organisms can induce the disease in humans [79]. The organisms spread from the port of entry to regional lymph nodes, where they cause formation of granulomas and caseous-type necroses that morphologically are indistinguishable from tuberculosis [80]. Further hematogenous and lymphatic spread in humans and other mammals can give rise to septicemia and dissemination of the organisms to bone marrow, spleen, and liver [80].

F tularensis is an intracellular parasite. Studies in mice have suggested that it enters the macrophage without triggering the respiratory burst [81]. After entry into the macrophage, the bacteria are contained in the phagosome. Later in the process, the bacteria escape the phagosome probably by membrane degradation, emerge into the cytoplasm, and subsequently induce apoptosis of the cell. On apoptosis, large numbers of organisms, ready to infect new cells, are released. The induction of apoptosis is a means of escaping the cell without generating an inflammatory response [82].

The ability to minimize inflammatory response seems to be a significant property of *F tularensis* [82]. Apart from avoiding the respiratory burst and causing cell death through apoptosis, the lipopolysaccharide of *Francisella* is much less pyrogenic than enterobacterial lipopolysaccharide, possibly because of a unique lipid A. No exotoxins or other secreted products have been identified in *Francisella* [82].

The genetic background for the higher virulence of the subspecies *F t tularensis* is unknown. The genome sequence of the highly virulent Schu S4 strain was published [83]. The genome sequence did not reveal any obvious explanations for the high virulence of the bacterium. A few notable features that may be significant for virulence were revealed, however: a set of genes encoding type IV pili, a type II secretion system, a surface polysaccharide, a putative poly-D-glutamic acid capsule, and an iron acquisition system. A putative pathogenicity island also was identified and found to be present as a duplicated 33.9-kb region containing 25 genes that lack homologues in other characterized bacterial species. Several genes of this region and a few others have by genetic disruption been shown to be important for virulence [82]. The first report of a defined mutant in *F t tularensis* was published in which a deletion of a 58-kd protein effectively attenuated the highly virulent Schu S4 strains in mice [84]. This protein is one of five members of a protein family identified in the Schu S4 genome sequence [83]. The function of the protein is unknown, and none of the five members of this protein family show any similarity to sequences in protein databanks [83]. This protein also is present in virulent type B strains. It is unknown whether the same degree of attenuation is mediated on loss of the protein in virulent type B strains.

The cell-mediated immune response is crucial for elimination of the infection and generally gives rise to protective immunity in humans 2 weeks after onset of the disease [80]. The humoral immune response is of only limited value in eliminating the bacteria. Agglutinating antibodies can be detected approximately 1 week after onset of detectable cell-mediated immunity

[80]. Infection induces long-lasting immunity in humans, but reinfection with a milder clinical course has been reported [76].

Clinical manifestations

The clinical picture in tularemia depends on the subspecies involved and the route of transmission, making certain clinical forms more common in certain parts of the world. Tularemia caused by *F t tularensis* is a severe disease, especially in immunocompromised patients, with a significant risk of rapid progression, septic shock, and fatal outcome. The reported lethality in the preantibiotic era in the United States varies from 3.6% to 33% [5,85]. Since the introduction of antibiotics, lethality of 2.2% to 3.8% has been reported [6,86]. None of the reports has taken into account, however, the relative frequencies of the two prevailing subspecies in the United States. During an outbreak of type A tularemia on Martha's Vineyard in 2000, 1 of 11 cases of respiratory tularemia had a fatal outcome [42]. Tularemia caused by subspecies other than *F t tularensis* is a milder disease, with almost no lethality even in the preantibiotic era. No treatment or appropriate but delayed therapy often leads to protracted disease, however, with fever, prostration, and suppurating lymph nodes.

The incubation period is usually 3 to 6 days, but a period ranging from a few hours to 2 or 3 weeks has been reported [6,85,86]. The onset of tularemia is usually abrupt with chills, fever, muscle pains, and headache [6,58]. The initial symptoms are similar in infections caused by *F t tularensis* and *F t holarctica*. A dry cough is common in all forms of disease, as are dermatologic manifestations, such as papular lesions and erythema nodosum [6,87]. Routine blood tests usually show moderately elevated C-reactive protein levels and a normal or slightly elevated white blood cell count [6,88]. In addition to the more general symptoms, tularemia can be divided into the following forms, according to more specific symptoms.

Ulceroglandular or glandular tularemia

Ulceroglandular or glandular tularemia (Figs. 1 and 2) is usually easily recognized, especially in areas where tularemia is endemic and where clinical staff is well acquainted with the disease. At the port of entry through the skin, a papule develops, often progressing to a slow-healing ulcer with crust formation. Simultaneously, the patient develops one or several enlarged and tender lymph nodes, usually axillary or inguinal, depending on the site of the primary lesion. Sometimes, and especially if not treated, the size of the glandules can be that of a hen's egg, and suppuration is common. After several weeks to months, if untreated, the swelling disappears, and the fistula heals. Ulceroglandular tularemia is usually the result of direct contact with infected animals or vector-borne infection. In the former case, the primary lesion typically is localized to one of the hands. In the latter, the most

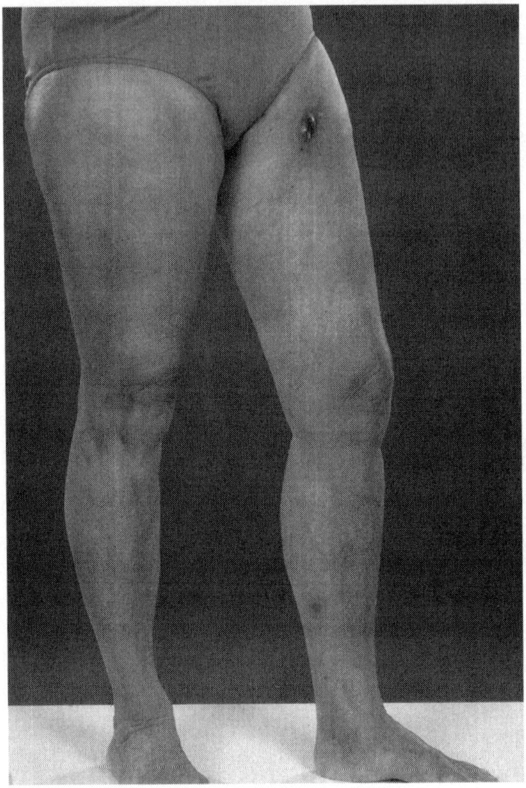

Fig. 1. Suppurating inguinal lymph node in a patient with ulceroglandular tularemia, 7 weeks after becoming ill. The primary lesion is seen on the lower leg. The patient was misdiagnosed initially, delaying treatment until after 5 weeks of disease.

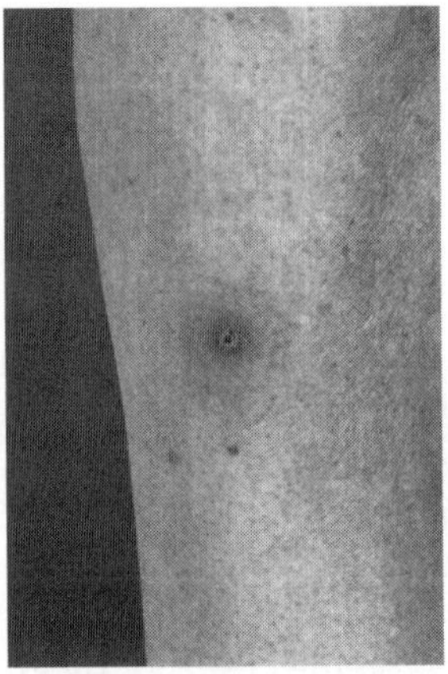

Fig. 2. Primary lesion on the lower leg of the patient in Fig. 1.

common localization is the lower leg in the case of transmission by mosquitoes or any part of the body in the case of infection by deerflies or ticks.

Glandular tularemia resembles the ulceroglandular form except for the absence of a visible primary lesion. It can be speculated that such cases could be the result of the organism's penetration through intact skin, but in the authors' experience, a minute primary lesion can be found in most cases. In the more than 250 cases of type B tularemia treated at the author's department over 6 years, only a handful of patients with glandular tularemia were seen in which no primary lesion could be identified. When a case of ulceroglandular or glandular tularemia appears in a nonendemic area, and the primary lesion is overlooked or absent, the differential diagnoses are several. Misdiagnosed tularemia in such cases can lead to extirpation of the lymph node on suspicion of tuberculosis or lymphoma.

Oropharyngeal tularemia

With oropharyngeal tularemia, after ingestion of contaminated food or water, the patient develops an ulcerative tonsillitis or pharyngitis, most often single-sided, with prominent swelling of adjacent lymph nodes. In some areas, this form seems to affect children to a larger extent than other forms of tularemia [69]. In nonendemic areas, the true diagnosis can easily be missed or delayed. A cluster of cases with ulcerative tonsillitis or pharyngitis with prominent enlargement of cervical lymph nodes should alert the physician to a diagnostic procedure aiming at tularemia and to an investigation of possible contaminated food or water supply.

Oculoglandular tularemia

Oculoglandular tularemia is unusual and is merely a special form of ulceroglandular tularemia, with the primary lesion found in the conjunctiva. A severe unilateral conjunctivitis in combination with swelling of preauricular lymph nodes should suggest a diagnosis of tularemia. In the case of oculoglandular tularemia, the bacteria are thought to be transmitted to the eye from the patient's own hands, perhaps after contact with infected animals or contaminated water [89].

Typhoidal tularemia

In addition to the general symptoms mentioned previously, there are no typical or focal signs that give clues to the diagnosis of typhoidal tularemia, apart from a prolonged high-grade fever and a relative bradycardia. Gastrointestinal symptoms and pulmonary infiltrates are common in patients with typhoidal tularemia. Diagnosis often is delayed or even possibly never made because the disease in many cases, and especially when caused by *F t holarctica,* is self-limited. Some patients with typhoidal tularemia caused by *F t tularensis* can develop a dramatic and life-threatening septic condition, however, particularly if they are immunocompromised. The typhoidal form of tularemia is, together with respiratory tularemia, the most serious form of tularemia. Typhoidal tularemia can be contracted through inhalation and through other transmission routes. Serious forms of tularemia sometimes can be complicated by meningitis, endocarditis, and rhabdomyolysis [90–93]. Tularemia should be considered and sought for in patients with fever of unknown origin.

Respiratory tularemia

Respiratory or pneumonic tularemia refers to patients with a clinical picture dominated by a respiratory infection, sometimes with severe respiratory insufficiency and necrotizing pneumonitis. Naturally, this form of tularemia usually is contracted through inhalation of the organism, but hematogenous spread to the lungs has been described, analogous to pneumonia in plague or typhoid fever. The radiologic picture in respiratory tularemia can show infiltrates and hilar adenopathy and pleural effusion [6,63,94]. In the authors' experience from respiratory tularemia caused by subspecies *holarctica*, the infiltrates are often discrete.

Diagnosis

The diagnosis of tularemia is based primarily on a thorough clinical examination and a clinical and epidemiologic history. Proper confirmatory testing and adequate therapy should be initiated after the history and physical examination.

Serology

Confirmation of tularemia is achieved most commonly through serology because other diagnostic means are less sensitive. Early and late sera should be obtained, to detect a seroconversion or significant increase in titers. The serum agglutination test, described by Francis [5], is still the prevailing serologic diagnostic method and provides an accurate diagnosis in most cases. Serology has some disadvantages, however. A significant increase in titers does not commonly occur until the third week of the disease or even later, delaying the diagnosis and occasionally the treatment [95]. The sensitivity is high, but single cases of tularemia have been described in which serologic tests repeatedly have been negative, whereas other tests, such as PCR, culture, and lymphocyte stimulation, have been positive [96].

False-positive results have been described in patients with brucellosis [5,97]. Repeated testing of patients with a documented episode of tularemia has shown a sustained high level of antibodies several years after the episode [5]. This reduces the usefulness of the agglutination test in endemic areas, unless parallel testing of acute and convalescence serum samples is possible. Enzyme-linked immunosorbent assay tests have been developed, but have no great advantage over agglutination tests because the IgM titers also remain elevated for years [80]. A strategy based on screening with enzyme-linked immunosorbent assay and confirmation by Western blot has been suggested for diagnosis [98]. The serologic tests do not discriminate between tularemia types A and B.

Culture

The pathogen can be cultured, most easily from ulcers, but sometimes also from blood, lymph node aspirates, or other clinical specimens. Because *Francisella* requires cysteine-rich media, such as modified Thayer-Martin medium, it does not grow readily on routine culture media [96]. Inoculation of samples into laboratory animals, usually guinea pigs, and subsequent culturing also is possible. The organism occasionally can be obtained from standard blood cultures [60,90,99]. In the authors' experience of tularemia caused by subspecies *holarctica,* a positive blood culture is achieved in less than 10% of patients. The high risk of laboratory infection makes culture hazardous, and consequently it is allowed only in biosafety level 3 (BSL 3) laboratories. For this reason, culture has not become a routine procedure in clinical practice. When tularemia is suspected, the laboratory should be informed of the suspicion, to ensure that adequate culture techniques and safety procedures are applied.

Polymerase chain reaction

A clinically useful PCR method, with high specificity and sensitivity when applied to samples from primary lesions in patients with ulceroglandular disease, has been developed [96,100,101]. The test is more sensitive than culture [96,101]. The assay, including sample preparation, is performed in a few hours, and the physician can obtain the laboratory result within 24 hours, even if sample transportation is required. From encrusted primary lesions, the sensitivity is greater than 90% when samples are collected properly from underneath the crust. In ulcerous lesions, the test has a sensitivity of about 70% [101]. The method does not differentiate between *F t tularensis* and *F t holarctica.* Rapid PCR tests that discriminate between type A and B tularemia could be available in the near future, however.

Skin test

Intracutaneous tests have been described and were formerly used in clinical practice. This method of testing the cellular immune response has not been standardized to the authors' knowledge and is of limited use today.

Lymphocyte stimulation

Cellular immunity is crucial in curing tularemia, and it is tempting to consider demonstration of cellular immune response development as a confirmation of diagnosis. Currently available methods are, however, time-consuming and not readily used for routine diagnosis [102]. A simplified method for lymphocyte stimulation has been developed [103]. Preliminary results from the authors' investigations of this method, adapted for tularemia, show promising results.

Immunofluorescence

Immunofluorescence can be used to identify the organism in tissue samples and consequently is used more often for diagnosis of tularemia in animals [104]. The method also can be used for confirmation of recovered isolates. To the authors' knowledge, it has not been evaluated in the hospital setting, but has occasionally been helpful in establishing an early diagnosis.

Treatment

As in most bacterial infections, the cornerstone of successful treatment is early diagnosis and institution of appropriate antimicrobial therapy. General principles for supportive care in critically ill patients apply, including prevention and management of septic shock and, if needed, the use of artificial ventilation. In most patients, however, the course is uneventful, and early defervescence should be expected if appropriate antibiotics are instituted early. If large lymph nodes already have developed, a sustained fever is often seen. The inflamed and enlarged lymph nodes should not be extirpated to avoid a secondary lymphedema. If the lymph node is fluctuating, drainage by puncture or incision is appropriate.

If fever reappears, it is more likely to be the effect of an immunologic reaction, usually associated with abscess formation within the lymph node, rather than a true relapse. Nevertheless, reinstitution of a new 14-day course of antibiotics is advocated because exclusion of a true relapse is difficult.

Ideally, decisions on antibiotic treatment regimens and other treatments should be based on randomized, controlled clinical trials. This approach is not, and probably never will be, possible for tularemia because there are few clinical centers that treat more than just a few cases. In areas where the disease is more common, it often appears in unforeseen outbreaks, during a short time span, making the planning of treatment studies difficult.

In North America, treatment traditionally has been based on streptomycin or gentamicin for 7 to 14 days, with only a small percentage of failures or relapses [85,105–107]. Streptomycin nowadays has a limited availability in many countries, leading to the use of gentamicin [108]. Data on the efficiency of other aminoglycosides are sparse, but treatment failures have been reported for tobramycin [105]. Treatment using aminoglycosides, other than gentamicin or streptomycin, is not recommended.

In Europe, where the milder form of tularemia occurs, treatment has been based on monotherapy with tetracyclines, most often doxycycline, 200 mg daily for 14 days. This treatment is usually effective, but treatment failures occur, and the risk of relapse tends to be higher after tetracycline than after aminoglycoside therapy. It is plausible that such relapses could be a consequence of the bacteriostatic effect of tetracyclines, in analogy with chloramphenicol, another bacteriostatic drug that is effective against tularemia, but has a high rate of relapses [105].

Generally, it is difficult to rank the efficiency of different antibiotics because no controlled studies have been performed. Additionally, most centers report only a few cases, and there is often a scarcity of information in the literature on the pretreatment duration of the disease in relation to the results of the treatment. Yet another problem is the difficulty of interpreting in vitro susceptibility testing because discrepancies seem to exist between minimal inhibitory concentration (MIC) values and the treatment outcome in patients. Third-generation cephalosporins sometimes have acceptable in vitro MIC values, but often fail when used in clinical treatment [109,110]. Chloramphenicol currently is not recommended because of the risk of relapse in addition to the risk of serious side effects. It can be considered, however, in the treatment of tularemia meningitis [108]. The usefulness of rifampin is still uncertain, bearing in mind the potential of rifampin to induce resistance [111]. North American strains are generally sensitive to macrolides, in contrast to European isolates [112]. Clinical data on macrolide efficiency are lacking, however, and macrolides currently are not recommended. Telithromycin, a ketolide, has shown promisingly low MIC values, but clinical experience is lacking [113]. Clindamycin and co-trimoxazole should not be used in the treatment of tularemia because MIC values are high, and evidence of efficiency is lacking [105,113].

Good results have been reported on fluoroquinolone treatment in tularemia. These drugs have very low MIC values for subspecies *tularensis* and subspecies *holarctica,* are bactericidal, and generate high concentrations intracellularly in macrophages [112,114–116]. Another advantage is the possibility to use oral preparations, which makes outpatient treatment simpler and more cost-effective. There has been general concern over the use of fluoroquinolones in children because of possible side effects. With the current growing experience of fluoroquinolone treatment in children, this group of antibiotics can be considered as a treatment alternative in children and adults [111]. The clinical use of quinolones in tularemia treatment has been reported only for infections caused by subspecies *holarctica* [57,111,112,115,117]. There is no clinical documentation on treatment of infections caused by the subspecies *tularensis* with quinolones, but there is no reason to believe that they would not work as well for subspecies *tularensis* as for subspecies *holarctica.* In the authors' experience with tularemia caused by the subspecies *holarctica,* ciprofloxacin and doxycycline are effective, but a few relapses have occurred after doxycycline treatment.

In the authors' opinion, fluoroquinolones should be the drug of first choice in mild-to-moderate forms of tularemia. In Europe, doxycycline is an acceptable alternative for treatment in adults and children older than 10 years old. As for treatment of many other intracellular pathogens, the duration of treatment should be at least 14 days, to minimize the risk of relapse. In severe forms (eg, in septic patients and patients with respiratory tularemia), gentamicin in combination with a quinolone is recommended. When a clinical response has been achieved, discontinuation of the aminoglycoside treatment could be considered, whereas the quinolone treatment should be continued for a minimum of 14 days. The most commonly used quinolone to date is ciprofloxacin. In a report on experimental infections in mice, treatment with gatifloxacin and moxifloxacin was superior to ciprofloxacin treatment [118]. In contrast, susceptibility testing of isolates of subspecies *holarctica* and *tularensis* has shown higher MIC values for moxifloxacin than for ciprofloxacin [112]. Until further experience is gathered, the authors regard ciprofloxacin as the quinolone of choice.

Prevention

Prevention must be directed at avoiding exposure to the most common local transmission routes. Protective gloves should be worn when in direct contact with wild rodents and lagomorphs. Handling of sick animals or carcasses should be avoided. In known foci of tularemia, other measures of protection include the use of chemical insect repellents; proper clothing to avoid bites from mosquitoes, deerflies, and ticks; and the prompt removal of ticks. Only water from protected wells should be used in endemic areas. In activities that create dust from potentially contaminated material in tularemia endemic areas, the use of a protective mask is advocated. There is no risk of human-to-human spread.

A live vaccine has been used to a wide extent in the former Soviet Union with good results, but this vaccine is currently not approved and is not generally available [43]. The live vaccine strain vaccine was derived from the Russian vaccine and has been used only to vaccinate at-risk personnel in the United States and Western Europe. There are several reasons why the live vaccine strain vaccine remains unlicensed [119]; the genetic background for the attenuation and for protection is unknown, and the live vaccine strain retains high virulence in mice and shows phase variation between one immunogenic and protective variant and another that does not generate protection. A new vaccine is needed, or further work needs to be undertaken to license the existing live vaccine strain vaccine.

Francisella tularensis as a potential agent for bioterrorism

Studies on human volunteers subjected to a minimal infective dose of *F tularensis* type A (10–50 bacteria of the highly virulent strain SchuS4) in the form of an aerosol of 0.7-μm particles, showed that 16 of the 20 exposed volunteers developed systemic evidence of infection, with an incubation period of 4 to 7 days [120]. The high attack rate by the respiratory route, the low infective dose, and the relative ease of production stimulated research on *F tularensis* as a potential biological weapon. In the period 1932 to 1945, Japanese research units examined the utility of *F tularensis* as a biological weapon. *F tularensis* has since been an organism of concern in defense plans against biologic attacks [121]. During World War II, tularemia outbreaks affecting tens of thousands of Soviet and German soldiers were reported, and the possibility of intentional use has been suggested, but not verified [122]. After the war, military studies of tularemia were continued. In a large state-funded biological weapons program of the 1950s, the US military developed weapons that could disseminate *F tularensis* aerosols. Studies on aerosol survival of *F tularensis* in wet and dry states at different temperatures and relative humidity have been published [123–125]. In addition, antibiotic-resistant strains were developed [126]. The USSR, as part of a program called Biopreparat, also incorporated an extensive research program for developing *F tularensis* into weapons [127]. In 1970, the World Health Organization published a report estimating that an aerosol dispersal of 50 kg of virulent *F tularensis* over a metropolitan area with 5 million inhabitants would result in 250,000 incapacitating causalities, including 19,000 deaths [128]. As the emphasis has shifted toward defending against biologic terrorism, the same features of this bacterium that attracted state-sponsored programs for development of biological weapons may pose a risk of use in a bioterrorism scenario. Outbreaks of suspected airborne tularemia might motivate an investigation of possible, intentional and unintentional, explanations for aerosolization of the bacteria [121,129].

In tularemia areas, detailed information on endemic strains of the organism would assist greatly in differentiating between naturally occurring cases and cases occurring from possible intentional release. A high-resolution multiple-locus variable-number tandem repeats analysis (MLVA) typing method for *F tularensis* targeting 25 different loci has been developed [130]. Apart from providing an excellent isolate discrimination, mLVA provides a powerful tool in understanding natural population structures and may be crucial in forensic attribution of suspected perpetrators in the possible event of bioterrorism activities.

Summary

Four subspecies of the zoonotic bacterium *F tularensis* have been described to date, with *F t tularensis* and *F t holarctica* being the subspecies causing most human tularemia cases. *F t holarctica* causes tularemia type B, a milder form of tularemia that appears over almost the entire Northern Hemisphere and that seems dependent on an aquatic life cycle. *F t tularensis,* the agent of the more severe tularemia type A that occurs in North America, has been divided into two major subpopulations. Each of the subpopulations occurs in different areas of North America and seems to be connected to different vectors. Despite more recent findings, several aspects of the ecology and epidemiology of tularemia still need to be clarified. Tularemia has emerged, or re-emerged, in new areas, showing the potential of *Francisella* for geographic propagation.

There are few, if any, zoonotic diseases with an epidemiology as complex as is the case with tularemia. Transmission to humans can occur by several routes, including vectors, direct contact, aerosol, food, and water. The clinical manifestations depend on the subspecies involved and on the route of acquisition. Different clinical forms of tularemia are recognized: ulceroglandular or glandular, oropharyngeal, oculoglandular, typhoidal, and respiratory. Laboratory diagnostics are based mainly on serology, culture, and molecular methods. More recent studies of tularemia have shed new light on the pathogenesis of this intracellular parasite, including its ability to minimize inflammatory response through different mechanisms.

Treatment of tularemia in North America traditionally has been based on aminoglycosides and in Europe on tetracyclines. Today, increasing experience with fluoroquinolones in the treatment of tularemia makes these agents alternatives in treatment of children and adults with tularemia. The low infective dose of *Francisella,* the high attack rate via the respiratory route, and the relative ease of production cause concern over its use in possible bioterrorism scenarios. Molecular typing methods will prove crucial tools in future research on the epidemiology of tularemia and in the event of bioterrorism. Today there are no commercially available vaccines, and prevention of tularemia has to be based on physical protection. The development of a new, highly protective vaccine is a high-priority research field.

References

[1] Francis E. Landmark article April 25, 1925: Tularemia. By Edward Francis. JAMA 1983; 250:3216–24.
[2] Scheel O, Sandvik T, Hoel T, et al. [Tularemia in Norway: a clinical and epidemiological review]. Tidsskr Nor Laegeforen 1992;112:635–7.
[3] Ohara S. Studies on yato-byo (Ohara's disease, tularemia in Japan). I. Jpn J Exp Med 1954; 24:69–79.
[4] Francis E. The occurrence of tularaemia in nature as a disease of man. Public Health Rep 1921;36:1731–53.
[5] Francis E. Symptoms, diagnosis and pathology of tularemia. JAMA 1928;91:1155–61.
[6] Evans ME, Gregory DW, Schaffner W, et al. Tularemia: a 30-year experience with 88 cases. Medicine (Baltimore) 1985;64:251–69.
[7] Sjostedt A. *Francisella,* vol. 2. 2nd edition. New York: Springer-Verlag; 2005.
[8] Gurycova D. First isolation of *Francisella tularensis* subsp. *tularensis* in Europe. Eur J Epidemiol 1998;14:797–802.
[9] Farlow J, Wagner DM, Dukerich M, et al. *Francisella tularensis* in the United States. Emerg Infect Dis 2005;11:1835–41.
[10] Lundquist M, Caspersen MB, Wikstrom P, et al. Discrimination of *Francisella tularensis* subspecies using surface enhanced laser desorption ionization mass spectrometry and multivariate data analysis. FEMS Microbiol Lett 2005;243:303–10.

[11] Whipp MJ, Davis JM, Lum G, et al. Characterization of a novicida-like subspecies of *Francisella tularensis* isolated in Australia. J Med Microbiol 2003;52(Pt 9):839–42.
[12] Hopla CE. The ecology of tularemia. Adv Vet Sci Comp Med 1974;18:25–53.
[13] Morner T. The ecology of tularaemia. Rev Sci Tech 1992;11:1123–30.
[14] Jellison WL. Tularemia in Montana. Mont Wildl 1971;5–24.
[15] Berdal BP, Mehl R, Meidell NK, et al. Field investigations of tularemia in Norway. FEMS Immunol Med Microbiol 1996;13:191–5.
[16] Abd H, Johansson T, Golovliov I, et al. Survival and growth of *Francisella tularensis* in *Acanthamoeba castellanii*. Appl Environ Microbiol 2003;69:600–6.
[17] Parker RR, Steinhaus EA, Kohls GM, et al. Contamination of natural waters and mud with *Pasteurella tularensis* and tularemia in beavers and muskrats in the northwestern United States. Bull Natl Inst Health 1951;193:1–161.
[18] Jellison WL. Tularemia in North America. 1930–1974. Missoula (MT): University of Montana; 1974.
[19] Greco D, Allegrini G, Tizzi T, et al. A waterborne tularemia outbreak. Eur J Epidemiol 1987;3:35–8.
[20] Tikhenko NI, Efremenko VI, Omarieva E, et al. [Outbreak of tularemia in the Republic of Dagestan]. Zh Mikrobiol Epidemiol Immunobiol 2001;(6 Suppl):68–72 [in Russian].
[21] Pazdiora P, Moravkova I, Nocarova D, et al. [A water-borne epidemic of tularemia in Chlumcany]. Epidemiol Mikrobiol Imunol 2002;51:23–5.
[22] Rogutskii SV, Khramtsov MM, Avchinikov AV, et al. [An epidemiological investigation of a tularemia outbreak in Smolensk Province]. Zh Mikrobiol Epidemiol Immunobiol 1997;2: 33–7.
[23] Helvaci S, Gedikoglu S, Akalin H, et al. Tularemia in Bursa, Turkey: 205 cases in ten years. Eur J Epidemiol 2000;16:271–6.
[24] Anda P, Segura del Pozo J, Diaz Garcia JM, et al. Waterborne outbreak of tularemia associated with crayfish fishing. Emerg Infect Dis 2001;7(3 Suppl):575–82.
[25] Reintjes R, Dedushaj I, Gjini A, et al. Tularemia outbreak investigation in Kosovo: case control and environmental studies. Emerg Infect Dis 2002;8:69–73.
[26] Pavlovsky EN. Tularemia. In: Levine ND, editor. Natural nidality of transmissible diseases. Urbana (IL): University of Illinois Press; 1966. p. 93–128.
[27] Martin T, Holmes IH, Wobeser GA, et al. Tularemia in Canada with a focus on Saskatchewan. Can Med Assoc J 1982;127:279–82.
[28] Bell JF, Stewart SJ. Chronic shedding tularemia nephritis in rodents: possible relation to occurrence of *Francisella tularensis* in lotic waters. J Wildl Dis 1975;11:421–30.
[29] Cabelli VJ, Hodapp FA, Ferguson EW, et al. The susceptibility of birds to tularaemia. Paper presented at Proceedings of the First International Symposium on Aerobiology, Berkeley (CA), 1963.
[30] Morner T, Mattsson R. Tularemia in a rough-legged buzzard (*Buteo lagopus*) and a ural owl (*Strix uralensis*). J Wildl Dis 1983;19:360–1.
[31] Tarnvik A, Priebe HS, Grunow R. Tularaemia in Europe: an epidemiological overview. Scand J Infect Dis 2004;36:350–5.
[32] Francis E. Sources of infection and seasonal incidence of tularemia in man. Public Health Rep 1937;52:103–13.
[33] Hubalek Z, Treml F, Halouzka J, et al. Frequent isolation of *Francisella tularensis* from *Dermacentor reticulatus* ticks in an enzootic focus of tularaemia. Med Vet Entomol 1996; 10:241–6.
[34] Petrisheva PA. Vectors of diseases of natural foci. Jerusalem: Israel Program for Scientific Translations; 1965.
[35] Olin G. The occurrence and mode of transmission of tularemia in Sweden. Acta Pathol 1942;19:220–47.
[36] Scoles GA. Phylogenetic analysis of the *Francisella*-like endosymbionts of *Dermacentor* ticks. J Med Entomol 2004;41:277–86.

[37] Sun LV, Scoles GA, Fish D, et al. Francisella-like endosymbionts of ticks. J Invertebr Pathol 2000;76:301–3.
[38] Barns SM, Grow CC, Okinaka RT, et al. Detection of diverse new *Francisella*-like bacteria in environmental samples. Appl Environ Microbiol 2005;71:5494–500.
[39] McChesney TC, Narain J. A five-year evaluation of tularemia in Arkansas. J Ark Med Soc 1983;80:257–62.
[40] Centers for Disease Control and Prevention. Tularemia—United States. 1990–2000. MMWR Morb Mortal Wkly Rep 2002;51:181–4.
[41] Chang MH, Glynn MK, Groseclose SL. Endemic, notifiable bioterrorism-related diseases, United States, 1992–1999. Emerg Infect Dis 2003;9:556–64.
[42] Feldman KA, Enscore RE, Lathrop SL, et al. An outbreak of primary pneumonic tularemia on Martha's Vineyard. N Engl J Med 2001;345:1601–6.
[43] Meshcheryakova IS. A history of the tularemia outbreaks and the experience of live vaccine use in Russia. Paper presented at Fourth International Conference on Tularemia, Bath (UK), 2003.
[44] Pang ZC. [The investigation of the first outbreak of tularemia in Shandong Peninsula]. Zhonghua Liu Xing Bing Xue Za Zhi 1987;8:261–3.
[45] Ebright JR, Altantsetseg T, Oyungerel R. Emerging infectious diseases in Mongolia. Emerg Infect Dis 2003;9:1509–15.
[46] Fedorov VP, Logachev AI, Peshkov BI, et al. [Detection of the agent of tularemia in the Mongolian People's Republic]. Zh Mikrobiol Epidemiol Immunobiol 1977;2:138–9.
[47] Arata A, Chamsa H, Farhang-Azad A, et al. First detection of tularaemia in domestic and wild mammals in Iran. Bull World Health Organ 1973;49:597–603.
[48] Ohara Y, Sato T, Homma M. Epidemiological analysis of tularemia in Japan (yato-byo). FEMS Immunol Med Microbiol 1996;13:185–9.
[49] Ohara Y, Sato T, Fujita H, et al. Clinical manifestations of tularemia in Japan—analysis of 1,355 cases observed between 1924 and 1987. Infection 1991;19:14–7.
[50] Ohara Y, Sato T, Homma M. Arthropod-borne tularemia in Japan: clinical analysis of 1,374 cases observed between 1924 and 1996. J Med Entomol 1998;35:471–3.
[51] Gurcan S, Otkun MT, Otkun M, et al. An outbreak of tularemia in Western Black Sea region of Turkey. Yonsei Med J 2004;45:17–22.
[52] Karadenizli A, Gurcan S, Kolayli F, et al. Outbreak of tularaemia in Golcuk, Turkey in 2005: report of 5 cases and an overview of the literature from Turkey. Scand J Infect Dis 2005;37:712–6.
[53] Munnich D, Lakatos M. Clinical, epidemiological and therapeutical experience with human tularaemia: the role of hamster hunters. Infection 1979;7:61–3.
[54] Vaissaire J, Mendy C, Le Doujet C, et al. [Tularemia: the disease and its epidemiology in France]. Med Mal Infect 2005;35:273–80.
[55] Christova I, Velinov T, Kantardjiev T, et al. Tularaemia outbreak in Bulgaria. Scand J Infect Dis 2004;36:785–9.
[56] Cerny Z. Changes of the epidemiology and the clinical picture of tularemia in Southern Moravia (the Czech Republic) during the period 1936–1999. Eur J Epidemiol 2001;17: 637–42.
[57] Perez-Castrillon JL, Bachiller-Luque P, Martin-Luquero M, et al. Tularemia epidemic in northwestern Spain: clinical description and therapeutic response. Clin Infect Dis 2001; 33:573–6.
[58] Christenson B. An outbreak of tularemia in the northern part of central Sweden. Scand J Infect Dis 1984;16:285–90.
[59] Eliasson H, Lindback J, Nuorti JP, et al. The 2000 tularemia outbreak: a case-control study of risk factors in disease-endemic and emergent areas. Sweden. Emerg Infect Dis 2002;8: 956–60.
[60] Eliasson H, Back E. Myositis and septicaemia caused by *Francisella tularensis* biovar holarctica. Scand J Infect Dis 2003;35:510–1.

[61] Tarnvik A, Sandstrom G, Sjostedt A. Epidemiological analysis of tularemia in Sweden 1931–1993. FEMS Immunol Med Microbiol 1996;13:201–4.
[62] Dahlstrand S, Ringertz O, Zetterberg B. Airborne tularemia in Sweden. Scand J Infect Dis 1971;3:7–16.
[63] Syrjala H, Kujala P, Myllyla V, Salminen A. Airborne transmission of tularemia in farmers. Scand J Infect Dis 1985;17:371–5.
[64] Petersen JM, Schriefer ME. Tularemia: emergence/re-emergence. Vet Res 2005;36:455–67.
[65] Payne L. Endemic tularemia, Sweden, 2003. Emerg Infect Dis 2005;11:1440–2.
[66] Avashia SB, Petersen JM, Lindley CM, et al. First reported prairie dog-to-human tularemia transmission, Texas, 2002. Emerg Infect Dis 2004;10:483–6.
[67] Petersen JM, Schriefer ME, Carter LG, et al. Laboratory analysis of tularemia in wild-trapped, commercially traded prairie dogs, Texas, 2002. Emerg Infect Dis 2004;10:419–25.
[68] Ohara H. Experimental inoculation of disease of wild rabbits into the human body, and its bacteriological study. The Japan Medical World 1926;11:299–304.
[69] Stewart SJ. Tularemia: association with hunting and farming. FEMS Immunol Med Microbiol 1996;13:197–9.
[70] Feldman KA. Tularemia. J Am Vet Med Assoc 2003;222:725–30.
[71] Taylor JP, Istre GR, McChesney TC, et al. Epidemiologic characteristics of human tularemia in the southwest-central states, 1981–1987. Am J Epidemiol 1991;133:1032–8.
[72] Markowitz LE, Hynes NA, de la Cruz P, et al. Tick-borne tularemia: an outbreak of lymphadenopathy in children. JAMA 1985;254:2922–5.
[73] Hubalek Z, Juricova Z, Halouzka J. *Francisella tularensis* from ixodid ticks in Czechoslovakia. Folia Parasitol (Praha) 1990;37:255–60.
[74] Klock LE, Olsen PF, Fukushima T. Tularemia epidemic associated with the deerfly. JAMA 1973;226:149–52.
[75] Feldman KA, Stiles-Enos D, Julian K, et al. Tularemia on Martha's Vineyard: seroprevalence and occupational risk. Emerg Infect Dis 2003;9:350–4.
[76] Overholt EL, Tigertt WD, Kadull PJ, et al. An analysis of forty-two cases of laboratory-acquired tularemia: treatment with broad spectrum antibiotics. Am J Med 1961;30:785–806.
[77] Jensen WA, Kirsch CM. Tularemia. Semin Respir Infect 2003;18:146–58.
[78] Parker RR, Spencer RR. Six additional cases of laboratory infection of tularaemia in man. Public Health Rep 1926;41:1341–55.
[79] Sjostedt A. Virulence determinants and protective antigens of *Francisella tularensis*. Curr Opin Microbiol 2003;6:66–71.
[80] Tarnvik A. Nature of protective immunity to *Francisella tularensis*. Rev Infect Dis 1989;11:440–51.
[81] Fortier AH, Green SJ, Polsinelli T, et al. Life and death of an intracellular pathogen: Francisella *tularensis* and the macrophage. Immunol Ser 1994;60:349–61.
[82] Sjostedt A. Intracellular survival mechanisms of *Francisella tularensis*, a stealth pathogen. Microbes Infect 2005;15:15.
[83] Larsson P, Oyston PC, Chain P, et al. The complete genome sequence of *Francisella tularensis*, the causative agent of tularemia. Nat Genet 2005;37:153–9.
[84] Twine S, Bystrom M, Chen W, et al. A mutant of *Francisella tularensis* strain SCHU S4 lacking the ability to express a 58-kilodalton protein is attenuated for virulence and is an effective live vaccine. Infect Immun 2005;73:8345–52.
[85] Giddens WR, Wilson JW Jr, Dienst FT Jr, et al. Tularemia; an analysis of one hundred forty-seven cases. J La State Med Soc 1957;109:93–8.
[86] Sanders CV, Hahn R. Analysis of 106 cases of tularemia. J La State Med Soc 1968;120:391–3.
[87] Syrjala H, Karvonen J, Salminen A. Skin manifestations of tularemia: a study of 88 cases in northern Finland during 16 years (1967–1983). Acta Derm Venereol 1984;64:513–6.

[88] Syrjala H. Peripheral blood leukocyte counts, erythrocyte sedimentation rate and C-reactive protein in tularemia caused by the type B strain of *Francisella tularensis*. Infection 1986;14:51–4.
[89] Guerrant RL, Humphries MK Jr, Butler JE, et al. Tickborne oculoglandular tularemia: case report and review of seasonal and vectorial associations in 106 cases. Arch Intern Med 1976;136:811–3.
[90] Tarnvik A, Sandstrom G, Sjostedt A. Infrequent manifestations of tularaemia in Sweden. Scand J Infect Dis 1997;29:443–6.
[91] Kaiser AB, Rieves D, Price AH, et al. Tularemia and rhabdomyolysis. JAMA 1985;253: 241–3.
[92] Klotz SA, Penn RL, Provenza JM. The unusual presentations of tularemia: bacteremia, pneumonia, and rhabdomyolysis. Arch Intern Med 1987;147:214.
[93] Tancik CA, Dillaha JA. Francisella tularensis endocarditis. Clin Infect Dis 2000;30: 399–400.
[94] Tarnvik A, Berglund L. Tularaemia. Eur Respir J 2003;21:361–73.
[95] Stralin K, Eliasson H, Back E. An outbreak of primary pneumonic tularemia. N Engl J Med 2002;346:1027–9.
[96] Johansson A, Berglund L, Eriksson U, et al. Comparative analysis of PCR versus culture for diagnosis of ulceroglandular tularemia. J Clin Microbiol 2000;38:22–6.
[97] Duenas AI, Ortega M, Garrote I, et al. [Laboratory diagnosis and serologic course in patients with tularemia]. Med Clin (Barc) 2000;114:407–10.
[98] Schmitt P, Splettstosser W, Porsch-Ozcurumez M, et al. A novel screening ELISA and a confirmatory Western blot useful for diagnosis and epidemiological studies of tularemia. Epidemiol Infect 2005;133:759–66.
[99] Provenza JM, Klotz SA, Penn RL. Isolation of *Francisella tularensis* from blood. J Clin Microbiol 1986;24:453–5.
[100] Sjostedt A, Eriksson U, Berglund L, et al. Detection of *Francisella tularensis* in ulcers of patients with tularemia by PCR. J Clin Microbiol 1997;35:1045–8.
[101] Eliasson H, Sjostedt A, Back E. Clinical use of a diagnostic PCR for *Francisella tularensis* in patients with suspected ulceroglandular tularaemia. Scand J Infect Dis 2005;37:833–7.
[102] Syrjala H, Herva E, Ilonen J, et al. A whole-blood lymphocyte stimulation test for the diagnosis of human tularemia. J Infect Dis 1984;150:912–5.
[103] Gaines H, Biberfeld G. Measurement of lymphoproliferation at the single-cell level by flow cytometry. Methods Mol Biol 2000;134:243–55.
[104] Morner T. The use of FA-technique for detecting *Francisella tularensis* in formalin fixed material: a method useful in routine post mortem work. Acta Vet Scand 1981;22: 296–306.
[105] Enderlin G, Morales L, Jacobs RF, et al. Streptomycin and alternative agents for the treatment of tularemia: review of the literature. Clin Infect Dis 1994;19:42–7.
[106] Mason WL, Eigelsbach HT, Little SF, et al. Treatment of tularemia, including pulmonary tularemia, with gentamicin. Am Rev Respir Dis 1980;121:39–45.
[107] Mitchell CL, Cross JT. Tularemia. Curr Treat Options Infect Dis 2002;4:429–35.
[108] Amsden JR, Warmack S, Gubbins PO. Tick-borne bacterial, rickettsial, spirochetal, and protozoal infectious diseases in the United States: a comprehensive review. Pharmacotherapy 2005;25:191–210.
[109] Cross JT, Jacobs RF. Tularemia: treatment failures with outpatient use of ceftriaxone. Clin Infect Dis 1993;17:976–80.
[110] Baker CN, Hollis DG, Thornsberry C. Antimicrobial susceptibility testing of *Francisella tularensis* with a modified Mueller-Hinton broth. J Clin Microbiol 1985;22:212–5.
[111] Johansson A, Berglund L, Gothefors L, et al. Ciprofloxacin for treatment of tularemia in children. Pediatr Infect Dis J 2000;19:449–53.
[112] Johansson A, Urich SK, Chu MC, et al. In vitro susceptibility to quinolones of *Francisella tularensis* subspecies *tularensis*. Scand J Infect Dis 2002;34:327–30.

[113] Maurin M, Mersali NF, Raoult D. Bactericidal activities of antibiotics against intracellular *Francisella tularensis*. Antimicrob Agents Chemother 2000;44:3428–31.
[114] Ikaheimo I, Syrjala H, Karhukorpi J, et al. In vitro antibiotic susceptibility of *Francisella tularensis* isolated from humans and animals. J Antimicrob Chemother 2000;46:287–90.
[115] Syrjala H, Schildt R, Raisainen S. In vitro susceptibility of *Francisella tularensis* to fluoroquinolones and treatment of tularemia with norfloxacin and ciprofloxacin. Eur J Clin Microbiol Infect Dis 1991;10:68–70.
[116] Russell P, Eley SM, Fulop MJ, et al. The efficacy of ciprofloxacin and doxycycline against experimental tularaemia. J Antimicrob Chemother 1998;41:461–5.
[117] Chocarro A, Gonzalez A, Garcia I. Treatment of tularemia with ciprofloxacin. Clin Infect Dis 2000;31:623.
[118] Piercy T, Steward J, Lever MS, Brooks TJ. In vivo efficacy of fluoroquinolones against systemic tularaemia infection in mice. J Antimicrob Chemother 2005;13:13.
[119] Sandstrom G. The tularaemia vaccine. J Chem Technol Biotechnol 1994;59:315–20.
[120] Saslaw S, Eigelsbach HT, Prior JA, et al. Tularemia vaccine study: II. Respiratory challenge. Arch Intern Med 1961;107:702–14.
[121] Dennis DT, Inglesby TV, Henderson DA, et al. Tularemia as a biological weapon: medical and public health management. JAMA 2001;285:2763–73.
[122] Alibek K. Biohazard: the chilling true story of the largest covert biological weapons program in the world, told from the inside by the man who ran it. New York: Random House; 1999.
[123] Cox CS. Aerosol survival of *Pasteurella tularensis* disseminated from the wet and dry states. Appl Microbiol 1971;21:482–6.
[124] Cox CS, Goldberg LJ. Aerosol survival of *Pasteurella tularensis* and the influence of relative humidity. Appl Microbiol 1972;23:1–3.
[125] Ehrlich R, Miller S. Survival of airborne *Pasteurella tularensis* at different atmospheric temperatures. Appl Microbiol 1973;25:369–72.
[126] SIPRI. The problem of chemical and biological warfare, vol. 2. CB weapons today. Stockholm: Almqvist & Wiksell; 1973.
[127] Davis CJ. Nuclear blindness: an overview of the biological weapons programs of the former Soviet Union and Iraq. Emerg Infect Dis 1999;5:509–12.
[128] WHO. Health aspects of chemical and biological weapons. Geneva: World Health Organization; 1970.
[129] Bossi P, Tegnell A, Baka A, et al. Bichat guidelines for the clinical management of tularaemia and bioterrorism-related tularaemia. Eur Surveill 2004;9:E9–10.
[130] Johansson A, Farlow J, Larsson P, et al. Worldwide genetic relationships among *Francisella tularensis* isolates determined by multiple-locus variable-number tandem repeat analysis. J Bacteriol 2004;186:5808–18.

ELSEVIER
SAUNDERS

Infect Dis Clin N Am
20 (2006) 313–327

INFECTIOUS
DISEASE CLINICS
OF NORTH AMERICA

Botulism: The Many Faces of Botulinum Toxin and its Potential for Bioterrorism

Rodrigo G. Villar, MD*, Sean P. Elliott, MD, Karen M. Davenport, MD

Department of Pediatrics and Steele Children's Research Center, University of Arizona Health Sciences Center, 1501 N. Campbell Avenue, Tucson, AZ 85724, USA

The neurotoxins produced by *Clostridium botulinum* are among the most potent poisons known. Botulinum toxin currently is used for an increasing number of medical conditions intentionally to weaken or alleviate spasticity of specific muscle groups. Concern about its use as a potential agent in bioterrorism attacks, however, also is growing. Awareness of the botulism syndromes is critical to allow prompt identification of cases and rapid delivery of antitoxin that may alleviate disease severity and to provide supportive care, especially in the event of respiratory failure. This article describes the microbiology, pharmacology, and epidemiology of *C botulinum* and its toxins; the recognized botulism syndromes; modes of transmission; and treatment. Additionally, it focuses on the potential use of botulinum toxin as a biological weapon, reviewing potential modes of toxin delivery; recognition of intentional attacks; laboratory methods for toxin detection; and possible methods for prevention, treatment, and control of botulism in the event of an intentional attack.

Microbiology and botulinum toxins

Clostridia are anaerobic gram-positive, spore-forming bacilli found worldwide in soils, marine and fresh water sediments, and the intestines of many animals [1]. For humans, the most important species of botulinum toxin–producing *Clostridium* species is *C botulinum*. Three other phylogenetically distinct species, *Clostridium baratii*, *Clostridium butyricum*, and

* Corresponding author.
E-mail address: rodrigo.villar@tmcaz.com (R.G. Villar).

0891-5520/06/$ - see front matter
doi:10.1016/j.idc.2006.02.003

Clostridium argentinense, however, also produce botulinum toxin [1,2]. *Clostridium* spores are extremely hardy and are able to survive up to 2 hours at 100°C. *Clostridia* vegetate and elaborate botulinum toxin in oxygen-poor, low-salt, low-sugar, and low-acidity environments. Toxin is denatured and inactivated by heating at 85°C for 5 minutes [3].

Specific strains of *C botulinum* produce one of seven immunologically distinct polypeptide toxins designated by the letters A through G. The toxin subtypes are defined by their inability to cross-neutralize each other (ie, anti-A antitoxin does not neutralize toxin types B–G) [4]. These toxins are zinc metalloproteases that cleave and inactivate specific cellular proteins essential to the release of neurotransmitter. The toxins are composed of polypeptides linked by disulfide bonds that undergo posttranslational cleavage by a clostridial trypsin-like protease into one heavy (100 kd) and one light (50 kd) chain. The heavy chain facilitates binding to gangliosides on the presynaptic motor neuron plasma membrane and internalization by receptor-mediated endocytosis. The light chain is a zinc-containing endopeptidase that blocks acetylcholine-containing vesicles from binding to the outer membrane of the neuron [5–7].

In the cytoplasm of the presynaptic neuron, the light chain binds irreversibly to specific synaptic fusion complex proteins known as SNARE proteins. The SNARE complex consists of synaptobrevin, SNAP-25, and syntaxin. The light chain from specific toxin subtypes targets and cleaves specific proteins in this complex. Toxin types A and E cleave SNAP-25; toxin types B, D, F, and G cleave synaptobrevin; and toxin type C cleaves both SNAP-25 and syntaxin. Cleavage of any of these membrane fusion proteins disrupts the fusion of endocytoplasmic acetylcholine-containing vesicles with the outer cell membrane and prevents neurotransmission [7–9]. The resultant lack of adequate concentrations of acetylcholine at the postsynaptic motor unit results in ineffective motor fiber contraction and the clinical appearance of the botulism syndromes [10]. The toxins affect all ganglionic synapses, parasympathetic synapses, and neuromuscular junctions.

Because the binding of the light chain to the SNARE complex is irreversible, new axonal sprouting and regeneration of SNARE complexes must occur for neurotransmission to resume and for muscular function to be restored. Although maximal effect of botulinum toxin appears 24 to 72 hours after exposure, muscle weakness and dysfunction may be present for many months [11].

Exact lethal doses for botulinum toxins have not been reported, but extrapolations from primate studies suggest that less than 0.1 μg of toxin delivered intravenously or intramuscularly, 0.7 to 0.9 μg if inhaled, and 70 μg if ingested orally may be enough to kill an adult human [8,12,13]. When converted to actual amounts of toxin, 100 U of type A toxin is equivalent to 20 U/ng of neuroprotein complex and represents approximately only about 0.3% of the estimated human lethal inhalational dose and 0.005% of the estimated lethal oral dose [8].

Botulinum toxins for therapeutic indications are available commercially from several distributors in single-use vials of lyophilized toxin. In the United States, commercial type A toxin is available, 100 U per vial from Allergan Pharmaceuticals, Irving, California and in Europe, 500 U per vial from Ipsen Pharmaceuticals, Berkshire, Great Britain). Both preparations contain human albumin and neither contains a preservative. The manufacturers recommend that vials be stored for up to 15 to 24 months at 2°C to 8°C and used within 4 to 8 hours following reconstitution if kept between 2°C and 8°C. For therapeutic uses, typical recommended doses of type A botulinum toxin range from 50 to 400 U per treatment site in adults (maximum total dose per patient per treatment of 400 U). Although much higher doses and total amounts have been used, there are no controlled studies to report a maximum dosing range [14]. Patients have developed botulism-like syndromes from therapeutic doses [15,16].

Botulinum toxin type B (Solstice Neurosciences, South San Francisco, California) is available in single-dose vials of 2500, 5000, and 10,000 units per vial. One unit corresponds to the calculated median lethal intraperitoneal dose in mice (Solstice Neurosciences) and typical recommended total dose per patient treatment ranges between 2500 and 5000 U. Type B toxin produces essentially the same clinical syndrome as type A toxin. This commercial product is not as widely used and is generally reserved for patients whose clinical response decreases after multiple exposures to type A toxin because of the development of antibodies.

Epidemiology

Spores of *C botulinum* are found worldwide with toxin-specific subtypes identified more frequently in certain geographic areas. In the United States, *C botulinum* strains that produce toxin types A and B occur more frequently in the lower 48 states, whereas type E–producing strains occur more frequently in Alaska and near the Great Lakes, likely associated with fish and marine animals. Types A, B, and E account for nearly all human cases of botulism. Types C and D most commonly cause disease in other animals including mammals and birds. Clinical botulism has been reported worldwide [1,2,4,17].

Clinical botulism syndromes

Botulism results from toxin absorption by a mucosal membrane (gut or lung) or from a wound; botulinum toxin does not penetrate intact skin. All described botulism syndromes have similar clinical manifestations that typically occur within 24 to 72 hours of toxin exposure. Signs and symptoms almost always include cranial nerve dysfunction followed by a descending motor paralysis that spares sensation and sensorium (Table 1). Prompt

Table 1
Clinical features of botulism, types A and B

	% cases
Symptom	
Dysphagia	96
Dry mouth	93
Double vision	91
Dysarthria	84
Fatigue	77
Arm weakness	73
Constipation	73
Leg weakness	69
Blurred vision	65
Dyspnea	60
Nausea	64
Vomiting	59
Sore throat	54
Dizziness	51
Abdominal cramps	42
Diarrhea	19
Paresthesia	14
Sign	
Alert mental status	90
Arm weakness	75
Ptosis	73
Leg weakness	69
Diminished gag reflex	65
Gaze paralysis	65
Facial palsy	63
Tongue weakness	58
Pupils dilated or fixed	44
Hyporeflexia or areflexia	40
Nystagmus	22
Ataxia	17

Outbreaks reported in the United States 1973–1974.

Data from Hughes JM, Blumenthal JR, Merson MH. Clinical features of type A and B food-borne botulism. Ann Intern Med 1981;95:442.

identification of cases is critical to provide antitoxin that may alleviate severity and provide supportive care, especially in the event of respiratory failure.

Foodborne botulism

Foodborne botulism occurs when preformed toxin is ingested. In cases of foodborne botulism, typically the food items that contain clostridial spores are undercooked and prepared in a manner that favors spore vegetation and toxin production. In the United States, vehicles most commonly implicated in foodborne botulism are home-canned foods and native Alaskan dishes. Such foods are prepared without adequate heat to kill *Clostridium* spores and stored in a low-acid, low-sugar, anaerobic environment between 4°C and 48°C that favors toxin production. Consumption of these foods without sufficient heating adequately to denature the preformed toxin leads to disease. Clinical manifestations usually occur between 24 and 72 hours after consumption of a contaminated food; however, symptom onset has been reported as long 5 days as after presumed exposure [18].

Infant botulism

In contrast to foodborne botulism where ingestion of food containing preformed toxin causes illness, infant botulism occurs when *C botulinum* colonizes the intestine of infants less than 1 year old and begins to produce toxin in vivo. The absorbed toxin produces the recognizable botulism syndrome demonstrated by poor sucking and swallowing, a change in the pitch or volume of the infant's cry, ptosis, loss of neck control, and progressive descending paralysis. *C botulinum* is not a normal member of the intestinal flora and reasons for colonization are not well understood. Ingestion of honey has been identified as a risk factor in up to 25% of these cases. Full recovery is expected with supportive care but may be compromised by complications of mechanical ventilation and associated secondary infections [19].

Wound botulism

Wound botulism has most frequently been described among intravenous drug users who inject polybacterial-contaminated "black tar" heroin under the skin, known as "skin popping." If tissue necrosis and abscess formation occur and produce an anaerobic environment, *Clostridia* may vegetate and elaborate toxin resulting in botulism. These patients demonstrate the typical cranial nerve dysfunction and descending paralysis seen in other botulism syndromes [20].

Adult intestinal toxemia botulism

Adult intestinal botulism follows a similar mechanism as infant botulism. *C botulinum* may colonize the intestine of certain adults with functional or anatomic abnormalities of the gastrointestinal tract and produce toxin in vivo [21,22]. Exposure to antimicrobials may lead to altered gastrointestinal flora and predispose to colonization with *Clostridia*. Absorbed toxin produces the botulism syndrome.

Inhalational botulism

Few cases of inhalation botulism have occurred and the inhalational route is not considered to be a natural mode of transmission. Inhalational botulism is expected to produce a clinical picture similar to foodborne botulism. Accidental inhalation of type A botulinum toxin among three veterinary laboratory workers in Germany in 1962 resulted in clinical botulism. These persons received antitoxin and had subsequent resolution of symptoms [23]. Inhalational botulism has been demonstrated experimentally in primates [24] and in mice. In addition to producing clinical botulism, inhaled type A botulinum toxin in mice has produced severe lung injury including alveolar hemorrhage and interstitial edema [25].

Iatrogenic botulism

The US Food and Drug Administration has approved the use of botulinum toxin type A for four medical applications: (1) alleviation of cervical dystonia, (2) primary axillary hyperhidrosis, (3) blepharospasm, and (4) strabismus. Botulinum toxin is used off-label, however, for a wide spectrum of disorders including spasticity in patients with cerebral palsy and other focal spastic disorders, achalasia, sialorrhea, anal sphincter spasticity, and for cosmetic modification [26]. Although rare, clinical botulism has occurred after therapeutic intramuscular injections of type A botulinum toxin used to treat spasticity [15,16,27,28]. In the reported cases, the doses used were within the recommended range for therapeutic purposes. The toxin may have entered the bloodstream and produced an increased effect with resultant botulism syndrome.

Botulinum toxin as a weapon

As with any potential biological weapon, major characteristics that need to be considered are ease of dissemination or transmission, potential for major public health impact, potential for public panic and social disruption, and requirements for public health preparedness [29]. For an efficient agent in a mass attack, the agent should be pathogenic, toxic at low doses, environmentally stable, transmissible by aerosol, and capable of causing significant morbidity or mortality [7,8]. Botulinum toxin meets several of these requirements and is considered a potential biological weapon threat. Any large attack with botulinum toxin could overwhelm health care resources if severely affected patients required intensive care and mechanical ventilation. Additionally, if many persons presented with a suspected botulism syndrome, the limited supply of antitoxin could rapidly be exhausted, first locally and then nationally. For use in an intentional attack, a bioterrorist has to produce, store, disseminate, and administer botulinum toxin in a manner that preserves the stability of the neurotoxic proteins. Any of the routes by which botulism may occur could provide potential methods for intentional attacks.

Intentional injected botulinum toxin

Intentional injection of botulinum toxin into an individual could produce lethal results if undiagnosed or untreated. Delivery of injected botulinum toxin to a large number of persons in a bioterrorist act likely would be impractical unless it was delivered by another injectable vehicle (eg, medications, fluids, and so forth). This mode of delivery requires the undetected addition of toxin to a vehicle during its manufacture, production, distribution, or delivery, and that the toxin remain stable in that vehicle. Many medications are prepared with chemical additives and maintain either an acidic or basic environment to inhibit microbial activity and are unfavorable environments for storing botulinum toxin. Although unlikely, such a widespread attack could be devastating if it were linked to a commonly used medication administered in large quantities daily. In this case, many persons could be affected before a botulism outbreak was detected and a product alert or recall could be instituted.

Commercial botulinum toxin is expensive and limited in supply. It is normally distributed under prescription and delivered by medical doctors. Widespread reports in the media have described its use outside controlled medical environments, however, particularly at exclusive "Botox parties" at which toxin is injected for cosmetic use. Additionally, non–human grade botulinum toxin has been misused or sold as a less expensive product for cosmetic use and found to produce tissue abscesses. Intentional overdosing or misuse of these products could cause weakness and even death.

Intentional aerosolized botulinum toxin

Because botulism and botulinum toxin are neither contagious nor transmitted from person to person, aerosol attack is the most likely scenario for the use of botulinum toxins. Delivery of botulinum toxin by the inhalational route could be expected to affect large numbers of people: 1 g of crystalline toxin, evenly dispersed and inhaled, could kill more than 1 million people [8]. Terrorists have already attempted to distribute botulinum toxin by aerosol in downtown Tokyo, Japan, and at United States military sites in Japan between 1990 and 1995 [7,8,30]. Four of the countries identified by the United States government as "state sponsors of terrorism" are thought to be developing botulinum toxin as a weapon [31]. After the 1991 Persian Gulf War, Iraq admitted to production of 19,000 L of concentrated botulinum toxin, 10,000 L of which was reportedly weaponized. This amount of toxin represents approximately three times the amount necessary to kill the entire human population by inhalation, and has never been fully accounted for [32].

It is unclear how effective botulinum toxin is as an aerosolized bioweapon because the toxin is easily denatured by environmental conditions and subject to constraints of concentration and stabilization for aerosol dissemination. Persistence of aerosolized botulinum toxin at a site of deliberate release depends on atmospheric conditions and the particle size of the aerosol. Extremes of temperature degrade the toxin: heat destroys the toxins in 30 minutes at 80°C and in several minutes at 100°C, whereas sunlight inactivates the toxins within 1 to 3 hours [33]. Also, aerosolized toxin has been estimated to decay at 1% to 4% per minute, depending on the weather and dispersal pattern [34]. A point-source aerosol release of botulinum toxin, however, is thought to have the potential to incapacitate or kill 10% of persons within a 0.5-km distance downwind of the release site [32].

The time to onset of inhalational botulism is unknown because so few cases are known. Monkeys showed signs of botulism 12 to 80 hours after significant exposure, and the three known accidental human cases developed symptoms approximately 72 hours after exposure [23,32]. Aerosol dissemination may not be difficult to identify because a large number of human cases would develop, sharing common geographic exposure and temporal association. Additionally, confirmation of an unusual toxin type (types C, D, F, or G) and lack of a common dietary exposure suggest deliberate aerosolized release of botulinum toxin. Unfortunately, recognition of such release by current methods likely would occur too late to prevent additional cases. Rapid detection of aerosolized botulinum toxin by ELISA, however, is a component of the United States military's Biologic Integrated Detection System for rapid recognition of biologic agents on the battlefield. Additional detection methods use ultraviolet and laser-induced fluorescence to detect biologic aerosol clouds at a distance up to 5 km [33].

Intentional foodborne botulinum toxin

Intentional contamination of widely distributed commercial or noncommercial foods can also provide a route for bioterrorists to deliver botulinum toxin. To be an effective vehicle for botulinum toxin, a contaminated food has to provide an environment in which the toxin can remain stable. Foods that have a low pH, high osmotic or sugar content, or particularly those that require cooking are inefficient vehicles because toxin denatures at temperatures $\geq$85°C for 5 minutes [1,2]. Commercially canned and preserved foods sold in the United States are prepared in a manner that reduces the risk of botulism; intentional contamination with toxin or *Clostridium* spores requires manipulation of the food at the origin of its preparation. To cause a commercial food item to be an efficient vehicle for botulism, a bioterrorist has to alter its ingredients or preparation practices to create a milieu capable of sustaining sporulation and toxin production or one preventing destruction of preformed toxin in ready-to-eat foods. Because outbreaks of botulism most frequently are associated with the consumption of home-canned foods, any outbreak associated with the consumption of commercial food products suggests an intentional source. To remain an effective bioweapon, such food has to be consumed without further cooking and before it naturally spoils and is discarded. Ingestion of foods contaminated with toxin or inactive spores is an unlikely and impractical route for botulism bioterrorism against a large number of persons. Although intentional delivery of food items contaminated with bacteria to cause illness has been used successfully [35], intentional contamination of most foods with *C botulinum* spores likely would not cause disease. Because of their ubiquitous presence in nature, inactive *Clostridium* spores probably are ingested frequently, but the required environment to sporulate and produce toxin rarely occurs inside the human body.

Intentional water contamination

Botulinum toxin has been listed as a potential threat to water supplies because of its stability in fluids. Although botulinum toxin has been shown to retain up to 50% of its activity for 5 to 70 days in various types of untreated water and beverages [36], there have been no reports of outbreaks from contamination of water supplies with the toxin. In 1973, however, a German biologist threatened to contaminate water supplies with *Bacillus anthracis* and botulinum toxin unless he was paid $8.5 million [37].

Five factors cited as barriers to deliberate contamination of modern water supplies include (1) dilution; (2) specific inactivation from chlorine or other disinfectants; (3) nonspecific inactivation by hydrolysis, sunlight, and microbes; (4) filtration; and (5) the relatively small quantity of water that is actually ingested [37]. It is unlikely for botulinum toxin effectively to contaminate a water supply because it is inactivated by sunlight, aeration, and chlorine. Even if botulinum toxin is introduced downstream from a water treatment facility it is unlikely to survive because of chlorine content and aeration. Contamination of natural water supplies probably is ineffective because of a limited amount of people affected who might drink untreated water before toxin inactivation. Although personal-use water purification devices without reverse osmosis fail to remove botulinum toxin, those with reverse osmosis capability, as used by the United States military, can eliminate the toxin [38]. Most water bottled in the United States is purified by reverse osmosis, but many international bottlers do not use this process. In some cities, 15% to 30% of residents report that they drink only bottled water [37]. Others have personal reverse osmosis purification systems. Toxin introduction to municipal water supplies or to bottled water or other beverages is a threat that should be considered if no other vehicle is recognized.

Diagnosis

Currently, the mouse bioassay is the standard method for quantification of toxin, and doses are often expressed in mouse intraperitoneal lethal dose units [1]. The mouse bioassay can also be used to differentiate the botulinum toxin serotypes. It requires pretreatment of mice with type-specific antitoxin. Control mice are not pretreated with antitoxin. Both groups of mice are then injected intraperitoneally with serum, stool supernatant, or other substance suspected to contain botulinum toxin. Mice are evaluated for 24 to 72 hours for signs of botulism or death. The limitations of this assay are that it is labor intensive, slow, and requires the use of live animals.

In the United States, most of this testing occurs at the Centers for Disease Control and Prevention (CDC) [3]. For testing of human patient specimens, samples of the patient's blood (20 mL in a "tiger" or "red" top tube), stool (25 g is ideal, if the patient is constipated sterile water enema can be used to obtain a sample), gastric contents or vomitus (20 mL), environmental or wound swabs, and suspected foods are sent to a reference laboratory under the guidance of state and federal health officials. Procedures for collecting, storing, and shipping samples can be accessed through the American Society of Microbiology website (Box 1). Other toxin detection methods less widely used include real-time polymerase chain reaction to detect a fragment of the neurotoxin gene [39]. The polymerase chain reaction assay may be useful in wound botulism and could have a role in toxin detection when *C botulinum* is present in tissues, foods, or other vehicles suspected of causing botulism [40,41]. Rapid mass spectrometry may also be useful to detect small amounts of toxin and even specific subtypes more quickly and with equal sensitivity to the mouse assay, especially when very low quantities of toxin are present [6]. ELISA testing also provides a rapid result but it is less sensitive and is currently being used as a fast screening technique.

Treatment

Clinical treatment is primarily supportive with frequent neurologic evaluation and close attention for respiratory insufficiency and failure. Treatment should avoid agents that may further inhibit the neuromuscular junction including aminoglycosides, clindamycin, polymyxin B, and magnesium-containing compounds. In addition to supportive care, antitoxin may

Box 1. Emergency contacts for cases of botulism

Contact state health department by 24-hour emergency line. If unable to establish contact quickly, call the Centers for Disease Control and Prevention Emergency Operations Center at 770-488-7100.

For suspected infant botulism occurring in any state, contact the California Department of Health Services, Infant Botulism Prevention Program at 510-540-2646.

Procedures for collecting, storing, and shipping samples from patents with suspected botulism can be found at the American Society for Microbiology website: http://www.asm.org/Policy/index.asp?bid=6342.

be effective in preventing progression of paralysis and leading to a less severe course. To be effective, antitoxin must be given as soon as the clinician suspects botulism exposure to neutralize circulating toxin before it binds irreversibly to sites on the presynaptic terminal. Antitoxin may be given when continued toxin exposure is suspected but is generally not recommended if a patient's exposure is greater than 72 hours.

Type-specific antitoxins exist with activity against any one of the seven toxin subtypes. Antitoxin binds the toxin and the antitoxin-toxin complex is cleared from circulation. Both human- and equine-derived antitoxin products are currently available. The trivalent antitoxin (against A, B, and E) is the current treatment in the United States. Because it is derived from an equine source, the risk of allergic reaction is significant and preparations to deal with anaphylaxis are needed. The current dosing regimen recommends a single vial of antitoxin diluted 1:10 in normal saline administered intravenously over 30 to 60 minutes [42]. The short-term effects of equine-derived antitoxin are generally well-tolerated; however, long-term effects are unknown. Human-derived botulinum antitoxin (formerly known as "botulinum immune globulin") is available from the California Department of Health Services for cases of infant botulism (see Box 1) [43].

Active immunization against botulinum toxin has been available since the early 1960s [44,45]. An effective pentavalent vaccine (A–E) containing formalin-inactivated botulinum toxin adsorbed to aluminum phosphate and preserved with thimerosal is currently distributed by the CDC. The immunization schedule consists of doses at 0, 2, and 12 weeks with an annual booster and is recommended typically only for laboratorians working with *C botulinum* [46]. A vaccine against toxin type F is in development [47]. Development of further immunization strategies based on toxoid, different protein subunits, and recombinant Hc fragments is limited. Administration of poly(lactide-co-glycolide) microspheres to entrap recombinant fragments of various toxin subtypes by subcutaneous, intramuscular, or intranasal routes may show promise as neutralizing agents [48–51]. Development of monoclonal antibodies against botulinum toxins may also provide passive immunization for postexposure protection [52].

Because botulinum toxins are zinc metalloproteases, strategies aimed at inhibiting enzyme function have also been explored. Zinc chelation is too broad an approach because many zinc-dependent enzymes would be affected. Synthesized proteins that bind specific toxin loci may function as effective toxin inhibitors and serve to protect exposed individuals [53,54].

In addition to antitoxin and supportive therapies, measures used to treat botulism include cleaning of any wound that potentially harbors clostridium spores and avoidance of antimicrobials except to treat secondary infections. In cases of foodborne botulism, activated charcoal, cathartics, and enemas may play a role in removing toxin-containing food from the body. Standard precautions are recommended for patients with botulism because toxin is not absorbed through the skin and there is no risk for person-to-person transmission. Once hospitalized, patients do not require isolation. The organism, *C botulinum*, itself does not directly cause illness in healthy hosts [55].

Protocols for suspected botulism cases

The public health response to cases of botulism should be similar for both naturally occurring and deliberately caused disease, both of which should be regarded as emergencies. The most important public health efforts are assurance of proper food preparation, storage, and consumption, and surveillance of cases for rapid detection and response. Any suspected case should trigger an epidemiologic and environmental investigation. Suspicion for a bioterrorist act must be raised if an outbreak involves such unusual circumstances as unexpected victims; large numbers of cases; or unusual routes, vehicles, locations, or clinical syndromes.

All cases of botulism, regardless of clinical subtype, constitute a public health emergency and public health authorities should be notified immediately on suspicion of a case. Clinicians suspecting a case of botulism should call their state health department to trigger surveillance and antitoxin release protocols. Health department personnel initiate epidemiologic and environmental investigations, discuss the case with a CDC consultant, arrange for specimen testing at a public health laboratory, and assist with shipment of antitoxin to the hospital where case-patients are located. Emergency contacts are listed in Box 1. Because supplies of antitoxin are limited and rapid delivery to patients is critical, antitoxin is maintained at a network of quarantine stations at major international airports in the United States. Botulinum antitoxin may only be obtained through the state health departments and CDC. CDC maintains a stock of bivalent anti-A and -B antitoxin and trivalent anti-A, -B, and -E antitoxin for cases involving foods suspected of containing type E toxin, such as fish. The US Army maintains a stock of investigational hexavalent (A–G) antitoxin [56]. In the event of a bioterrorist attack with multiple toxin types, procurement of polyvalent antitoxin requires coordination through the military.

Summary

Botulinum toxin is an extremely potent poison that has the potential to be used as a bioweapon. The clinical syndrome of botulism with cranial nerve dysfunction and descending paralysis likely occurs regardless of the route of toxin delivery. Botulism occurring with unusual temporal or geographic associations, large numbers of affected people, or atypical presentations should alert health care providers to consider bioterrorism. A high index of suspicion followed by clinical diagnosis and newer diagnostic tests can help identify botulism rapidly to allow prompt identification of a source, limit exposures, treat exposed or affected individuals, and control outbreaks. All cases of botulism are emergencies that require immediate notification of public health officials.

References

[1] Hatheway CL. Toxigenic clostridia. Clin Microbiol Rev 1990;3:66–98.
[2] Hatheway C. Clostridium: the spore bearing anaerobes. In: Collier L, Balows A, Sussman M, editors. Topley and Wilson's microbiology and microbial infections. New York: Oxford University Press; 1998. p. 731–82.
[3] CDC. Botulism in the United States, 1899–1996. In: CDC Handbook for epidemiologists, clinicians, and laboratory workers. Atlanta: CDC; 1996. Available at: http://www.cdc.gov/ncidod/dbmd/diseaseinfo/files/botulism_manual.htm#XV.
[4] Hatheway C. Clostridium botulinum. In: Bartlett JG, Blacklow NR, editors. Infectious diseases. Orlando: WB Saunders; 1991. p. 1583–6.
[5] Schiavo G, Matteoli M, Montecucco C. Neurotoxins affecting neuroexocytosis. Physiol Rev 2000;80:717–66.
[6] Barr JR. Botulinum neurotoxin detection and differentiation by mass spectrometry. Emerg Infect Dis 2005;11:1578–83.
[7] Caya JG, Agni R, Miller JE. *Clostridium botulinum* and the clinical laboratorian: a detailed review of botulism, including biological warfare ramifications of botulinum toxin. Arch Pathol Lab Med 2004;128:653–62.
[8] Arnon SS, Schechter R, Inglesby TV, et al. Botulinum toxin as a biological weapon: medical and public health management. JAMA 2001;285:1059–70.
[9] Montecucco C. Clostridial neurotoxins: the molecular pathogenesis of tetanus and botulism. Curr Top Microbiol Immunol 1995;195:221–42.
[10] Goonetilleke A, Harris JB. Clostridial neurotoxins. J Neurol Neurosurg Psychiatry 2004; 75(Suppl 3):35–9.
[11] Hughes JM, Blumenthal JR, Merson MH. Clinical features of type A and B foodborne botulism. Ann Intern Med 1981;95:442–5.
[12] Scott AB, Suzuki D. Systemic toxicity of botulinum toxin by intramuscular injection in the monkey. Mov Disord 1988;3:333–5.
[13] Herrero BA, Ecklung AE, Streett CS. Experimental botulism in monkeys: a clinical pathological study. Exp Mol Pathol 1967;6:84–95.
[14] Kinnett D. Botulinum toxin A injections in children: technique and dosing issues. Am J Phys Med Rehabil 2004;83:S59–64.
[15] Tugnoli V, Eleopra R, Quatrale R, et al. Botulism-like syndrome after botulinum toxin type A injections for focal hyperhidrosis. Br J Dermatol 2002;147:808–9.
[16] Beseler-Soto B, Sanchez-Palomares M, Santos-Serrano L, et al. Iatrogenic botulism: a complication to be taken into account in the treatment of child spasticity. Rev Neurol 2003;37: 444–6.
[17] Hatheway CL. Botulism: the present status of the disease. Curr Top Microbiol Immunol 1995;195:55–75.
[18] Villar RG, Shapiro RL, Busto S, et al. Outbreak of type A botulism and development of a botulism surveillance and antitoxin release system in Argentina. JAMA 1999;281:1334–8, 1340.
[19] Shapiro RL, Hatheway C, Swerdlow DL. Botulism in the United States: a clinical and epidemiologic review. Ann Intern Med 1998;129:221–8.
[20] Passaro DJ, Werner SB, McGee J. Wound botulism associated with black tar heroin among injecting drug users. JAMA 1998;279:859–63.

[21] Chia JK, Clark JB, Ryan CA, et al. Botulism in an adult associated with food-borne intestinal infection with *Clostridium botulinum*. N Engl J Med 1986;315:239–41.
[22] Arnon SS. Botulism as an intestinal toxemia. In: Blaser MJ, Smith PD, Ravdin JI, et al, editors. Infections of the gastrointestinal tract. New York: Raven Press; 1995. p. 257–71.
[23] Holzer E. Botulism caused by inhalation. Med Klin 1962;57:1735–8.
[24] Franz DR, Pitt LM, Clyton MA, et al. Efficacy of prophylactic and therapeutic administration of antitoxin for inhalational botulism. In: DasGupta BR, editor. Botulinum and tetanus neurotoxins: neurotransmission and biomedical aspects. New York: Plenum Press; 1993. p. 473–6.
[25] Taysse L, Daulon S, Calvet J, et al. Induction of acute lung injury after intranasal administration of toxin botulinum a complex. Toxicol Pathol 2005;33:336–42.
[26] Montecucco C, Molgo J. Botulinal neurotoxins: revival of an old killer. Curr Opin Pharmacol 2005;5:274–9.
[27] Bakheit AM, Ward CD, McLellan DL. Generalised botulism-like syndrome after intramuscular injections of botulinum toxin type A: a report of two cases. J Neurol Neurosurg Psychiatry 1997;62:198.
[28] Cobb DB, Watson WA, Fernandez MC. Botulism-like syndrome after injections of botulinum toxin. Vet Hum Toxicol 2000;42:163.
[29] CDC. Recognition of illness associated with the intentional release of a biologic agent. MMWR Surveill Summ 2001;50:893–7.
[30] Zilinskas RA. Iraq's biological weapons: the past as future. JAMA 1997;278:418–24.
[31] Clarke S. Bacteria as potential tools in bioterrorism, with an emphasis on bacterial toxins. Br J Biomed Sci 2005;62:40–6.
[32] Arnon SS, Schechter R, Inglesby TV, et al. Botulinum toxin as a biological weapon: medical and public health management. JAMA 2001;285:1059–70.
[33] Kortepeter M, Christopher G, Cieslak T, et al, editors. Medical management of biological casualties handbook. Frederick (MD): USAMRIID; 2001.
[34] Dorsey EL, Beebe JM, Johns EE. Responses of Air-borne *Clostridium botulinum* toxin to certain atmospheric stresses. Technical Memorandum 62. Frederick (MD): US Army Biological Laboratories; 1964.
[35] Torok TH, Tauxe RV, Wise RP. A large community outbreak of salmonellosis caused by intentional contamination of restaurant salad bars. JAMA 1997;278:389–95.
[36] Kazdobina IS. Stability of botulinum toxins in solutions and beverages. Gig Sanit 1995;1:9–12.
[37] Khan AS, Swerdlow DL, Juranek DD. Precautions against biological and chemical terrorism directed at food and water supplies. Public Health Rep 2001;116:3–14.
[38] Horman A, Nevas M, Lindstrom M, et al. Elimination of botulinum neurotoxin (BoNT) type B from drinking water by small-scale (personal-use) water purification devices and detection of BoNT in water samples. Appl Environ Microbiol 2005;71:1941–5.
[39] Akbulut D, Grant KA, McLauchlin J. Improvement in laboratory diagnosis of wound botulism and tetanus among injecting illicit-drug users by use of real-time PCR assays for neurotoxin gene fragments. J Clin Microbiol 2005;43:4342–8.
[40] Lindstrom M, Keto R, Markkula A, et al. Multiplex PCR assay for detection and identification of *Clostridium botulinum* types A, B, E, and F in food and fecal material. Appl Environ Microbiol 2001;67:5694–9.
[41] Akbulut D, Grant KA, McLauchlin J. Development and application of real-time PCR assays to detect fragments of the *Clostridium botulinum* types A, B, and E neurotoxin genes for investigation of human foodborne and infant botulism. Foodborne Pathog Dis 2004;1:247–57.
[42] Goldfrank LR. Botulinum antitoxin. In: Goldfrank's toxicologic emergencies. New York: McGraw-Hill; 2002. p. 1112–4.
[43] Arnon SS. Infant botulism. In: Feigin RD, Cherry JD, editors. Textbook of pediatric infectious diseases. Philadelphia: WB Saunders; 1998. p. 1570–7.

[44] Bramwell VW, Eyles JE, Oya Alpar H. Particulate delivery systems for biodefense subunit vaccines. Adv Drug Deliv Rev 2005;57:1247–65.
[45] Fiock MA, Cardella NF. Studies on immunity to toxins of *Clostridium botulinum*. IX. Immunologic response of man to purified pentavalent ABCDE botulinum toxoid. J Immunol 1963;90:697–702.
[46] Ellis RJ. Immunobiologic agents and drugs available from the Centers for Disease Control: Descriptions, recommendations, adverse reactions, and serologic response. Atlanta: Centers for Disease Control, Public Health Service, US Department of Health and Human Services; 1982.
[47] Siegel LS. Evaluation of neutralizing antibodies to type A, B, E, and F toxins in sera from human recipients of botulinum pentavalent (ABCDE) toxoid. J Clin Microbiol 1989;27: 1906–8.
[48] Whalen RL, Dempsey DJ, Thompson LM, et al. Microencapsulated vaccines to provide prolonged immunity with a single administration. ASAIO J 1996;42:M649–54.
[49] Holley JL, Williamson JE, Eyles JE. Use of poly-L-lactide microspheres for the delivery of a *Clostridium botulinum* type F subunit vaccine. In: Proceedings of the 10th European Workshop Conference on Bacterial Protein Toxins, Bohon, Belgium, June 24–9, 2001.
[50] Jathoul AP, Holley JL, Garmory HS. Efficacy of DNA vaccines expressing the type F botulinum toxin Hc fragment using different promoters. Vaccine 2004;22:3942–6.
[51] Park JB, Simpson LL. Progress toward development of an inhalation vaccine against botulinum toxin. Expert Rev Vaccines 2004;3:477–87.
[52] Mowry MC, Meagher M, Smith L, et al. Production and purification of a chimeric monoclonal antibody against botulinum neurotoxin serotype A. Protein Expr Purif 2004;37: 399–408.
[53] Anne C, Turcaud S, Blommaert AG, et al. Partial protection against botulinum B neurotoxin-induced blocking of exocytosis by a potent inhibitor of its metallopeptidase activity. Chembiochem 2005;6:1375–80.
[54] Anne C, Turcaud S, Quancard J, et al. Development of potent inhibitors of botulinum neurotoxin type B. J Med Chem 2003;46:4648–56.
[55] Sobel J, Tucker N, Sulka A, et al. Foodborne botulism in the United States, 1990–2000. Emerg Infect Dis 2004;10:1606–11.
[56] Hibbs RG, Weber JT, Corwin A, et al. Experience with the use of an investigational F(ab')2 heptavalent botulism immune globulin of equine origin during an outbreak of type E botulism in Egypt. Clin Infect Dis 1996;23:337–40.

ELSEVIER
SAUNDERS

Infect Dis Clin N Am
20 (2006) 329–357

INFECTIOUS
DISEASE CLINICS
OF NORTH AMERICA

Smallpox as a Bioterrorist Weapon: Myth or Menace?

Dennis J. Cleri, MD[a,b,*], Richard B. Porwancher, MD[c,d], Anthony J. Ricketti, MD[a,b], Luz S. Ramos-Bonner, MD[b], John R. Vernaleo, MD[e]

[a]*Department of Medicine, Seton Hall University School of Graduate Medical Education, South Orange, NJ 07079, USA*
[b]*Department of Medicine, St. Francis Medical Center, 601 Hamilton Avenue, Trenton, NJ 08629, USA*
[c]*Department of Medicine, UMDNJ–Robert Wood Johnson Medical School, Piscataway, NJ 08854, USA*
[d]*Division of Infectious Diseases, St. Francis Medical Center, 601 Hamilton Avenue, Trenton, NJ 08629, USA*
[e]*Division of Infectious Diseases, Wycoff Heights Medical Center, 374 Stockholm Street, Brooklyn, NY 11237, USA*

> "The story of the human race is war. Except for brief and precarious interludes, there has never been peace in the world."—Winston Churchill, *The World Crisis and My Early Life*.

Smallpox (*Poxvirus variolae*) is a member of the Poxviridae family, genus *Orthopoxvirus*. Poxviridae are linear double-stranded DNA viruses consisting of two subfamilies, Chordopoxvirinae (infecting vertebrates) and Entomopoxvirinae (infecting insects) [1–12]; they replicate in cytoplasm, have no RNA phase, and most commonly use a virus-encoded, DNA-dependent RNA polymerase transcriptase and DNA polymerase replicase [2,4–9,11]. Historically, smallpox has been the most important poxvirus infection, first documented in early hieroglyphics dating from 3700 BC and believed to be the cause of death of Ramses V in 1157 BC [1,6].

Chordopoxvirinae consist of *Orthopoxvirus, Parapoxvirus, Avipoxvirus, Leporipoxvirus, Molluscipoxvirus, Suipoxvirus, Capripoxvirus,* and *Yatapoxvirus*. The first disease description attributed to *Parapoxvirus* (the genus that includes pseudocowpox and orf viruses), scabby mouth disease in sheep, was published

* Corresponding author. Department of Medicine, St. Francis Medical Center, 601 Hamilton Avenue, Trenton, NJ 08629, USA.
E-mail address: dcleri@che-east.org (D.J. Cleri).

doi:10.1016/j.idc.2006.03.005

in 1787 [7]. Diseases attributed to at least one member each of *Avipoxvirus, Leporipoxvirus, Molluscipoxvirus,* and *Suipoxvirus* genera were first published in the nineteenth century, whereas diseases caused by *Capripoxvirus* and *Yatapoxvirus* genera were published in the twentieth century [2–12].

Besides variola, members of the *Orthopoxvirus* genus include vaccinia virus, monkeypox virus, and cowpox virus, all of which readily infect humans and have animal hosts [6]. In contrast to the other poxviruses, there is no animal reservoir for variola virus [13]. The remaining members of this genus (camelpox virus, ectromelia virus, raccoonpox virus, taterapox virus, volepox virus, skunkpox virus, and Uasin Gishu disease virus—causing papular skin lesions in horses) infect animals, but uncommonly infect humans [6]. Other poxviruses that infect humans are orf virus, bovine papular stomatitis virus and pseudocowpox virus (genus *Parapoxvirus*), tanapox and yabapox, and molluscum contagiosum virus [14–16].

Variola may exist as intracellular mature virions, which are released by cell lysis and enter new host cells by fusion with vesicles created by surface invaginations. Extracellular enveloped virions possess a lipoprotein envelope absent in the intracellular mature virion. Extracellular enveloped virions facilitate cell-to-cell spread through endocytosis [15,16].

Because of its large size, vaccinia virus is not amenable to high-resolution electron microscopy image reconstruction. Using atomic force microscopy, the complex structural relationship between the viral genome and intact virion and the importance of the intracellular mature virion undergoing cell entry have been elucidated [17]; this structure, in addition to immunologic studies, indicates that immunity against the intracellular mature virion is far more important than the extracellular enveloped virion [18,19].

History of smallpox

Variola virus is believed to have evolved at least 10,000 years ago from African rodent poxviruses. Because of the absence of an animal reservoir, the first agricultural communities in the Nile and Mesopotamia river basins needed to reach a population of 200,000 (about 3000 BC) before they could sustain smallpox endemicity [1,13,20]. From Africa, the disease spread and became endemic in India. Sanskrit medical texts describe a disease consistent with smallpox in India in 1500 BC Alexander the Great's army probably became infected with smallpox in the lower Indus valley [1]. During this early period, the *Artharva Veda* describe Brahmin priests traveling throughout the land praying to the smallpox Hindu goddess, Shitala mata (wife of Shiva the Destroyer) to spare the population. The disease impacted so many populations of the ancient world that it was common for each to worship their own smallpox goddess; she was variously known as Mariyammai, Shital Devi, Devi mata, Thakurani, Patragale, Mariatale, Rugboi, and Jyeshtha [21].

From 430 BC to 29 BC, smallpox spread from Egypt to Libya and Ethiopia and from Greece to Persia. "Hunpox" was introduced into China about

250 BC, although the disease may have been present in China in 1700 BC [22,23]. The Roman legions returning from Mesopotamia (165–80 BC) brought smallpox to Rome. The plague of Antoninus (AD 166–180), now believed to be smallpox, killed almost one third of the population on the Italian peninsula [22]. The disease spread through Europe and became endemic on the Iberian Peninsula and Mauritania in 710 AD. Written descriptions of smallpox appeared in China in the fourth century AD and in southwest Asia in the tenth century AD [13]. Bishop Marius of Avenches first used the term *variola* from the Latin words for "spotted" (*varius*) and "pimple" (*varus*) [13].

Some of the most famous smallpox survivors were Queen Elizabeth I, George Washington, Andrew Jackson (whose brother died of the disease), and Abraham Lincoln who became ill shortly after the Gettysburg Address [24,25]. The powerful and famous who succumbed to smallpox included Roman emperor Marcus Aurelius, Prince William II of Orange (Denmark), Louis XV of France (1774), Queen Mary II of England, the Duke of Gloucester (last heir to the throne of England in the Stuart lineage), Tsar Peter II, Panchen Lama of Tibet, and Omaha Chief Blackbird (along with two thirds of his tribe). The most famous physician who contracted and died of smallpox was Thomas Sydenham in 1869 [25]. Smallpox even had its own patron saint—St. Nicasius of Rheims, who survived the disease, but was beheaded on his church steps in 452 AD [1,25–27].

A historical review of smallpox epidemics documents the loss of tens of millions of lives [1]. Smallpox was introduced to the New World by Spanish conquistadors, killing one third of the native population [22]. Three million died in India in 1769 [25]. At about the same time in Europe, smallpox caused one third of all blindness and 400,000 deaths per year, most being children and young adults [23].

This formidable illness often altered the course of human history. It was believed to have played a significant role in the defeat of Athens in the Peloponnesian War (430 BC, also ascribed to measles, typhus, and plague) and the Abyssininan (Ethiopian) army defeat at Mecca during the "Elephant War" (569–570 AD), indirectly described in the Koran. An epidemic in Greenland (1430) killed the entire Norman colony. Smallpox stopped the English-Iroquois assault on Montreal (1649), contributed to the American defeat at Quebec (1776), and prevented the Spanish-French fleet from invading England (1779) [22,25,27]. From 1775 through 1782, smallpox ravaged Central and North America from Mexico, north through the Canadian North-West Territories, Quebec, and Hudson Bay [28]. The use of smallpox as a bioterrorist weapon is discussed later.

A success story: the medical conquest of smallpox

Early attempts at treatment of smallpox included purgatives, bleeding, palm oil, herbal liniments (West Africa), wrapping patients in red cloth, opening pustules with gold or silver needles, and administration of antimony and mercury compounds. Red objects of all sorts were believed to have therapeutic efficacy—red candies, red pictures hanging in the sickroom, and swabbing the first pustule with fuchsin or other red pigments. In 1901, Finsen "successfully" used red light to treat 150 smallpox victims with only one failure [23,29].

The practice of cutaneous inoculation of material from scabs or pus from smallpox patients probably began in India about 1000 BC, based on translations of the *Atharva Veda*. By 1000 AD, insufflation (inhaling powder made from dried smallpox scabs) was widely practiced; it was first described in China in 1643 by Yu T'ien-Chih. By the late seventeenth century, Chinese inoculation methods also included (1) plugging the nose with smallpox scabs in cotton or the contents of a vesicle in cotton; (2) blowing powdered scabs into the nose, similar to insufflation; and (3) dressing a healthy child for days in the undergarments of an infected child [1,30]. Even before the Chinese practice of "insufflating" material from smallpox victims became known in England, rural peasants in Poland, Scotland, Denmark, and Greece practiced cutaneous inoculation of smallpox-infected material, also known as "buying the smallpox" [26].

In 1717, Lady Mary Wortley Montague, wife of the British Ambassador to the Ottoman Empire and herself scarred by smallpox at a young age, observed the practice of cutaneous inoculation of smallpox-infected material in Constantinople and had her own son inoculated in 1718. She brought the method (called *variolation*) back to England in 1721. Because the medical establishment was skeptical of the procedure, Lady Montague convinced the Prince of Wales to have the method publicly tested on six prisoners awaiting hanging. All survived and were pardoned [26].

Smallpox vaccine is the oldest vaccine known to humans. When variolation was first introduced in London in 1721, smallpox had a mortality of 1 in 6; within a few years, mortality was reduced to 1 in 50 (James Jurin, 1722, and Zabdiel Boylston, 1726). By 1765, refinements in the variolation technique had reduced mortality to 1 in 500 [31]. Cutaneous inoculation, rather than respiratory, seems to have attenuated the clinical course. Research on viral pathogenesis suggests a possible role for cutaneous T cell defenses in altering the subsequent illness [23,26,32].

Before Jenner's publication of *Variolae Vaccinae* in 1798, Fewster presented his paper, "Cowpox and Its Ability to Prevent Smallpox" at the London Medical Society in 1765. Bose (Gottingen, Germany, 1769), Plett (Holstein, 1791), and Jensen (Holstein, 1791) all had claimed to inoculate individuals with cowpox (also known as *Poxvirus bovis*) [26]. In 1774, simultaneous outbreaks of smallpox in Yetminster (Dorset) and cowpox on the Elford farm in Chetnole prompted the farmer, Benjamin Jetsey, to inoculate his pregnant wife and three children, ages 1 to 3, with cowpox. Although his wife developed fever and severe swelling of her arm, she fully recovered and delivered a normal healthy infant. Fifteen years later Jetsey inoculated his sons with smallpox-infected material to prove they were immune. In 1797, he moved to Worth Matravers on the Isle of Purbeck, where he performed vaccination on many of the villagers. Although Jetsey's contribution was acknowledged later by Jenner, Jetsey himself admitted that he was not the first person to employ cowpox vaccination in his vicinity [1,26,32].

Although Jenner was the first to associate angina pectoris with coronary artery disease, this achievement has been all but forgotten because he proved that inoculation with cowpox conferred immunity to smallpox, and that cowpox could be inoculated from person to person [1,26,30]. The latter property allowed the de Balmis expedition (1803–1806) to transport the vaccine by sea to Spanish colonies in the New World and Asia through arm-to-arm vaccination of orphaned children onboard their vessels [13,33]. Jenner's first attempt at cowpox inoculation involved the 8-year-old son of one of his employees, James Phipps. Using material from a milkmaid with cowpox, Jenner was able to induce protection against smallpox. One month later, he inoculated Phipps with pus from a case of smallpox (May–July 1796) to show he was immune. In 1798, Jenner repeated the experiment on more children, including his own son. Cowpox was a relatively rare disease, so he was forced to use material from equine "grease" disease, which is now believed to be extinct. Jenner's work initially was treated with skepticism by the British medical establishment, and in 1798 he decided to publish a medical monograph on his own. As the value of Jenner's methods gained recognition in Europe and America, so too did Jenner's place in history. He was moved to build a home for his famous patient, James Phipps, which later became the Edward Jenner Museum [1,26].

Cowpox virus comes from a rodent reservoir and infects cattle, cats, foxes, and other mammals. It is believed that cats act as an intermediary host for human infection. The rodent virus, cowpox, still is found in Europe and Asia, but has not been seen in exported cattle. Some of Jenner's strains of "cowpox" probably were contaminated with smallpox virus. High rates of reassortment are known to occur within poxvirus-infected cells, as shown by Shope fibroma virus (the cause of benign fibromas in rabbits) and myxoma virus leading to malignant rabbit fibroma virus. Reassortment also occurs between capripoxviruses (the cause of sheep pox, goatpox, and lumpy skin disease in cattle). The DNA sequencing of vaccinia, variola, monkeypox, and cowpox viruses indicates that cowpox and vaccinia are the most closely related [1,16,34]. It is unclear whether Jenner's vaccine consisted solely of cowpox or a strain with genes from smallpox and cowpox.

In 1799, Waterhouse of Harvard Medical School obtained a copy of Jenner's self-published monograph and a sample of cowpox and in 1800 inoculated his own family. In 1803, Dunning coined the term *vaccination* (*vacca* is Latin for "cow"), and Pasteur adopted the term to refer to all immunizations [1]. In 1801, Thomas Jefferson began vaccinating Native Americans. The start of government-sponsored vaccination programs in America marked the beginning of the worldwide decline in smallpox incidence. In 1939, Great Britain became free of smallpox.

"Success in war depends upon the golden rule of war. speed—simplicity—boldness"—Lieutenant General George S. Patton, Jr, inscribed in his field notebook [35].

In 1947, 12 cases of smallpox were reported in New York City leading to a massive vaccination program; prompted in part by the New York City outbreak, the World Health Organization (WHO) decided to attempt eradication of the disease worldwide. Beginning in 1966, Henderson from the WHO led the "Target Zero" campaign (1966–1977). Thousands of field workers tracked down every case of smallpox around the world and instituted the "ring vaccination" strategy to isolate the infected individuals with a "wall" of immune individuals [15,20]. The last case of endemic variola major was reported in Bangladesh in 1975, and the last case of endemic variola minor was seen in Somalia in 1977. A laboratory accident in Birmingham, England, resulted in a single case of smallpox and a suicide in 1979 [1,15,20].

Routine civilian vaccination ceased in the United States in 1971 and was suspended by the US military in 1990. The WHO declared the world free of smallpox in 1979–1980, and in 1983, the vaccine manufacturer, Wyeth, discontinued distribution. What was once the most feared viral disease on the planet became the first epidemic human disease to be eradicated [1,20].

Epidemiology and physical properties

Humans are the only natural reservoir and source of smallpox virus. There is no subclinical persistent state, no reactivation of infection (as with herpesvirus and varicella virus), no animal reservoir, and no "natural" environmental source, although the virus may persist in dust for 2 years. An aerosol release of the virus would result in inactivation within 48 hours. The virus is resistant to heat, drying, cold, and common disinfectants. Variola stops multiplying at 41°C and must be heated to 55°C for at least 30 minutes before it is inactivated. Variola and vaccinia remain infectious after lyophilization and exposure to temperatures of −180°C [1,36–42].

Natural infection is acquired by inhalation of airborne droplets from an infected patient's oral, nasal, or pharyngeal mucosa. Inhalation of just a few virions is sufficient to produce infection [36–42]. Direct exposure to infected materials, contaminated clothing, and blankets also can result in infection. Respiratory spread of infection over long distances (eg, from one hospital floor to another), although infrequent, has been reported [1,43].

Using the US blood supply as a vector to spread smallpox has been considered a potential bioterrorist threat. In vitro studies have shown that vaccinia virus may be removed from plasma products by filtration. Because of the relatively large size of the pathogenic poxviruses, filtration of plasma likely would be able to prevent the spread of incubating monkeypox and smallpox from donated blood and blood products [1,37]. Real-time polymerase chain reaction followed by melting analysis has been developed to differentiate variola virus from other orthopoxviruses in donated blood and blood products [44].

Pathophysiology

The virus enters the respiratory tree and infects macrophages during the first 72 hours of the asymptomatic incubation phase. Macrophages use the Wiskott-Aldrich syndrome protein to induce an actin tail, giving vaccinia and variola virus a selective dissemination advantage [1,16,45]. The virus is transported to local lymph nodes, where they multiply over the next 96 hours and become blood-borne [1,16]. A second viremia occurs after replication in the spleen, bone marrow, and lymph tissue. At this stage, the patient is toxic. Leukocytes with viable virus localize in dermal and mucosal vessels. Oral, pharyngeal, and sometimes gastrointestinal lesions ulcerate, and a maculopapular rash becomes vesiculopustular in normal hosts [1,14–16,36,39–42]. Flat lesions without pustules may develop in immunocompromised patients, however, and is often, but not invariably, fatal. Hemorrhagic disease with petechial skin lesions, bleeding from mucosal surfaces, severe toxemia, and early death are seen in some (probably immunocompromised) adults and pregnant women [1,36,37,39–42].

Cytopathology is suggestive, but not diagnostic, of smallpox. B-type inclusion bodies (Guarnieri bodies) are seen where there is viral replication of all the poxviruses. These may be seen with the light microscope with hematoxylin and eosin stain (light basophilic granular bodies). They are best visualized in the epithelial cells at the base of the vesicles or pustules with May-Grunwald Giemsa stain (appearing magenta red).

A-type inclusion bodies are produced by some, but not all, *Orthopoxvirus* species (cowpox; ectromelia virus; and raccoon, vole, and skunk poxviruses) and some *Avipoxvirus* species. A-type inclusion bodies have different designations: Downie bodies with cowpox infection, Marchal bodies with ectromelia virus infection, and Borrel bodies in fowlpox (*Avipoxvirus* genus) infections.

Electron microscopy can visualize negatively staining poxvirus that are compatible with variola, vaccinia, molluscum contagiousum, and monkeypox, but cannot differentiate among them. Negative electron microscopy staining identifies herpesviruses (varicella and herpes simplex 1 and 2) [1,14–16].

Clinical presentation

Incubation period

The average incubation period is 10 to 12 days (range 6–22 days) [1,36,37,40,41,45,46]. Shorter incubation periods may be seen with intrauterine infections and entry portals other than the respiratory tract. Antiviral chemotherapy, vaccinia immunoglobulin, and any form of partial immunity may lengthen the incubation period [1,36,37].

Contagious period

Patients generally are not contagious during the incubation period [1,36,37,40,41,46,47]. Patients may become contagious, however, 1 to 2 days before the onset of symptoms or coincident with the oral enanthema (often 24 hours before the onset of the rash). Viral shedding is greatest from the onset of the enanthema through the first 10 days of the rash. Patients are contagious until all scabs and crusts are shed. Close contacts have attack rates of 37% to 88% [1,37–42,46,47].

Prodrome

The prodrome commonly lasts 48 to 72 hours, although it may be prolonged 5 days; it begins with the sudden onset of fever and chills, often accompanied by lumbar pain, headache, and malaise and less frequently nausea, vomiting, abdominal pain, and delirium. Children may experience seizures. Diarrhea occurs when the mucous membranes of the gastrointestinal tract are involved [1,37]. There may be a transient erythematous or petechial rash lasting only 12 hours that can be mistaken for measles [36,37,40]. Table 1 presents additional signs and symptoms. The WHO divides the subsequent clinical course into four categories, based on the appearance of the rash: (1) ordinary, (2) modified, (3) flat, and (4) hemorrhagic [1,36,40].

Typical (ordinary) smallpox—variola major

A centrifugal rash appears 2 to 3 days after the onset of the toxemic symptoms and quickly following the enanthema—at first maculopapular on the face, hands, and forearms. The early lesions are shotty and cannot be obliterated by pressure. During the next 24 to 48 hours, the rash becomes vesicular and then pustular. The lesions themselves are round, firm, and in the same general stage of evolution in any given area. There is an increased density of lesions over bony prominences and areas of trauma and pressure. The palms, soles, trunk, and upper thighs are involved next. If the patient survives, by day 8 or 9, the rash crusts, and scabs fall off as the patient recovers. Many of the crusted lesions leave a depressed depigmented scar.

The overall mortality for variola major is 30% (range 15–50%) in an unvaccinated population and 3% mortality in a vaccinated population. Watson noted more than 200 years ago that the density of the lesions was directly related to survival [31]. Patients characterized as having "discrete smallpox" (lesions on the face well separated) have 15% mortality. Patients with "confluent smallpox" (merging lesions) have 50% mortality [1,36,37,40,41,47,48].

Table 1
Clinical presentations of smallpox (variola major)

Clinical designation	Symptoms	Rash	Immune status	Mortality (%)
Ordinary	Fever, rigors, backache, malaise, prostration, headache, delirium (15%), occasional abdominal pain	Discrete, confluent	Nonimmune for all	15, 30
				50
		(Overall)		(20–50)
Modified (vaccine-modified)	Less severe symptoms	Discrete	Previously immunized—partially immune	Rare
Flat (malignant)	Symptoms more severe, persistent fever, abdominal pain more frequent; death occurs between the 7th and 15th day from encephalitis or hemorrhage	Dusky erythema evolves into pleomorphic or petechial rash; papules are not well formed; lesions may be discrete or confluent	Discrete-immunized	45.4
			Discrete-unimmunized	85
			Confluent-immunized	79.1
			Confluent-unimmunized	99.3
			Overall	
			Immunized	64.5
			Unimmunized	97
Hemorrhagic (fulminate)	Prodrome is prolonged and severe; patients are febrile, restless, and toxic; fevers are persistently high	Dusky rash appears on chest followed by diffuse petechiae and bleeding from mucous membranes; rare patients who survive >10 days develop confluent hemorrhagic vesiculation	Immunized	98.3
			Unimmunized	96.2
Variola sine eruptione (variola sine exanthemata)	Pharyngeal form	Spotty enanthema over soft palate, uvula, and pharynx	Immunized	0
	Influenza-like form	Rash rare	Immunized but low degree of immunity	0
	Pulmonary disease	Severe symptoms, cyanosis, bilateral infiltrates	Low or no immunity	Not available

From Cleri DJ, Villota FJ, Porwancher RB. Smallpox, bioterrorism, and the neurologist. Arch Neurol 2003;60:490; with permission.

Modified smallpox—vaccino-modified (variola minor, alastrim, amaas)

Modified smallpox is seen in partially immune patients or patients infected with the less virulent, variola minor strains of the virus. The disease is clinically less severe, and deaths are rare. The patient has the common prodrome, although it may be so mild as to go unnoticed. The disease often is confused with influenza until the rash develops. When smallpox was endemic, modified smallpox and chickenpox often were confused. Modified smallpox and variola minor also have been confused with variola major, scabies, acne, and syphilis [1,36,40].

The rash of modified smallpox follows a typical pattern beginning 3 to 5 days after the prodrome, but may occur later than normal. In contrast to chickenpox, the rash does not appear in crops. There is an abbreviated clinical course: papular stage, 2 days; vesicular stage, 1 day; pustular stage, 3 to 4 days; and crusting beginning on day 6 or 7. Complications are rare, but include boils, blepharitis, conjunctivitis, and keratitis with ulceration [1].

Flat "malignant" smallpox

Ten percent to 20% of variola major patients present with flat "malignant" smallpox, the lethal form of disease. Patients are most commonly unvaccinated children. After a severe prodrome, poorly formed papules and a dusky erythema develop over the face, followed by the arms, back, and upper torso. As the patient's clinical condition worsens, the rash becomes pleomorphic or petechial. Patients who develop discrete vesicles are more likely to survive. Patients who die often have what looks like "vesiculating sunburn." Death usually occurs between day 7 and 15 from encephalitis or hemorrhage. Autopsies reveal extensive organ necrosis. Mortality is particularly high among unvaccinated patients [1,36,37,40].

Hemorrhagic "fulminate" smallpox

The hemorrhagic form of smallpox occurs in adults and pregnant women, few of whom survive. The prodrome is prolonged and severe. Patients are toxic, are restless, and have high fevers throughout the disease. An early-onset dusky rash appears on the face and chest. The disease mimics viral hemorrhagic fevers with diffuse petechiae and bleeding from the mucous membranes. Patients die by day 7 without a maculopapular rash. Rare patients who survive to day 10 develop a maculopapular rash or confluent hemorrhagic vesiculation. The mortality is greater than 95% regardless of vaccination status [1,36].

Variola sine eruptione—variola sine exanthemata

Three forms of smallpox present without a rash: pharyngeal, influenza-like, and pulmonary. In the pharyngeal form, patients usually are previously immunized and develop an uneven spotty enanthema over the soft palate and uvula. Although the influenza-like form occurs in previously immunized patients, they generally have a suboptimal response to the vaccine. A few patients with the flulike variety develop a mild rash without sequelae. Variola sine eruptione becomes life-threatening in the pulmonary form. Symptoms are severe, and patients are often cyanotic. Chest x-rays reveal bilateral lower lobe infiltrates with bilateral hilar adenopathy [1,36,37,40,46].

Centers for Disease Control and Prevention assistance with diagnosis

Information for health care providers is available through the main CDC website (http://www.cdc.gov). Smallpox images may be viewed directly at http://www.bt.cdc.gov/agent/smallpox/smallpoximages.asp. An online diagnostic algorithm is available at http://www.bt.cdc.gov/agent/smallpox/diagnosis/riskalgorithm/. A clinical evaluation tool for adverse reactions to smallpox vaccine may be accessed at http://www.bt.cdc.gov/agent/smallpox/vaccination/clineval.

All suspected smallpox cases should be reported to individual state health departments. All state health departments have the capacity to perform rapid varicella diagnostics by direct fluorescent antibody or polymerase chain reaction to assist differentiating chickenpox from smallpox (communication via Internet [bqs1@cdc.gov] from BH Stover, Clinician Communication Team, CDC, April 6, 2005). Local and state health departments arrange for specimen transportation to the CDC if further testing is needed. Instructions for specimen collection are found at http://www.bt.cdc.gov/agent/smallpox/response-plan/files/guide-d.pdf. Only previously vaccinated individuals using personal protection equipment should collect and handle specimens.

Smallpox complications

Encephalopathy

Most patients have some degree of encephalopathy. Most complain of "splitting" headaches and spinal pain. Neuropsychologic manifestations include hallucinations, delirium, depressive psychosis, "melancholia," and manic depression. These may persist into convalescence. Perivenular demyelination has been observed in patients dying from smallpox [1,15,34,36,37,40,46,47,49].

Ocular complications—variola residua

In modern times, 10% to 20% of smallpox patients developed ophthalmologic complications. The most common was conjunctivitis, which usually developed 5 days after the onset of the rash, but cleared without complication. Occasional patients developed painful pustules on the bulbar conjunctiva. When smallpox was epidemic, corneal ulceration was common, often leading to secondary bacterial infection and perforation. Luckier patients healed with corneal scars. Because complications were often bilateral, blindness resulted from enucleation or adherent leukoma (perforation blocked by the iris) [1,36,50]. One third of all blindness was due to smallpox.

Smallpox osteomyelitis—osteomyelitis variolosa

Osteomyelitis variolosa and viral arthritis affected 2% to 5% of children with symptomatic disease. This was not the result of secondary bacterial invasion. Viral particles may be found in bone lesions. X-ray surveys of children during epidemics showed bony involvement in about 20% [1,36,48].

Smallpox in pregnancy and neonates

Pregnant women have a propensity to develop hemorrhagic smallpox. An Indian study of 225 unvaccinated pregnant women found 75% mortality compared with 24% to 25% mortality for unvaccinated nonpregnant women [51]. An African outbreak in 1946 led to 46% mortality in unvaccinated pregnant women. Vaccinated pregnant women still had 20.7% mortality for smallpox compared with 3% to 4% for vaccinated nonpregnant women and men.

Fetal death and premature delivery are common, even in mild maternal cases of smallpox. One study involving 46 patients showed 81% mortality (fetal death or neonatal death after premature delivery) [51]. Intrauterine infection includes infants who develop symptomatic disease at 2 to 3 weeks of age. Autopsy studies of fatal cases show disseminated necrosis of the skin, thymus, lungs, liver, kidneys, intestines, and adrenals. Guarnieri bodies (intracytoplasmic inclusion bodies) are seen in the decidual cells of the placenta [51].

Diagnosis

Differentiating smallpox from chickenpox

Similarities between smallpox and chickenpox include (1) overlapping prodromes and febrile syndromes; (2) incubation periods; (3) rash evolution periods; (4) rash present on the palms and soles; and (5) similar complications, including bacterial superinfection, scarring, pneumonia, and encephalitis. Patients with smallpox are more likely to have had vaccination against chickenpox, a centrifugal rather than central rash distribution, round rather than oval lesions, deep lesions, and lesions on the palms and soles. Varicella lesions often show differing stages of maturation within the same area, whereas smallpox lesions tend to be at the same stage. A Tzanck preparation of the base of an unroofed vesicle may reveal multinucleated giant cells typical of herpesvirus infection. Immunofluorescent antibody studies of vesicle fluid for varicella antigen are often helpful. Prior smallpox vaccination may cause the patient to have a milder presentation, further confusing the diagnosis [1,14,16,38,40–42].

Differential diagnosis

Diseases that may be confused with smallpox are listed in Table 2. The papulovesicular rashes that may be confused with smallpox include acne, chickenpox, generalized vaccinia, generalized herpes simplex, eczema vaccinatum, insect bites, and monkeypox. Less likely to be confused with smallpox are drug eruptions (maculopapular rashes and papulovesicular rashes), secondary syphilis, vaccine reactions (maculopapular rashes), and viral hemorrhagic fevers (maculopapular and hemorrhagic rashes). Tissue diagnosis using polymerase chain reaction to look for smallpox viral DNA is available through the CDC and state departments of health [30,46,52,53].

Procedures to follow for suspected cases

Aerosol release of smallpox virus is capable of causing infection in susceptible hosts for approximately 48 hours; after that, airborne virus is likely inactivated. Smallpox exposure may not become clinically evident for at least 2 weeks and may not be suspected for an additional few days until the rash takes on a more typical appearance. In a population without significant background immunity, 30% to 50% mortality would be expected in unimmunized patients, and each generation of disease may expand individuals infected by 3 to 30 fold [42].

All individuals with suspected cases must be placed in strict isolation and offered supportive therapy. Any patient with a presumptive diagnosis of smallpox should be reported to local or state health departments, who in turn report them to the CDC. Under most, if not all, circumstances, these health officials direct the response.

Table 2
Diseases commonly confused with smallpox

Disease	Typical rash
Acne	Papulovesicular
Chickenpox	Papulovesicular
Drug eruptions	Papulovesicular or maculopapular
Generalized vaccinia and eczema vaccinatum	Papulovesicular
Insect bites	Papulovesicular
Monkeypox (prevalence may be increased with the cessation of smallpox vaccination [103])	Papulovesicular
Secondary syphilis	Maculopapular
Vaccine reactions	Maculopapular
Viral hemorrhagic fever (may be confused with hemorrhagic smallpox)	Maculopapular and hemorrhagic

Data from Breman JG, Henderson DA. Diagnosis and management of smallpox. N Engl J Med 2002;346:1300–7; and Borio LL, Ingles T, Peters CJ, et al. Hemorrhagic fever viruses as biological weapons: medical and public health management. JAMA 2002;287:2391–405.

Should a real case of smallpox occur, one would anticipate the following public health response. All individuals with face-to-face contact with the index case after disease onset would receive smallpox vaccination; exposed individuals also would record daily evening temperatures and watch for new symptoms for 22 days after the last exposure. From day 6 through day 22, exposed individuals would be quarantined at home, and if fever greater than 38°C (>101°F) develops, they would be isolated in an appropriate facility until a definitive diagnosis could be made. Close contacts of these new patients would be vaccinated. A bifurcated needle method may be preferred [54]. In patients with a normal immune response, vaccination probably would prevent or mitigate the disease if given within the first 4 to 7 days after exposure [1,15,42]. In the event of mass exposure, isolation in tertiary facilities would not be practical; these individuals would be isolated at home because little more than supportive care could be offered in the hospital [42]. Aggressive ring vaccination would be key to successful containment, although mass vaccination of the public may become necessary in more severe circumstances.

There are *no* absolute contraindications to postexposure prophylaxis [46,55]. Contraindications for pre-exposure prophylaxis are immunosuppression, HIV infection, eczema, pregnancy, and household or sexual contact with an individual with known contraindications. For individuals with contraindications who are exposed to smallpox, simultaneous administration of vaccinia immunoglobulin (0.6 mL/kg intramuscularly given in multiple sites over 24–36 hours) may mitigate complications [46,55].

Complications of vaccination

The frequency of fatal and nonfatal complications of vaccinia prophylaxis is presented in Tables 3 and 4. Smallpox vaccine results in more complications than most vaccines used today. Mild reactions (satellite lesions, fever, muscle aches, lymphadenopathy, fatigue, headache, nausea, rashes, and soreness at the vaccination site) are common and cause one third of

Table 3
Fatal complications of vaccinia prophylaxis

Vaccination status	No. vaccinated	Postvaccinial encephalitis (No.)		Vaccinia Necrosum (No.)		Eczema Vaccinatum (No.)	
		Cases	Fatalities	Cases	Fatalities	Cases	Fatalities
Primary vaccination	5.6 million	16	4	5	2	58	0
Revaccination	8.6 million	0	0	6	2	8	0
Contacts	Unknown	0	0	0	0	60	1

Data from Lane JM, Ruben FL, Neff JM, et al. Complications of smallpox vaccination, 1968: national surveillance in the United States. N Engl J Med 1969;281:1201–8.

Table 4
Nonfatal complications of vaccinia prophylaxis

Vaccination status	No. vaccinated	Generalized vaccinia (No.)	Accidental infection (No.)	Other complications[a]	Grand total fatal and nonfatal events including those from Table 3
Primary vaccination	5.6 million	131	142	66	418
Revaccination	8.6 million	10	7	9	40
Contacts	Unknown	2	44	8	114

[a] Erythema multiforme, painful primary take, bacterial superinfection, miscellaneous rashes, and burns.

Data from Lane JM, Ruben FL, Neff JM, et al. Complications of smallpox vaccination, 1968: national surveillance in the United States. N Engl J Med 1969;281:1201–8.

vaccinees to miss school or work. Adverse reactions are 10 times more common and death is 4 times more common in first-time vaccinees than repeat vaccinees. During the 1968 vaccination campaign, the rates of serious complications were as follows: death, 1 per 1 million vaccinations; progressive vaccinia, 1.5 per 1 million vaccinations; eczema vaccinatum, 39 per 1 million vaccinations; and generalized vaccinia, 241 per 1 million vaccinations [56].

Postvaccinal encephalitis

Encephalitis is one of the most severe complications of smallpox vaccination and usually is seen in young children and first-time vaccinees. The incidence of postvaccinal encephalitis varies from 0 to 103 per 100,000 in children younger than 2 years old and from 2 to 1219 per 100,000 in children older than 2 years. Most affected children are younger than 4 years old [58]. The wide range in the incidence of encephalitis may be related to differences among the vaccinia strains used for immunization. A marked decrease in neurologic complications was noted when the Lister strain of vaccinia virus became more widely used for prophylaxis. During the 1968 vaccination campaign, there were 16 cases of encephalitis and 4 deaths among 5,594,000 primary vaccinees. No cases of encephalitis were reported among the 8,574,000 patients revaccinated [1,13,40,57,58].

Neurologic symptoms in children younger than age 2 years begin 6 to 10 days after the initial vaccination. Signs and symptoms include fever, headache, malaise, irritability, hyperactivity, somnolence, apnea, vomiting, generalized or jacksonian seizures, sixth cranial nerve palsy, hemiplegia, Guillain-Barré syndrome, aphasia, stiff neck, opisthotonos, and coma. Death from encephalitis may occur in only a few days; patients who recover often have significant sequelae (mental retardation or paralysis) [1,13,36].

Older children (>2 years old) and adults with encephalitis develop signs and symptoms later (11–15 days after vaccination). Complaints include fever, vomiting, malaise, lethargy, personality changes, paraparesis, headache, and anorexia. As patients deteriorate, they become confused and drowsy, develop focal or generalized seizures, and finally become comatose. Mortality rates range from 10% to 35% with death occurring in 7 days. Survivors often have upper motor neuron paralysis and cognitive dysfunction. Pathologic changes are similar to changes seen in measles encephalitis and after rabies vaccination. Patients who fully recover do so within 2 weeks of the onset of symptoms [13,36,40,59].

Although vaccinia virus has been cultured from the blood, brain, and cerebrospinal fluid of patients with postvaccinal encephalitis, the role of antiviral therapy for treatment is uncertain; cidofovir shows in vitro and in vivo activity against vaccinia virus, but there has been no clinical experience with this agent [60–62]. The timing of postvaccinal encephalitis, a minimal cerebrospinal fluid inflammatory response, and histologic evidence of demyelination all are consistent with a postviral immune-mediated process. Although vaccinia immunoglobulin has not proved effective for encephalitis, some experts have suggested benefit from use of steroids [60].

Decompressive hemicraniectomy and durotomy have been employed successfully for the treatment of massive cerebral edema associated with acute encephalomyelitis refractory to medical therapy; the authors suggest that this technique might be used for smallpox vaccine–related encephalitis when medical treatment fails to control cerebral edema [63]. The principal effort to decrease neurologic complications from immunization has focused on the development of new smallpox vaccines with fewer side effects (see later).

Vaccinia necrosum—progressive vaccinia

Vaccinia necrosum is a life-threatening complication seen in immunocompromised patients. Initially, the vaccination take seems normal, but the lesion fails to regress over the next 10 days to 3 weeks. Progressive local necrosis follows without lymphadenopathy, erythema, or systemic toxicity. Eventually, satellite lesions may develop at distant sites. One third of patients die from this complication. In 1968, of the 5.6 million primary vaccinees, there were 5 cases of vaccinia necrosum and 2 fatalities. Of the 8.6 million repeat vaccinees, there were 6 cases and 2 fatalities [1,13,36,40,58]. Intramuscular vaccinia immunoglobulin may decrease mortality.

Eczema vaccinatum

Atopic and eczematous patients may develop eczema vaccinatum after vaccination or exposure to a vaccinee. After a 5-day incubation period, a maculopapular or pustular eruption may develop at eczematous or previously eczematous sites. Patients are toxic with high fever and lymphadenopathy. Of the 5.6 million primary vaccinees in the 1968 study, there were 58 cases and no fatalities. Of the 8.6 million repeat vaccinees, there were 8 cases and no fatalities. During the 1968 study, 60 contacts of vaccinees developed eczema vaccinatum, and 1 contact died; these secondary cases underscore the importance of screening close contacts of potential vaccinees before vaccination. Death may be due to secondary bacterial infections or disseminated vaccinia. Treatment with vaccinia immunoglobulin reduces mortality [1,13,36,40,46,58].

Ocular complications

Autoinoculation of the face or eyelids occurs in 6 in 10,000 vaccinations [36]. The most common eye complications are vaccinia conjunctivitis and blepharitis. The progression from vesicle to pustule to crusting is similar to that seen at the primary vaccination site. Occasionally, patients are left with a depigmented scar. Corneal complications are rare (1.2 per 1 million primary vaccinees) and represent 6% to 37% of all ocular involvement. Keratitis is more common in primary vaccinees. Clinically, patients may have superficial punctate keratitis, interstitial or stromal keratitis, disciform keratitis with keratitic precipitates, or necrosis and perforation. Of patients with keratitis, 18% have permanent sequelae (madarosis, punctate stenosis, and cicatricial lid changes). Follow-up of patients with corneal vaccinia reveals rare residua—mild corneal scarring, ghost vessels, and subepithelial opacities with chronic conjunctivitis [1,36,50]. Although there is no approved treatment for ocular complications of vaccinia keratitis, topical trifluridine or vidarabine may be considered [1]; vaccinia immunoglobulin is relatively contraindicated.

Multiple branch retinal arteriolar occlusions with encephalopathy resulting in sudden temporal visual field loss have been reported 10 days after vaccination [64]. In this patient, there were retinal infarcts in the inferior macula, multiple cotton-wool spots over the posterior pole, and focal white matter lesions on MRI; the patient was treated with hyperbaric oxygen with improvement.

Other complications

Between 1907 and 1975, there were 12 nosocomial outbreaks of vaccinia involving 85 patients [1]; these cases underscore the contagious potential of vaccinia virus. Rare complications include an urticarial rash beginning 7 to 12 days after vaccination, erythema nodosum leprosum, vaccinial osteomyelitis, thrombocytopenia, arthritis, pericarditis, and malignant melanoma in the vaccination scar [1,13,36,40]. Two cases of folliculitis originally were diagnosed as erythema multiforme; both patients had received anthrax vaccine 2 weeks before smallpox vaccine [65].

A study of laboratory workers who had received the vaccine revealed the most common complaint was pruritus at the vaccination site. Primary vaccinees, especially individuals younger than 30 years old, had more subjective and objective complaints than repeat vaccinees; these included joint pain (25% versus 11%), muscle pain (46% versus 19%), fatigue (43% versus 29%), swelling at the vaccination site (58% versus 33%), generalized itching (31% versus 17%), abdominal pain (11% versus 2%), headache (40%

versus 25%), backache (17% versus 7%), and fever ($\geq$37.7°C) (20% versus 9%). All differences were statistically significant [66].

Myopericarditis

Between 1953 and 1999, there were 7 fatal and 59 nonfatal cases of postvaccinal myopericarditis reported in the medical literature. A more recent review of 540,824 US military personnel revealed that noncardiac complications secondary to smallpox vaccination were below anticipated levels, whereas cardiac complications were higher than expected [67–69]; 67 military personnel developed myopericarditis an average of 10 days after smallpox vaccination. ST segment elevations were noted in 57%, and cardiac enzymes peaked within 8 hours of clinical presentation. Of patients, 86% had complete recovery, whereas 14% experienced persistent atypical, nonlimiting chest discomfort [68]. Treatment with steroids has been described by some authors as "uniquely beneficial in myopericarditis related to smallpox vaccination" [69].

Postvaccinal myopericarditis patients may have a presentation similar to acute coronary syndrome, but lack cardiac risk factors and focal wall motion abnormalities on echocardiogram; elevations of troponin I and creatine kinase also develop earlier than in patients with acute coronary syndrome [70].

Nonfatal complications

Table 4 presents nonfatal complications. In a study by Vellozzi and coworkers [71], superinfection was reported in 48 of 36,043 vaccinees; the authors believed that some cases exhibiting larger than normal smallpox vaccination reactions may have been mistakenly diagnosed as bacterial infections [71].

Fetal and neonatal complications

Fatal bullous erythema multiforme occurs in 1 of 1 million vaccinated infants. High-grade viremia 8 to 9 days after vaccination may be fatal in 24 hours. Vaccinia immunoglobulin is advised for moderate-to-severe complications of smallpox vaccination (0.6 mL/kg intramuscularly every 48 hours until no new lesions appear); however, vaccinia immunoglobulin is not effective against postvaccinal encephalitis, possibly because of an autoimmune etiology [1,51,55].

Vaccinia in pregnancy

Pregnancy has been considered a relative contraindication to pre-exposure prophylaxis. In one study of 366 women who aborted after revaccination, vaccinia virus was isolated from only 12 (3.2%) of the products of conception; the reason for abortion in this setting is unclear [51]. In the twentieth century, 50 cases of fetal vaccinia virus infection were reported. In one report of 20 pregnant women vaccinated between 3 and 24 weeks' gestation, all delivered prematurely an average of 8 weeks after vaccination, and only three infants survived. Clinically, congenital vaccinia is similar to congenital variola. There are large circular necrotic skin lesions and multiple areas of focal necrosis in the placenta and internal organs [1,36,51].

Military Vaccination Program and Selective Civilian Vaccination Program of 2002–2004: neurologic adverse events

Between 2002 and 2004, the Department of Defense vaccinated 590,400 individuals and the Department of Health and Human Services vaccinated 64,600 adults using the New York City Board of Health strain of vaccinia (Dryvax; Wyeth Pharmaceuticals, Pearl River, NY) [72]. There were 435,000 primary vaccinees (66%). The national Vaccine Adverse Event Reporting System received 2060 reports; 214 of these were related to neurologic side effects. Of patients with neurologic side effects, 80% were younger than 50 years old, and 53% were primary vaccinees. Fifty-four percent of reactions occurred within 1 week of vaccination, and 80% occurred within 30 days. Headache (44% of adverse reactions; 14.3 per 100,000 vaccinations) was the most common symptom, often accompanied by fever and chills.

Thirty-nine serious neurologic adverse events were reported, including 13 patients with meningitis, 11 with Bell's palsy, 9 with seizures, 3 with encephalitis or myelitis, and 3 with Guillain-Barré syndrome. None of the neurologic events occurred more frequently than expected for a normal population [72]. The temporal relationship of vaccination and neurologic events suggests, however, that vaccination was causal.

Treatment of smallpox

Treatment of smallpox is supportive. Parenteral cidofovir (the nucleotide analogue of deoxycytidine monophosphate) is licensed for the treatment of cytomegalovirus, but also is active against herpesviruses, poxviruses, molluscum contagiosum, and variola virus. It is mutagenic and nephrotoxic, but has proved effective for postexposure prophylaxis for cowpox, vaccinia, and monkeypox. Theoretically, it could be used for the complications of smallpox or vaccination or postexposure prophylaxis, but there is no human clinical experience. More practical oral forms are under development [1,15,36,46,73,74]. Resistant cytomegalovirus has been isolated from treated patients, and cidofovir resistance may be induced in camelpox, cowpox, monkeypox, and vaccinia viruses [75]. Other investigational treatments include the kinase inhibitor imatinib mesylate (Gleevec) used to treat chronic myelogenous leukemia and cycloSal-nucleoside monophosphate derivatives of pronucleotides of acyclic nucleoside analogues of acyclovir-related drugs [76,77].

Newer vaccines

Older smallpox vaccines were produced in the skin of calves and sheep, and viral stocks were passed in calves, sheep, and rabbits. Contamination of viral stocks with "adventitious agents," such as *Brucella* spp., *Mycobacterium* spp., *Bacillus anthracis, Clostridium* spp., *Mycoplasma,* and viruses (eg, cowpox, bovine viruses, endogenous retroviruses, papillomavirus, herpesviruses, leporipoxviruses, and spongiform agents) is a significant concern. A review by Murphy and Osburn [78] enumerated the many hurdles faced by agencies in testing for adventitious agents and developing protocols to maintain sterility.

Replication of vaccinia virus, although it provides an excellent immune response, is responsible for most of the postvaccinal adverse events [79,80]. Modified vaccinia virus Ankara has been suggested as an alternate for Dryvax. Modified vaccinia virus Ankara is a nonreplicating virus with an excellent safety record, but poorer immunogenicity than Dryvax. It has been suggested to use it alone or in combination with Dryvax [79]. Other candidate vaccines include Lancy-Vaxina virus, LC16m8 virus, plasmid DNA encoding vaccinia antigens, a nonreplicating vaccinia virus combined with *Mycobacterium bovis* bacillus Calmette-Guérin, and single extracellular enveloped virus protein [81–84]. The efficacy of these new vaccines is unknown, but immunogenicity and toxicity in humans can be measured. Immunogenicity is measured using cutaneous reactions, neutralizing antibody titers, and cytotoxic T cell responses. The virulence of new strains as measured by a mouse model is positively correlated with human toxicity, as determined by phase I clinical trials. Alternative vaccines can be screened using immunogenicity as a proxy for efficacy and mouse virulence as a proxy for toxicity [85].

Smallpox and bioterrorism

History

Smallpox was used as a weapon against the native populations of South America by the Spanish conquistadors. Pizarro gave gifts of smallpox-contaminated clothing spreading the disease and contributing to the conquest of the Incas (1532–1533). During the French and Indian War (1754–1767), Lord Jeffrey Amherst passed to the Indians (led by Ottawa Chief Pontiac) loyal to the French blankets from smallpox victims during the siege of Fort Pitt (1763) [38]. Smallpox became epidemic, killing 50% of the targeted tribes, weakening their defense particularly at Fort Carillon, resulting in the loss of the war.

In 1980, the WHO recommended cessation of routine smallpox vaccination because it was believed that no naturally occurring disease existed anywhere in the human population. All smallpox virus stocks were to be destroyed except for those kept by the two WHO Collaborating Centers: the CDC in Atlanta, Georgia, and the State Research Center for Virology and Biotechnology (the Vektor Institute) in Novosibirsk, Siberia [37]. Despite treaties, the Soviet Union maintained a stockpile of 20 tons of smallpox and may have accidentally caused an outbreak in the region of the Aral Sea [52]. It is possible that "subnational" groups and other nations still may have stocks of virus [36].

The *Washington Post* in 2002 reported that the Central Intelligence Agency identified four nations that had clandestine smallpox virus stocks [86]. Other potential sources of smallpox virus are viral samples purloined from the massive Soviet stocks; smallpox victims (corpses) buried permafrost; and totally synthetically constructed virus from using published databases containing smallpox gene sequences [52]. These recombinant techniques have led to artificial synthesis of poliovirus and the 1918 strain of influenza virus [87–89].

The potential for using smallpox as a bioterrorist weapon increased when routine smallpox vaccination ceased (1971 in the United States and 1980 worldwide), and immunity of the world population waned. Releasing smallpox in the United States could result easily in more than 1 million deaths before it is contained and significant economic and social disruption [90,91]. A crash mass vaccination program has the potential to produce a significant number of inadvertent infections in immunocompromised, atopic, and eczematous patients [1,36,38,47,92–94]. The possible availability of weaponized smallpox and the certain catastrophic consequences of its release have led to government-sponsored programs to vaccinate first responders and selected health care professionals and to support disaster planning.

Response to attack

Ring vaccination consists of complete isolation of symptomatic patients diagnosed with smallpox and rapid vaccination of all contacts [93], sometimes combined with mass vaccinations of the at-risk populations; aggressive application of this approach was responsible for the WHO's success in eliminating naturally occurring smallpox [1]. The world's population was largely immune to smallpox at that time, however, and it is uncertain whether these results can be replicated should a new outbreak occur. Various computer models that purportedly predict the effectiveness of ring or mass vaccination depend on the virus' reproductive number (ie, the number of secondary cases caused by each primary case—the "R_0") [91]. The R_0 for smallpox has been estimated from 2 to 38 [1,91,95,96]. The rates of transmission may vary by season, availability of susceptible contacts, and type of contact [1,91,96]. Face-to-face contact is the most efficient way to spread smallpox. Distant airborne spread and fomite spread of infection also have been documented [1,13,15,46,47,91,96].

Computer models indicate that choosing ring versus mass vaccination strategies depends on the R_0, the initial number of infected cases, and the timing of the public health intervention; these models assume uniform distribution of initial smallpox cases, uniform transmission rates (R_0), and public health resources. Models using the aforementioned assumptions have suggested that ring vaccination coupled with vaccination of first responders would effectively control an outbreak. The authors are less sure that their assumptions are valid. For densely populated areas with significant numbers of nonimmune individuals, a high R_0, and delays in public health interventions, mass vaccination may be preferable to ring vaccination [97–99].

Ring vaccination and regional quarantine had been successful in populations with partial immunity to smallpox. Teams, sometimes in the thousands, descended on regions where an index case or cases were identified, isolated the cases, vaccinated the contacts and sometimes the entire local population, and educated the public. There is no evidence that ring vaccination would be effective in controlling a smallpox outbreak today. Today's world is a highly mobile world of international-intercontinental air travel, with most populations lacking effective smallpox immunity. Many elderly have waning immunity to smallpox, but often have disease or treatment that might render them susceptible (cancer, chemotherapy, organ transplantation). The release of smallpox virus by one or several vehicles, especially on the African continent with the HIV epidemic, would overwhelm any response rapidly. There would be widely variable transmission rates from group to group and area to area, making ring vaccination successful in some and a failure in other locations [90,95]. Even successful quarantining has adverse outcomes: increased risk of disease transmission in the quarantined area, mistrust of the government that may lead to violence, and ethnic bias altering public health decisions [100].

In 2002, President Bush announced plans to vaccinate 500,000 health care workers and first responders with the eventual goal of having 10 million emergency responders vaccinated by mid-2003. Nationwide, only 40,000 first responders and health care workers were vaccinated [101]. Vaccinating or revaccinating first responders and essential personnel (transit workers, public health staff, emergency management staff, all health care workers at facilities that may see infected patients, mortuary workers) should occur for all individuals without contraindications [1,42].

Of the first 33,444 civilian health care and public health workers vaccinated, there were 9 cases of generalized vaccinia (8 suspected and 1 confirmed), 31 inadvertent nonocular inoculations (29 suspected and 2 confirmed), and 10 myocarditis/pericarditis cases (7 suspected and 3 probable). Additionally, there were 45 serious adverse events requiring hospitalization temporally associated with vaccination, but not "causally associated with vaccination," and 369 minor adverse events (self-limited responses to smallpox vaccination). There were no cases of vaccinia transmitted to contacts, and one dose of vaccinia immunoglobulin was released [102].

On the local and regional level, government agencies should use the Standardized Emergency Management System framework for managing the response to a smallpox emergency. The Incident Command System of

Table 5
Arguments for and against pre-exposure prophylaxis for smallpox

For pre-exposure prophylaxis	Against pre-exposure prophylaxis
Estimates of casualties in a bioterrorist attack would outnumber by manifold the known morbidity and mortality from the vaccine; economic damage would be severe	Cannot quantify the risk of smallpox being used as a biological weapon; cost of inoculation program would be significant
Screening for contraindications to vaccine (eg, HIV, pregnancy) would limit the inadvertent administration of vaccine to the immunocompromised	Risk of inoculating immunocompromised or those in whom the vaccine is contraindicated; expense of screening would be significant
Special care can be taken to see that immunocompromised patients are not exposed to vaccinees; the risk of vaccinees spreading vaccinia virus via droplets is small [104]	Risk of exposing immunocompromised patients to the vaccine virus via exposure to healthy vaccinees; family disruption likely in some cases
Herd immunity would protect the immunocompromised or other individuals who should not or could not be vaccinated by limiting secondary smallpox cases	Defined morbidity and mortality of vaccine in normal individuals without a defined benefit ratio because of inability to quantify risk of attack
Historical data indicate that the basic reproductive number, the R_0 for smallpox (see text for explanation), may be highly variable and depend on population characteristics	The basic reproductive number, R_0, may be much lower than some models predict, making ring vaccination practical
As more healthy individuals are immunized, vaccinia immunoglobulin could be produced in sufficient quantity to treat any complications of vaccine	Lack of ready availability of effective drugs or vaccinia immunoglobulin to treat complications of vaccine; cost of treating vaccine complication is high
If the US is the primary target, limiting the spread of the disease here also helps limit secondary spread to populations that have not been immunized	There are no data to suggest that a ring vaccination strategy would not work in a population that is largely susceptible to smallpox
If another nation becomes the primary target, spread to an unimmunized US population is likely considering legitimate travel and legal and illegal immigration that would be impossible to control	In the absence of a readily available and rapid diagnostic test that can differentiate vaccinia from smallpox, accidental vaccinia infection causing generalized vaccinia, vaccinia necrosum, or eczema vaccinatum may be confused with smallpox, triggering unnecessary public anxiety and an unneeded public health response
There are no data to suggest that a ring vaccination and regional quarantine strategy would work in a population that is largely susceptible to smallpox	

Data from Refs. [13,46,92–94,103,104].

From Cleri DJ, Villota FJ, Porwancher RB. Smallpox, bioterrorism, and the neurologist. Arch Neurol 2003;60:493; with permission.

Standardized Emergency Management System consists of (1) management, (2) operations, (3) planning/intelligence, (4) logistics, and (5) finance/administration. The authors believe that a carefully executed voluntary pre-exposure prophylaxis program for all health care providers, first responders, and members of the general public who request vaccination should be instituted (Table 5). A concomitant increase in the availability of vaccinia immunoglobulin would be required for this program [1,36,93,95,96]. Extensive education and ready availability of rapid laboratory diagnostic techniques, such as polymerase chain reaction, are necessary to differentiate the inevitable cases of generalized vaccinia, vaccinia necrosum, and eczema vaccinatum from smallpox and varicella [36,46]. Smallpox vaccine provides some protection from monkeypox. With the cessation of smallpox vaccination, monkeypox is re-emerging as a possible "poor man's" smallpox look-alike and a potential weapon that may be stand-alone or used in conjunction with smallpox. Clinical differentiation of this disease in its early stages is difficult, if not nearly impossible, and rapid laboratory diagnosis is essential [1,103].

A successful voluntary pre-exposure prophylaxis program would (1) limit or eliminate smallpox as a bioterrorist weapon in the United States; (2) limit, but not eliminate, the morbidity and mortality associated with a hastily executed vaccination program; (3) enhance the effectiveness of any ring vaccination program in the event of an attack; (4) allow for herd immunity to buffer or prevent the exposure of individuals in whom vaccination is contraindicated; and (5) send a strong message regarding the determination of the United States to resist enemies' threats [36]. Any prophylactic program may result in the vaccination of individuals unaware of their medical contraindications. Additionally, there are innate risks to otherwise healthy individuals who receive the vaccine, but develop untoward reactions. Protection from vaccine-related lawsuits and compensation for patients harmed by the vaccine are essential components of any program. While awaiting the introduction of safer vaccines against smallpox, health care workers remain obligated to protect the public using all available means. History would judge us harshly if we failed to protect most of the people because of fear of harming the few [1,36].

References

[1] Cleri DJ, Ricketti AJ, Villota FJ, et al. Smallpox, monkeypox, other pox diseases and vaccination. Infect Dis Pract Clin 2005;29:395–406.

[2] Skinner MA, Laidlaw SM, Boulanger D. Avipoxvirus. In: Tidona CA, Darai G, editors. The Springer index of viruses. Berlin: Springer-Verlag; 2002. p. 864–8.

[3] Kitching RP. Capripoxvirus. In: Tidona CA, Darai G, editors. The Springer index of viruses. Berlin: Springer-Verlag; 2002. p. 869–72.

[4] Kerr PJ, McFadden G. Leporipoxvirus. In: Tidona CA, Darai G, editors. The Springer index of viruses. Berlin: Springer-Verlag; 2002. p. 873–9.

[5] Bugert JJ, Melquiot N. Molluscipoxvirus. In: Tidona CA, Darai G, editors. The Springer index of viruses. Berlin: Springer-Verlag; 2002. p. 880–4.

[6] Moss B, Senkevich TG. Orthopoxvirus. In: Tidona CA, Darai G, editors. The Springer index of viruses. Berlin: Springer-Verlag; 2002. p. 885–95.
[7] Mercer A, Fleming S. Parapoxvirus. In: Tidona CA, Darai G, editors. The Springer index of viruses. Berlin: Springer-Verlag; 2002. p. 896–901.
[8] Ness TL, Moyer RW. Suipoxvirus. In: Tidona CA, Darai G, editors. The Springer index of viruses. Berlin: Springer-Verlag; 2002. p. 902–6.
[9] Essani K, Bejcek BE, Paulose M. Yatapoxvirus. In: Tidona CA, Darai G, editors. The Springer index of viruses. Berlin: Springer-Verlag; 2002. p. 907–10.
[10] Bergoin M. Entomopoxvirus A. In: Tidona CA, Darai G, editors. The Springer index of viruses. Berlin: Springer-Verlag; 2002. p. 911–3.
[11] Arif BM, Moyer RW. Entomopoxvirus B. In: Tidona CA, Darai G, editors. The Springer index of viruses. Berlin: Springer-Verlag; 2002. p. 914–8.
[12] Federici BA. Entomopoxvirus C. In: Tidona CA, Darai G, editors. The Springer index of viruses. Berlin: Springer-Verlag; 2002. p. 919–21.
[13] Henderson DA, Borio LL, Lane JM. Smallpox and vaccinia. In: Plotkin SA, Orenstein WA, editors. Vaccines. 4th edition. Philadelphia: Saunders; 2004. p. 123–53.
[14] Fenner F. Poxviruses. In: Field BN, Knipe DM, Howley PM, editors. Fields virology, vol. 2. 3rd edition. Philadelphia: Lippincott-Raven; 1996. p. 2673–702.
[15] Esposito JJ, Fenner F. Poxviruses. In: Knipe DM, Howley PM, editors-in-chief. Fields virology, vol. 2. 4th edition. Philadelphia: Lippincott Williams & Wilkins; 2001. p. 2885–921.
[16] Moss B. Poxviridae: the viruses and their replication. In: Knipe DM, Howley PM, editors-in-chief. Fields virology, vol. 2. 4th edition. Philadelphia: Lippincott Williams & Wilkins; 2001. p. 2849–83.
[17] Malkin AJ, McPherson A, Gershon PD. Structure of intracellular mature vaccinia virus visualized by in situ atomic force microscopy. J Virol 2003;77:6332–40.
[18] Morikawa S, Sakiyama T, Hasegawa H, et al. An attenuated LC16m8 smallpox vaccine: analysis of full-genome sequence and induction of immune protection. J Virol 2005;79: 11873–91.
[19] Viner KM, Isaacs SN. Activity of vaccinia virus-neutralizing antibody in the sera of smallpox vaccinees. Microbes Infect 2005;7:579–83.
[20] Drexler M. Bioterror. In: Secret agents—the menace of emerging infections. Washington, DC: Joseph Henry Press; 2002. p. 231–74.
[21] Hopkins DR. The kiss of the goddess. In: The greatest killer—smallpox in history. Chicago: The University of Chicago Press; 2002. p. 139–62.
[22] Drexler M. Disease in disguise. In: Secret agents—the menace of emerging infections. Washington, DC: Joseph Henry Press; 2002. p. 1–18.
[23] Tucker JB. Smallpox and civilization. In: Scourge—the once and future threat of smallpox. New York: Atlantic Monthly Press; 2001. p. 5–22.
[24] Hopkins DR. The destroying angel. In: The greatest killer—smallpox in history. Chicago: The University of Chicago Press; 2002. p. 234–94.
[25] Hopkins DR. Chronology. In: The greatest killer—smallpox in history. Chicago: The University of Chicago Press; 2002. p. 311–7.
[26] Hopkins DR. The most terrible of all the ministers of death. In: The greatest killer—smallpox in history. Chicago: The University of Chicago Press; 2002. p. 22–102.
[27] Hopkins DR. The spotted death. In: The greatest killer—smallpox in history. Chicago: The University of Chicago Press; 2002. p. 164–203.
[28] Fenn EA. Pox Americana—the great smallpox epidemic of 1775–1782. New York: Hill & Wang; 2001.
[29] Hopkins DR. Erythrotherapy and eradication. In: The greatest killer—smallpox in history. Chicago: The University of Chicago Press; 2002. p. 295–310.
[30] Plotkin SL, Plotkin SA. A short history of vaccination. In: Plotkin SA, Orenstein WA, editors. Vaccines. 4th edition. Philadelphia: Saunders; 2004. p. 1–15.
[31] Boylston AW. Clinical investigation of smallpox in 1767. N Engl J Med 2002;346:1326–8.

[32] Ku CC, Zerboni L, Ito H, et al. Varicella-zoster virus transfer to skin by T cells and modulation of viral replication by epidermal cell interferon-alpha. J Exp Med 2004; 200:917–25.
[33] Franco-Paredes C, Lammoglia L, Santos-Preciado JI. The Spanish royal philanthropic expedition to bring smallpox vaccination to the New World and Asia in the 19th century. Clin Infect Dis 2005;41:1285–9.
[34] Fenner F. Poxviruses. In: Fields BN, Knipe DM, Howley PM, editors-in-chief. Fields virology, vol. 2. 3rd edition. Philadelphia: Lippincott Williams & Wilkins; 1996. p. 2673–702.
[35] Axelrod A. The golden rule of war. In: Patton on leadership—strategic lessons for corporate warfare. Paramus (NJ): Prentice Hall Press; 1999. p. 135.
[36] Cleri DJ, Villota FJ, Porwancher RB. Smallpox, bioterrorism, and the neurologist. Arch Neurol 2003;60:489–94.
[37] Tudor V, Strati I. The clinical picture. In: Smallpox: Cholera. Tunbridge Wells, Kent: Abacus Press; 1977. p. 34–71.
[38] Rotz LD, Cono J, Damon I. Smallpox and bioterrorism. In: Mandell GL, Bennett JE, Dolin R, editors. Mandell, Douglas, and Bennett's principles and practice of infectious diseases, vol. 2. 6th edition. Philadelphia: Churchill Livingstone; 2005. p. 3612–7.
[39] Damon I. Orthopoxviruses: vaccinia (smallpox vaccine), variola (smallpox), monkeypox, and cowpox. In: Mandell GL, Bennett JE, Dolin R, editors. Mandell, Douglas, and Bennett's principles and practice of infectious diseases, vol. 2. 6th edition. Philadelphia: Churchill Livingstone; 2005. p. 1742–51.
[40] Neff JM. Poxviridae. In: Mandell GL, Douglas RG, Bennett JE, editors. Principles and practice of infectious diseases, vol. 2. New York: John Wiley & Sons; 1979. p. 1341–52.
[41] Earle DP. Exanthematous and other virus diseases. In: Hunter GW, Swartzwelder JC, Clyde DF, editors. Tropical medicine. 5th edition. Philadelphia: Saunders; 1976. p. 81–94.
[42] Henderson DA, Inglesby TV, Bartlett JG, et al. Smallpox as a biological weapon—medical and public health management. JAMA 1999;281:2127–37.
[43] Berting A, Goerner W, Spruth M, et al. Effective poxvirus removal by sterile filtration during manufacture of plasma derivatives. J Med Virol 2005;75:603–7.
[44] Schmidt M, Roth WK, Meyer H, et al. Nucleic acid test screening of blood donors for orthopoxviruses can potentially prevent dispersion of viral agents in case of bioterrorism. Transfusion 2005;45:290–2.
[45] Guerra S, Aracil M, Conde R, et al. Wiskott-Aldrich syndrome protein is needed for vaccinia virus pathogenesis. J Virol 2005;79:2133–40.
[46] Breman JG, Henderson DA. Diagnosis and management of smallpox. N Engl J Med 2002; 346:1300–7.
[47] Kortepeter M, Christopher G, Cieslak T, et al. Smallpox. In: USAMRIID's medical management of biological casualties handbook. 4th edition. Fort Detrick (MD): Operational Medicine Department, US Army Medical Research Institute of Infectious Diseases; 2001. p. 44–8.
[48] Reeder MM, Palmer PES. Smallpox osteomyelitis (osteomyelitis variolosa). In: The radiology of tropical medicine with epidemiological, pathological and clinical correlation. Baltimore: Williams & Wilkins; 1981. p. 765–73.
[49] Johnson RT. Postinfectious demyelinating diseases. In: Viral infection of the nervous system. 2nd edition. Philadelphia: Lippincott-Raven; 1998. p. 181–210.
[50] Roger FC. Eye diseases. In: Manson-Bahr PEC, Bell DR, editors. Manson's tropical diseases. 19th edition. London: Bailliere Tindall; 1987. p. 1133–82.
[51] McMillan JA. Smallpox and vaccinia. In: Remington JS, Klein JO, Wilson CB, et al, editors. Infectious diseases of the fetus and newborn infant. 6th edition. Philadelphia: Saunders; 2006. p. 927–32.
[52] Darling RG, Burgess TH, Lawler JV, et al. Virologic and pathogenic aspects of variola virus (smallpox) as a bioweapon. In: Lindler LE, Lebeda FJ, Korch GW, editors. Biological

weapons defense—infectious diseases and counterterrorism. Totowa (NJ): Humana Press; 2005. p. 99–120.
[53] Borio LL, Ingles T, Peters CJ, et al. Hemorrhagic fever viruses as biological weapons: medical and public health management. JAMA 2002;287:2391–405.
[54] Balicer RD, Davidovitch N, Huerta M, et al. Smallpox vaccination techniques: considerations and unresolved issues. Harefuah 2005;144:51–6.
[55] Centers for Disease Control and Prevention. CDC vaccinia (smallpox) vaccine: recommendations of the Advisory Committee on Immunization Practices (ACIP). MMWR Morb Mortal Wkly Rep 2001;50(RR10):1–25.
[56] Belongia EA, Naleway AL. Smallpox vaccine: the good, the bad, and the ugly. Clin Med Res 2003;1:87–92.
[57] Tudor V, Strati I. The complications of smallpox vaccination. In: Smallpox: cholera. Tunbridge Wells, Kent: Abacus Press; 1977. p. 143–8.
[58] Lane JM, Ruben FL, Neff JM, et al. Complications of smallpox vaccination, 1968: national surveillance in the United States. N Engl J Med 1969;281:1201–8.
[59] Sejvar J, Boneva R, Lane JM, et al. Severe headaches following smallpox vaccination. Headache 2005;45:87–8.
[60] Miravalle A, Roos KL. Encephalitis complicating smallpox vaccination. Arch Neurol 2003;60:925–8.
[61] Gurvich EB, Vilesova IS. Vaccinia virus in postvaccinal encephalitis. Acta Virol 1983;27: 154–9.
[62] Anguolo JJ, Pimenta-De-Campos E, de Salles-Gomez LF. Post-vaccinal meningoencephalitis. JAMA 1964;187:151–3.
[63] Refai D, Lee MC, Goldenberg FD, et al. Decompressive hemicraniectomy for acute disseminated encephalomyelitis: case report. Neurosurgery 2005;56:872.
[64] Landa G, Marcovich A, Leiba H, et al. Multiple branch retinal arteriolar occlusions associated with smallpox vaccination. J Infect 2005;52:7–9.
[65] Oh RC. Folliculitis after smallpox vaccination: a report of two cases. Milit Med 2005;170: 133–6.
[66] Baggs J, Chen RT, Damon IK, et al. Safety profile of smallpox vaccine: insights from the laboratory worker smallpox vaccination program. Clin Infect Dis 2005;40:1133–40.
[67] Halsell JS, Riddle JR, Atwood JE, et al. Myopericarditis following smallpox vaccination among vaccinia-naive US military personnel. JAMA 2003;289:3306–8.
[68] Eckart RE, Love SS, Atwood JE, et al. Incidence and follow-up of inflammatory cardiac complications after smallpox vaccination. J Am Coll Cardiol 2004;44:201–5.
[69] Cassimatis DC, Atwood JE, Engler RM, et al. Smallpox vaccination and myopericarditis: a clinical review. J Am Coll Cardiol 2004;43:1503–10.
[70] Eckart RE, Shry EA, Jones SO 4th, et al. Comparison of clinical presentation of acute myocarditis following smallpox vaccination to acute coronary syndromes in patients $<$ 40 years of age. Am J Cardiol 2005;95:1252–5.
[71] Vellozzi C, Averhoff F, Lane JM, et al. Superinfection following vaccination (vaccinia), United States: January 2003 through January 2004. Clin Infect Dis 2004;39:1660–6.
[72] Sejvar JJ, Labutta RJ, Chapman LE, et al. Neurologic adverse events associated with smallpox vaccination in the United States, 2002–2004. JAMA 2005;294:2744–50.
[73] Hayden FG. Antiviral drugs (other than antiretrovirals). In: Mandell GL, Bennett JE, Dolin R, editors. Mandell, Douglas, and Bennett's principles and practice of infectious diseases, vol. 1. 6th edition. Philadelphia: Churchill Livingstone; 2005. p. 514–50.
[74] Kern ER, Hartline C, Harden E, et al. Enhanced inhibition oforthopoxvirus replication in vitro by alkoxyalkyl esters of cidofovir and cyclic cidofovir. Antimicrob Agents Chemother 2002;46:991–5.
[75] Smee DF, Sidwell RW, Kefauver D, et al. Characterization of wild-type and cidofovir-resistant strains of camelpox, cowpox, monkeypox and vaccinia virus. Antimicrob Agents Chemother 2002;46:1329–35.

[76] Sauerbrei A, Meier C, Meerbach A, et al. In vitro activity of cycloSal-nucleoside monophosphates and polyhydroxycarboxylates against orthopoxviruses. Antiviral Res 2005;67:147–54.
[77] Reeves PM, Bommarius B, Lebeis S, et al. Disabling poxvirus pathogenesis by inhibition of Abl-family tyrosine kinases. Nat Med 2005;11:731–9.
[78] Murphy FA, Osburn BI. Adventitious agents and smallpox vaccine in strategic national stockpile. Emerg Infect Dis 2005;11:1086–9.
[79] Slifka MK. The future of smallpox vaccination: is MVA the key? Med Immunol 2005;4:2.
[80] Coulibaly S, Bruhl P, Mayrhofer J, et al. The nonreplicating smallpox candidate vaccines defective vaccinia Lister (dVV-L) and modified vaccinia Ankara (MVA) elicit robust long-term protection. Virology 2005;341:91–101.
[81] Kim SH, Yeo SG, Jang HC, et al. Clinical responses to smallpox vaccine in vaccinia-naive and previously vaccinated populations: undiluted and diluted Lancy-Vaxina vaccine in a single-blind, randomized, prospective trial. J Infect Dis 2005;192:1066–70.
[82] Otero M, Calarota SA, Dai A, et al. Efficacy of novel plasmid DNA encoding vaccinia antigens in improving current smallpox vaccination strategy. Vaccine 2005;Aug [Epub ahead of print].
[83] Ami Y, Izumi Y, Matsuo K, et al. Priming-boosting vaccination with recombinant *Mycobacterium bovis* bacillus Calmette-Guerin and a nonreplicating vaccinia virus recombinant leads to long-lasting and effective immunity. J Virol 2005;79:12871–9.
[84] Fang M, Cheng H, Dai Z, et al. Immunization with a single extracellular enveloped virus protein produced in bacteria provides partial protection from a lethal orthopoxvirus infection in a natural host. Virology 2006;345:231–43.
[85] Monath TP, Caldwell JR, Mundt W, et al. ACAM2000 clonal Vero cell culture vaccinia virus (NYCBOH)—a second generation smallpox vaccine for biological defense. Int J Infect Dis 2004;8:S31–44.
[86] Lawler JV, Burgess TH. Smallpox. In: Roy MJ, editor. Physician's guide to terrorist attack. Totowa (NJ): Humana Press; 2004. p. 197–220.
[87] Cello J, Paul AV, Wimmer E. Chemical synthesis of poliovirus cDNA: generation of infectious virus in the absence of natural template. Science 2002;297:1016–8.
[88] Hammerschmidt S, Hacker J, Klenk HD. Threat of infection: microbes of high pathogenic potential—strategies for detection, control and eradication. Int J Med Microbiol 2005;295:141–51.
[89] Lim M-K. Hostile use of the life sciences. N Engl J Med 2005;353:2214–5.
[90] O'Toole T, Mair M, Inglesby TV. Shining light on "Dark Winter." Clin Infect Dis 2002;34:972–83.
[91] Enserink M. How devastating would a smallpox attack really be? Science 2002;296:1592–5.
[92] Nafziger SD. Smallpox. Crit Care Clin 2005;21:739–46.
[93] Kim-Farley RJ, Celentano JT, Gunter C, et al. Standardized emergency management system and response to a smallpox emergency. Prehosp Disast Med 2003;18:313–20.
[94] Durrheim DN, Muller R, Saunders V, et al. Australian public and smallpox. Emerg Infect Dis 2005;11:1748–50.
[95] Bicknell WJ. The case for voluntary smallpox vaccination. N Engl J Med 2002;346:1323–4.
[96] Meltzer MI, Damon I, LeDuc JW, et al. Modeling potential responses to smallpox as a bioterrorist weapon. Emerg Infect Dis 2001;7:959–69.
[97] Lau CY, Wahl B, Foo WK. Ring vaccination versus mass vaccination in event of smallpox attack. Hawaii Med J 2005;64:34–6.
[98] Ohkusa Y, Tanguchi K, Okubo I. Prediction of smallpox outbreak and evaluation of control-measure policy in Japan, using a mathematical model. J Infect Chemother 2005;11:71–80.
[99] Kretzschmar M, van den Hof S, Wallinga J, et al. Ring vaccination and smallpox control. Emerg Infect Dis 2004;10:832–41.

[100] Barbera J, Macintyre A, Gostin L, et al. Large-scale quarantine following biological terrorism in the United States—scientific examination, logistic and legal limits, and possible consequences. In: Henderson DA, Inglesby TV, O'Toole T, editors. Bioterrorism—guidelines for medical and public health management. Chicago: AMA Press; 2002. p. 221–32.
[101] Kaiser J. Report faults smallpox vaccination. Science 2005;305:1540.
[102] Centers for Disease Control and Prevention. Update: adverse events following civilian smallpox vaccination—United States, 2003. MMWR Morbid Mortal Wkly Rep 2003;52: 360–3.
[103] Nalca A, Rimoin AW, Bavari S, et al. Reemergence of monkeypox: prevalence, diagnostics, and countermeasures. Clin Infect Dis 2005;41:1765–71.
[104] Klote MM, Ludwig GV, Ulrich MP, et al. Absence of oropharyngeal vaccinia virus after vacccinia (smallpox) vaccination. Ann Allergy Asthma Immunol 2005;94:682–5.

ELSEVIER
SAUNDERS

Infect Dis Clin N Am
20 (2006) 359–393

INFECTIOUS
DISEASE CLINICS
OF NORTH AMERICA

Viral Hemorrhagic Fevers: Current Status of Endemic Disease and Strategies for Control

Dennis J. Cleri, MD[a,b,*], Anthony J. Ricketti, MD[a,b], Richard B. Porwancher, MD[b,c], Luz S. Ramos-Bonner, MD[b], John R. Vernaleo, MD[d]

[a]*Department of Medicine, Seton Hall University School of Graduate Medical Education, 400 South Orange Avenue, South Orange, NJ, USA*
[b]*Department of Medicine, Seton Hall University School of Graduate Medical Education at St. Francis Medical Center, 601 Hamilton Avenue, Trenton, NJ 08629, USA*
[c]*Department of Medicine, UMDNJ-Robert Wood Johnson Medical School, 47 Paterson Street, New Brunswick, NJ, USA*
[d]*Division of Infectious Diseases, Wycoff Heights Medical Center, 374 Stockholm Street, Brooklyn, NY 11237, USA*

The United States Army Medical Research Institute of Infectious Diseases lists four RNA viral families as the prime etiologic agents for viral hemorrhagic fevers (VHF): (1) the Arenaviridae (Argentine, Bolivian, Brazilian, and Venezuelan hemorrhagic fevers; and Lassa fever); (2) the Bunyaviridae (Hantavirus genus, Congo-Crimean hemorrhagic fever (CCHF) from the Nairovirus genus, and Rift Valley fever virus from the Phlebovirus genus) [1]; (3) the Filoviridae (Ebola and Marburg viruses); and (4) Flaviviridae (dengue and yellow fever) [2]. References 3 through 13 list the most important characteristics and classify the Arenaviridae viruses, Bunyaviridae viruses, Filoviridae viruses, and Flaviviridae viruses, respectively [3–13].

The threat posed by viral hemorrhagic fever viruses

The VHF agents pose a real threat as terror weapons for the following reasons:

1. Except for Marburg and Ebola viruses, they are widely distributed in nature
2. Many are naturally spread by airborne means

* Corresponding author.
E-mail address: dcleri@che-east.org (D.J. Cleri).

doi:10.1016/j.idc.2006.02.001

3. Humans are widely susceptible to serious and often life-threatening infections
4. The differential diagnosis encompasses a wide variety of organisms (rickettsial disease, leptospirosis, relapsing fever, malaria, typhoid, shigellosis, sepsis, and others), making the initial recognition of a VHF virus attack difficult to distinguish
5. There is great similarity in the clinical presentations of the VHFs, making them nearly impossible to differentiate without sophisticated and time-consuming laboratory analysis
6. VHFs that respond to antiviral therapy need to be treated immediately, but clinically cannot be separated from the viral pathogens that lack specific therapy
7. Limited prophylactic and therapeutic options [14]
8. Isolation and identification of VHF agents frequently require a biosafety 4 level laboratory
9. Life-saving supportive therapy often requires an intensive care bed, which is impractical in a mass casualty situation

Fortunately, few VHFs (CCHF, Lassa fever, Andes viruses, Ebola virus, and Marburg virus) exhibit secondary human-to-human spread especially in the nosocomial setting [14–22].

This article presents the virology, pathology, clinical presentation, and control measures available for a limited number of VHF agents to assist the practitioner in the early recognition and therapeutic options for these threats.

Virology and pathology

The Arenaviridae

Arenaviruses are spherical or pleomorphic enveloped single-stranded bisegmented RNA ambisense viruses that use virion RNA-dependent RNA polymerase for replication. The first arenavirus was isolated in 1933 (the lymphocytic choriomeningitis virus), and the first arenavirus hemorrhagic fever virus was isolated in 1958 (Junin virus, the cause of Argentine hemorrhagic fever) [3,23,24]. Machupo virus was isolated from cases of Bolivian hemorrhagic fever in 1965, and Lassa virus was isolated in 1970 [3]. There are 18 arenavirus species, with at least seven causing hemorrhagic fever: (1) Lassa fever virus–Lassa fever, (2) Junin virus–Argentine hemorrhagic fever, (3) Machupo virus–Bolivian hemorrhagic fever, (4) Guanarito virus–Venezuelan hemorrhagic fever, (5) Sabia virus–hemorrhagic fever with extensive hepatic necrosis, (6) Whitewater Arroyo virus–hemorrhagic fever with liver failure, and (7) Oliveros virus–hemorrhagic fever [19,25,26].

Arenaviruses cause chronic asymptomatic infection in rodents. Persistent rodent infection is caused by both molecular mechanisms and failure of the host's immune system. Congenital neonatal infection results in high-titer lifelong viral infection and abundant urinary excretion (up to 10^5 plaque-forming units per milliliter urine). During the acute infection, there is no cytopathic effect and most rodent cells remain infected for life [19,27].

Humans and nonreservoir hosts inhale aerosols containing the virus. The virus has been shown to enter by gastrointestinal and respiratory epithelial cells through the apical plasma membrane [24,28]. The cellular receptor for the Old World arenaviruses Lassa fever virus and lymphocytic choriomeningitis virus seems to be α-dystroglycan. α-Dystroglycan is a cell surface receptor that is the link between the extracellular matrix and the actin-based cytoskeleton [29].

After attachment, there is local viral replication. The virus spreads to hilar lymph nodes, lung, and other organs. There is no pulmonary consolidation, but interstitial infiltrates and edema do occur. Initially, macrophages are infected. This is followed by widespread epithelial involvement [19,30].

In fatal cases, fulminant viremia is believed to be caused by failure or delay in the cellular immune response. The pathogenicity of Lassa virus is related to its resistance to interferon. In one study, however, the interferon sensitivity of the Lassa virus isolate did not correlate with its lethality [31].

Pichinde virus, because it does not infect humans, has been used in the guinea pig model to mimic human Lassa fever [19]; 7 days after infection, during the initial viremia, there is weight loss (up to 25%) and fever. Macrophages are the cells that are primarily infected. Epithelial cells then become infected with little involvement of endothelial cells. Focal necrosis of the liver and adrenal glands, mild interstitial pneumonitis, marginal zone necrosis in the splenic white pulp, and intestinal villous blunting are seen histologically. The guinea pigs develop progressive decreasing cardiac output not caused by carditis, but from release of soluble inflammatory mediators (ie, tumor necrosis factor-α) [19].

In the Balb/c neonatal mouse model, Pichinde viral infection is fatal in most mice. In surviving mice, the virus was gradually cleared but could be detected for up to 9 months in the kidneys and brain. The animals had high antibody titers and major histocompatibility group restricted cytotoxic T-cell activity. Pichinde virus experiments require a biosafety level 2 laboratory [32].

Pirital virus coexists in the same region of Venezuela as Guanarito virus (the cause of Venezuelan hemorrhagic fever) and was originally isolated from the cotton rat (*Sigmodoni alstoni*) [33]; this virus provides another model that mimics fatal human Lassa fever infection in Syrian golden hamsters (*Mesocricetus auratus*). The golden hamsters develop interstitial pneumonitis, splenic lymphoid depletion and necrosis, and multifocal hepatic necrosis without a great deal of inflammatory infiltration. Special staining with in situ terminal deoxynucleotidyl transferase–mediated 2′-deoxyuridine 5′-triphosphate (dUTP) nick-end labeling stain demonstrates hepatocytes undergoing apoptosis or necrapoptosis. This model requires a biosafety level 3 laboratory [34].

South American hemorrhagic fever patients develop bleeding secondary to severe thrombocytopenia, caused in part by interferon-induced maturation arrest of megakaryocytes. Lassa fever is more likely to cause hepatic failure than thrombocytopenia. Risk of death from Lassa fever is correlated with high aspartate transaminase serum levels [19].

The Bunyaviridae

The Bunyaviridae are a family of animal and plant viruses consisting of 51 species (47 definite and 4 tentative), divided into five genera; four genera infect animals and one infects plants [4–8,35,36]. The virus was first isolated from *Aedes* mosquitoes in 1943 during a yellow fever epidemic [36].

The Bunyaviridae are spherical enveloped viruses (80–120 nm in diameter) [4]. The genome consists of a large (designated L), medium (M), and small (S) single-stranded negative-sense RNA with the same complimentary nucleotides at the 3′ and 5′ ends. Within each genus, the terminal nucleotide sequence is conserved, but differs significantly from genus to genus within the Bunyaviridae family. All members of the family contain viral sense RNA, whereas Phlebovirus and Tospovirus genera also contain complimentary sense RNA. Bunyavirus, Hantavirus, and Nairovirus genera use negative-sense coding, whereas Phlebovirus (includes Rift Valley fever) and Tospovirus (plant diseases) genera use ambisense coding [35].

Bunyavirus genus

Bunyavirus pathology is exemplified by that of California encephalitis, La Crosse, and Jamestown Canyon viruses. The cycle begins with an asymptomatic amplifying infection in natural vertebrate hosts (adult chipmunks, squirrels, foxes, and woodchucks for La Crosse virus; white-tailed deer for Jamestown virus; and snowshoe hares for snowshoe hare virus). Mosquitoes (ie, *Aedes triseriatus* in La Crosse virus, *Culiseta inorata* in Jamestown virus) become infected after feeding on these animals. The virus replicates in the mosquito midgut, then disseminates to all organs including the ovaries and mosquito salivary gland. The mosquito bite, in turn, infects humans. Mosquito ovarian infection is important in maintaining the virus in the mosquito population.

In humans, virus spreads from subcutaneous tissue to skeletal muscle where it replicates, and then secondarily spreads by lymphatics to distant skeletal and cardiac muscle where another round of replication takes place. From here, the virus disseminates to the central nervous system where it replicates in neurons and glial cells. This is followed by neuronal cell necrosis. Death occurs in 3 to 4 days. Brain lesions (principally the cerebral cortex and brainstem) consist of edema, perivascular cuffing, glial nodules, and leptomeningitis with some areas of focal necrosis [36].

Phlebovirus genus

In 1908, Doerr demonstrated that phlebotomus fevers were caused by a filterable agent [7]. The Phlebovirus that causes Rift Valley fever was first isolated from a newborn lamb in 1930 during an epidemic in sheep that caused both abortions and high mortality. "Sandfly fever" Sicilian and Naples viruses were isolated from American troops in Palermo in 1943 and Naples in 1944. Similar diseases were described during the Napoleonic Wars and again in 1905.

"Abortion storms" were described as early as 1931 as Rift Valley fever swept through herds of cattle and sheep. More recent abortion storms have been attributed to equine herpesvirus type 1 (especially Army 183 F–fetal strain); *Coxiella burnetii*; Thogoto virus (transmitted by Ixodid ticks); *Neospora caninum*; and one strain of equine arteritis virus [37–44]. It is important to be aware that abortion storms may be an early sign of a zootic or a bioterrorist attack with a hemorrhagic fever virus or other agents. Unfortunately, only 25% of abortion storm etiologic agents are ever identified [45].

Rift Valley fever infection is initiated by the bite of an infected mosquito. The inoculated virus is trapped in the local lymph nodes where it replicates and becomes the source for the primary viremia. The major organs are infected, and the second round of replication takes place in distant lymph nodes, spleen, liver, adrenals, lungs, and kidneys. Necrotic foci develop in the liver and in the brain of patients with clinical encephalitis. In hemorrhagic fever, thrombocytopenia and fibrin deposits in major organs are seen [36].

Punta toro virus infection in hamsters has become an experimental model for Rift Valley fever. In this model, the liver injury is responsible for the hemorrhagic complications. Viral replication directly causes apoptosis. Cellular viability decreases 12 hours after infection. Caspases 3/7 are activated, phosphatidylserine translocation and DNA fragmentation occur between 48 to 72 hours. Viral infection alone without systemic inflammatory reaction induces the hemorrhagic disease and suggests targets for therapeutics [46].

Nairovirus genus

The Nairovirus genus consist of tick-borne viruses with few being transmitted by culicoides flies and mosquitoes (CCHF: ticks [some species of *Hyalomma*, *Dermacentor*, and *Rhipicephalus*] and flies; Nairobi sheep disease: ticks, flies, mosquitoes) [36]. CCHF worldwide distribution mirrors *Hyalomma* ticks more closely than other species. The disease has been reported throughout sub-Saharan Africa, South Africa, Madagascar, the Middle East, European Russia, Pakistan, Afghanistan, the central Asian republics, Bulgaria, the former Yugoslavia, northern Greece, and Xijiang province of northern China [16,36,47]. CCHF and nairoviruses survive through various tick life-stages (transstadial transmission) and from tick generation to generation (transovarian transmission). Vertebrates (including ground-feeding birds in European Russia, Bulgaria, and Greece) provide blood-meals for infected ticks, become infected, and the viral source for uninfected ticks (viral amplification) [16,36,47]. Sheep, goats, cattle, ostriches, large wild herbivores, hares, and hedgehogs are known to amplify CCHF, and sheep and goats are known to amplify the other nairoviruses.

In Africa, the distribution of nairovirus infection follows the distribution of the tick host, *Rhipicephalus appendiculatus*. In the Middle East and India, the distribution of human infection follows the *Haemaphysalis intermedia* ticks and the closely related Ganjam virus [36].

Nairovirus reproduces in spleen, liver, and kidneys; and in sheep, goat, and suckling mouse infections, the vascular endothelium becomes the primary viral target. Edema and necrosis of the capillary walls of the mucosa of the intestine, gallbladder, and female genital tract is seen with the development of hemorrhage and inflammation [36]. In humans, local viral replication follows spread by blood and lymphatics to all major organs, especially the liver. There is edema, hemorrhage, and necrosis; diffuse intravascular coagulation (DIC); and thrombocytopenia with the expected abnormalities of the coagulation profile. IgM and IgG responses are detectable by Day 9 in survivors and are absent in most fatal cases [36].

Hantavirus genus

The *Hantavirus* genus first came to medical attention in 1934 with the publication of a case of hemorrhagic fever with renal syndrome [5]. Between 1951 and 1953, 3000 cases of an acute febrile illness, 33% with hemorrhagic manifestations, were reported among the United Nation's troops during the Korean War. First known as Korean hemorrhagic fever, now it is commonly referred to as hemorrhagic fever with renal syndrome (HFRS) [36]. *Apodemus agrarius* (the field mouse) was found to be the reservoir. The virus, first isolated in 1978, was designated the Hantaan virus after the Hantaan River (Korea) where many of the original cases were described. *Rattus norvegicus* and *R rattus* were the hosts of Seoul virus, the cause of urban HFRS [5,36]. In Scandinavia, nephropathia epidemica, a renal disease with mild or without hemorrhagic manifestations, was caused by Puumala virus spread from *Clethrionomys glareolus*, the bank vole. The only insectivore to harbor a hantavirus is the *Suncus murinus*, the Indian tree shrew. Prospect Hill virus was the first hantavirus causing human disease to be described in the Americas (*Microtus pennsylvanicus* [meadow vole] host). Severe HFRS of the Balkans was caused by Dobrava virus associated with *Apodemus flavicollis*. At least three subfamilies and 28 species of hantaviruses cause either HFRS or hantavirus pulmonary syndrome (HPS) [5,36,48].

In 1993, in the southwestern United States (Four Corners region, the meeting point of New Mexico, Arizona, Colorado, and Utah) an outbreak of an influenza-type illness that rapidly progressed to respiratory failure, shock, and death in 2 to 10 days (HPS) was found to be caused by the hantavirus Sin Nombre, with a reservoir in the deer mouse, *Peromyscus maniculatus* [49]. In Argentina, *Akodon azarae* is the most abundant rodent with a hantavirus seroprevalence of 9.3% [27].

The first outbreak of HPS in Central America (Los Santos, Panama) occurred in 1999 to 2000 with 11 cases, nine confirmed by serology and three fatalities. Household and neighborhood serologic studies found seropositivity of 13%, but no suggestion of person-to-person spread [50]. Western Venezuela is the home of the Maporal virus (closely related to South American HPS viruses) that infects the fulvous pygmy rice rat (*Oligoryzomys fulvescens*) [51].

Since that discovery, 10 different hantaviruses with 10 different rodent reservoirs have been shown to cause HPS throughout North and South America [5,36]. Identification of high-risk areas is essential for controlling human infection. Bayou virus is the second leading cause of HPS in the United States. Its rodent hosts include *Oryzomys palustris* (most commonly infected species, 16% seroprevalence rate), *Sigmodon hispidus*, *Peromyscus leucopus*, *Reithrodontomys fulvescens*, and *Baiomys taylori*. The heaviest male rodents had the highest seroprevalence. Seroprevalence is higher in the coastal prairie (20%) than old-fields (10.5%), and is directly related to host population densities [52].

The first cases of HPS in Maranhao State, Brazil, have been identified and the viruses designated as the Anajatuba and the Rio Mamore viruses (isolated from *Oligoryzomys fornesi* and *Gikicgukys scuyreys*) [53,54]. Two cases of HPS appeared in two areas of central Bolivia after dense forest was destroyed and replaced with pastures and sugarcane. *Oligoryzomys microtis* and *Calomys callosus* were identified as the rodent reservoirs associated with human disease [55]. It is interesting to note that neither HPS nor HFRS have been reported in Australia despite the fact that Hantavirus antibody–positive rodents have been found across the continent [56].

Hantavirus establishes an asymptomatic infection in its natural rodent reservoir that persists for months or years. In at-risk areas, the disease is spread (horizontally) by scratching, biting, or infected aerosols among the rodents. The virus spreads to all organs but particularly concentrates in the kidneys and lungs, with high rates of replication in the salivary glands. Virus is shed in urine, feces, and saliva, peaking 2 to 10 weeks after infection, and continuing for life, although in reduced quantity with rising antibody titers. There is no cell death observed in the infected animal-hosts. Seroprevalence studies in endemic areas have found *R norvegicus* to be the most frequently infected species (Kinmen study: *R norvegicus*, 50%; *Mus musculus*, 20%; *R flavipectus*, 2%) [57].

Most hantavirus infections are asymptomatic or go undetected. In India, there have been no reports of either HPS or HRFS [58]. A study of 152 patients with febrile illness found 23 (14.7%) seropositive by enzyme immunoassay for IgM directed against hantavirus. Eighteen (82%) of 22 patients were positive by indirect immunofluorescence assay. In the same study, 5.7% of healthy blood donors were positive by enzyme immunoassay, and 40% of these patients were positive by immunofluorescence assay [58]. A similar survey on Kinmen (an island between China and Taiwan) found a seroprevalence of 8.23% among scrub typhus-negative individuals [57].

HPS and HFRS infect humans after inhalation of infected rodent excreta. There is no cytopathologic effect in infected human cells. The lethal pathology seems to be immune modulated and a direct result of viral induction of cell apoptosis [29,46,59]. Other Bunyaviridae infections (Akabane and Aino viruses, the causes of abortion, stillbirths, and congenital defects in cattle, sheep, and goats) also result in the induction of apoptosis [60].

Paradoxically, serologic tests on individuals with frequent occupational contact with rodents had little or no evidence of exposure to Sin Nombre virus (the cause of HPS); Whitewater Arroyo virus (an Arenaviridae); or Ampari virus [61].

HFRS patients have acute tubulointerstitial nephritis. Puumala virus–associated HFRS results in interstitial infiltration of lymphocytes, plasma cells, monocyte-macrophages, neutrophils, and eosinophilic granulocytes. In HPS and HFRS there is a general increased production of cytokines [36].

Monocytes and macrophages play an important role in HPS and HFRS pathophysiology. Viral infection causes HFRS-infected cells to undergo complex metabolic changes with a resultant (infected cell) increase in bactericidal activity against *Staphylococcus aureus* [62].

The Filoviridae

Ebola and Marburg make up the two genera of the filoviridae [9,10,63]. Both genera are enveloped, single-stranded negative-sense RNA viruses. Ebola is bacilliform, bent-pin shaped; Marburg is filamentous shaped. Ebola virus was first isolated and identified in 1976, with its genetic sequence published in 1989. Marburg virus was first described in 1967, and its gene sequence was published in 1992 [9,10]. There are four species of Ebola virus (Zaire, Sudan, Reston, and Cote d'Ivoire) and one species of Marburg virus [63,64].

The macaque develops disease similar to humans after inhalation or injection of the virus. The Zaire species is the most virulent (60%–90% case fatality rate [65,66]) and the Reston species is the least virulent. The viral infection produces viral cytopathology, cytokine-mediated vascular leaks, and impairment of the host response. Macrophages and monocytes are some of the earliest cells infected, damaging the host's immune response and facilitating the spread of the virus.

Human pathology

Patients dying of either Ebola or Marburg hemorrhagic fevers exhibit necrosis of parenchymal cells of the liver, spleen, kidneys, ovaries, and testes. In the liver, there is hepatocellular necrosis with intact, hyalinized, ghost-like cells amid cellular debris filled with virions. Intact hepatocytes display intracytoplasmic inclusion bodies, which represent aggregates of viral nucleocapsids. There is injury to the microvasculature (Kupffer cells and capillary endothelium) with increased endothelial permeability that contributes to the shock and bleeding. There is lymphoid depletion in the spleen and lymph nodes with vascular follicular necrosis [64].

In fatal cases, there is no antibody response. In survivors and patients with a protracted course, the patients develop a delayed humoral response

[16]. Peters and coworkers [66] provide a detailed summary of the pathologic effects of the filoviruses. The viruses suppress the induction of interferon by VP35 protein, and block interferon action by VP24 protein [67].

Transmission of disease is person-to-person. Aerosol spread to nonhuman primates has been documented. It is believed that droplet spread is the common person-to-person vehicle among infected humans; aerosol spread is probably rare. Handling infected monkeys has been implicated in some cases. The source in nature remains unknown, although recent evidence of asymptomatic infection in fruit bats has been reported [64,65,68].

The Flaviviridae

In 1900 in Cuba, Walter Reed and James Carroll of the US Army Medical Corp proved Dr. Carlos Finlay's theory that yellow fever was transmitted by mosquitoes. Yellow fever virus was the first flavivirus to be isolated (1927) and grown in vitro (1932). There are 73 species of flaviviruses. The Flaviviridae are spherical, enveloped, single-stranded positive-sense RNA viruses [11–13,69–71]. The Flaviviridae consist of three genera: (1) Flavivirus (dengue virus, Ilheus virus, Japanese encephalitis virus, Kyasanur Forest disease virus, Kunjin virus, louping ill virus, Murray Valley encephalitis virus, Omsk hemorrhagic fever virus, Powassan virus, Rocio virus, St Louis encephalitis, tick-borne encephalitis, Wesselsbron disease, West Nile fever, yellow fever, and Zika disease); (2) Hepacivirus (hepatitis C virus); and (3) Pestivirus (Bovine viral diarrhea viruses, border disease virus, classical swine fever virus, and various animal pestiviruses) [11–13,72,73].

Mosquito-borne flavivirus hemorrhagic fevers

Natural transmission of flaviviruses may take place by transfer of virus from host to host by contaminated mouthparts of mosquitoes. More likely, either the arthropod or mosquito acquires the virus through a blood meal; the virus replicates in the epithelial cells lining the mesenteron (midgut); the replicated virus escapes to the hemocele and infects the salivary gland; and is secreted in the saliva during the next feeding, infecting a new host [70,74]. With dengue viruses, the virus may enter a number of mosquito ova, directly infecting mosquito progeny.

Dengue virus

Dengue virus survives in two hosts: the vector and the reservoir. *A aegypti* and other *Aedes* species are the most common mosquito vectors. *A aegypti* requires 10^5/mL viral titers in humans to become infected after a blood meal. This helps select out for strains of virus that rapidly reproduce [70,74].

In nonhuman primates, the virus replicates principally in monocytes in skin, lymph nodes, spleen, liver, lung, and thymus. Dengue fever is self-limited with skin lesions showing swelling of endothelial cells of small vessels, perivascular edema, and monocyte infiltration. Dengue hemorrhagic fever is the result of sequential infection. The primary pathophysiologic change in dengue hemorrhagic fever is vascular permeability, leakage of plasma into the extravascular compartment, hemoconcentration, and hypotension.

It is believed that immune reaction to a second infection with dengue virus results in dengue hemorrhagic fever. Pre-existing antibodies to dengue virus are heterologous, do not neutralize the virus, and permit the virus to replicate freely in the macrophage. A second theory contends that the virus mutates [70,74].

Chimeric dengue, tick-borne encephalitis, and West Nile virus (live-attenuated) vaccines are now under development [75]. Other control methods under consideration have been the introduction of sterile male mosquitoes to facilitate the displacement of the insect from the habitat [76].

Yellow fever virus

Yellow fever virus is transmitted to humans from infected humans or infected primates by tree-hole breeding mosquitoes (*Haemagogus janthinomys*, *Haemagogus* sp, *Saabethes chloropterus*, *Aedes* sp) usually during the tropical wet season and early dry season. As with other hemorrhagic fever viruses, the mosquito introduces the virus into the skin where it replicates locally and then spreads into the regional lymph nodes. The virus then disseminates by the bloodstream to the liver, spleen, bone marrow, and myocardium. The hallmark of the disease is steatosis, apoptosis, and necrosis mainly in the midzonal region of the liver [77]. Kupffer cells are infected followed by hepatocytes in the midzone of the liver. Midzonal necrosis develops. The appearance of Councilman's bodies is indicative of hepatocyte apoptosis with minimum mononuclear infiltrates [78]. There is a predominance of apoptosis over necrosis with contributions from a variety of activated lymphocytes and various cytokines, notably transforming growth factor-β [77].

Yellow fever vaccine is a live-attenuated vaccine given every 10 years for those at risk and produces immunity in 95% of recipients [79,80]. Experimental compound ZX-2401 inhibits yellow fever virus, dengue virus, bovine viral diarrhea virus, banzi virus, and West Nile virus and may become a candidate chemotherapeutic agent [81].

Tick-borne flavivirus hemorrhagic fevers

Kyasanur Forest disease (India). In humans, the virus produces parenchymal degeneration of the liver and kidneys, hemorrhagic pneumonia, increase in the reticuloendothelial tissue in the liver and spleen, and marked erythrophagocytosis. Macaques develop fatal infections with lymph tissue necrosis and some primates develop encephalitis with chromatolysis of neurons and focal demyelination.

The primary vector is the *Haemaphysalis spinigera* tick, although 10 species of ixodid ticks have also been implicated. Ticks transmit the virus among themselves by transstadial and transovarial transmission. Bats and ground-dwelling birds may be reservoirs. Cows, goats, and sheep have also become infected, but their epidemiologic importance is unknown [70,82].

Omsk hemorrhagic fever (Siberia). Dermacentor reticulates and *Ixodes apronophorus* are suspected vectors, and the *Arvicola terrestris* is believed to be the host [70].

Clinical presentations and management

Managing VHFs involves basic diagnostic, therapeutic, prophylactic, and infection control concepts, and a practical monitoring system for contacts. Guidelines must be understandable, practical, and make clear recommendations concerning any controversial treatments [17,83]. It is recommended that these guidelines include the following for possible VHF bioterrorism incidents:

1. Identify the patient and develop a complete differential diagnosis (which most often includes malaria, typhoid, gastroenteritis, meningococcemia, or other diseases). Examples of case definitions may be found on page 248 of reference 84 [84].
2. Notify public health authorities (in the United States and its territories, this is done through the local or state health departments).
3. Clinical laboratories must be organized and prepared through quality assurance activities properly to handle, test, and forward when indicated suspect specimens [85]. Confirm or eliminate the diagnosis by either viral isolation, identification of viral antigens by ELISA or polymerase chain reaction (PCR), or use of the modern antibody testing. All viral isolation specimens should be sent to a biosafety level 4 laboratory.
4. Isolate the patient and institute and strictly enforce infection control measures (strict isolation, negative pressure rooms). Intensive care is likely to be required. Adequate numbers of isolation beds where an "intensive" level of care may be delivered should be preplanned [86,87]. Details of the 11 specific protective measures recommended to prevent nosocomial spread of VHF viruses (including the use of the N-95 mask or powered air-purifying respirators) may be found in reference 14, page 210 [14]. Special training is necessary for laboratory workers handling patient specimens, postmortem practices, and environmental decontamination (linens, beds, hospital rooms, and so forth).
5. Identify at-risk contacts and institute prophylaxis where available and if recommended by public health authorities. At the present time, ribavirin prophylaxis is controversial [14].
6. On-going monitoring must be instituted for all at-risk contacts. A self-monitoring system is preferred because it is less labor- and resource-intensive [83].
7. Aggressively manage the patient with supportive therapy.

8. Provide specific antiviral therapy where available. Begin ribavirin pending the identification of the etiologic agent. Continue treatment if an arenavirus or a bunyavirus is identified. Discontinue therapy if flavivirus or filovirus or other viruses that do not respond to ribavirin are identified [14].
9. There is no licensed vaccine except for Yellow fever. Ribavirin prophylaxis is controversial because it may only delay the onset of disease [14].

The Arenaviridae

Lassa virus: Lassa fever

Lassa fever virus, of the Arenaviridae [88], was discovered 30 years ago and is endemic in West equatorial Africa. Serosurveys reveal antibody prevalence of 8% to 52% in Sierra Leone, 4% to 55% in Guinea, and 21% in Nigeria [89]. In Sierra Leone, Guinea, and Nigeria, the United Nations Development Program estimates that there are 59 million seronegative at-risk individuals, 3 million first-time infections per year, 3 million reinfections per year, and 67,000 deaths per year [89]. The *Matomys natalensis* rodent is its principle host in savannah and forest regions (11% antibody positive) and *Mus musculus* its principle host in coastal and urban areas (5% antibody positive) [90]. *M natalensis* caught near homes are 0% to 80% seropositive. Five percent to 22% of susceptible individuals seroconvert each year; the ratio of illness to infection is 9% to 26%; and 5% to 14% of those who seroconvert is febrile. Mortality rates are estimated at 1% to 2% of all those infected [91].

The peak incidence is believed to be in the dry season (January–March), but in Sierra Leone it overlaps with the rainy season (May–November). The incidence of disease in tropical endemic regions may drop off into the rainy season because of difficulty with travel [89]. The virus causes 5000 deaths among the 100,000 to 300,000 people per year it infects. Most infections are mild or asymptomatic (80%) and but there is a 1% overall mortality and a 15% to 20% mortality for patients requiring hospitalization.

Lassa fever may present anywhere in the world that is accessible to air travel [89,92,93]. Guidelines need to be clear and practical; international aspects need to be considered including the need for "reliable risk assessment to be performed before patients are medically evacuated"; and self-monitoring should be considered, because active surveillance is resource intense [83].

Although the incubation period is from 5 days to 3 weeks, most cases present within 7 to 14 days after exposure. The onset of the disease is gradual with fever, malaise, and myalgia. The patient develops conjunctival injection, pharyngitis with white and yellow exudates or ulcers, cough, chest pain, and abdominal pain with nausea and vomiting. Patients with mild disease improve within 10 days.

Severely ill patients develop facial and laryngeal edema, cyanosis, mild bleeding, and shock. In some patients severe disease is commonly complicated by pleural and pericardial effusions. These patients are noted to have mild thrombocytopenia and dysfunctional platelets. The patients' white blood cell counts are normal or reduced, and commonly with Lassa fever there is a mild elevation of aspartate transaminase levels. In some patients hepatitis is severe [16,17].

Thirty percent of patients develop permanent late sensorineural deafness. Sudden onset of deafness has been associated with Lassa virus seropositivity. There is no relationship between severity of illness, initial hearing loss, and eventual recovery [89]. Patients with neurologic complications (tremors, confusion, seizures, and coma) often die.

Pregnant women have the highest mortality rates (16%). Lassa virus crosses the placenta and commonly results in abortion, particularly in the third trimester. Overall mortality is between 1% and 2%. In hospitalized patients, the mortality is 15% to 20%. Poor prognostic signs include pharyngitis, tachypnea, bloody diarrhea, and high fever.

In children, 100% have fever and 60% have a cough and vomiting. The highest overall prevalence is among 5- to 9-year-old age group (41%). More girls develop clinical disease [94].

Differential diagnosis of Lassa hemorrhagic fever includes malaria, typhoid, other VHFs, meningococcemia, and sepsis. In Sierra Leone, fever, pharyngitis with exudates or ulcers, chest pain, and proteinuria were likely to be Lassa fever in 80% of cases [16,17]. On admission, most patients have antibodies against the virus (53% IgG and 67% IgM). Positive ELISAs for Lassa virus antigen combined with IgM antibody is 88% sensitive and 90% specific for the diagnosis of acute Lassa fever [89].

Lassa fever is acquired by rodent excreta that is either inhaled or contaminates food, or by person-to-person transmission. It is essential that precautions be taken with those who recover from the disease, because viremia is present into the second week of the clinical illness and virus is found in urine for 3 to 9 weeks and in semen for 2 to 3 months. There are no data as to the relative risk of sexual transmission [89,92].

Diagnosis is made by isolating the virus from blood, throat swabs, or urine in biosafety level 4 laboratory. ELISA detects Lassa virus antigen that may be confirmed by reverse transcriptase (RT)–PCR by Day 3 of illness. Specific antibody testing by IgM ELISA is also available and has replaced the indirect fluorescent antibody tests [16,89]. Other laboratory abnormalities include lymphocytopenia and thrombocytopenia that peaks between 10 and 11 days [89].

For prophylaxis and treatment of Lassa fever including pregnant women [14,16,17,84,87,95], high-dose intravenous ribavirin is recommended, 2 g intravenous loading dose followed by 1 g intravenously every 6 hours for 4 days. This is followed by 0.5 g intravenously every 8 hours for 6 days. It is recommended that women stop breast-feeding. Another recommended intravenous regimen is an initial dose of 30 mg/kg followed by 15 mg/kg every 6 hours for 4 days, followed by 7.5 mg/kg every 8 hours for 6 days. Oral ribavirin doses are, 2 g loading dose followed by 4 g/d in four divided doses for 4 days followed by 2 g/d for six doses. Oral ribavirin is believed to be only half as effective as intravenous therapy. Intravenous ribavirin, if given within 6 days of the beginning of symptoms, reduces mortality by 90% [89]. Postexposure prophylaxis with ribavirin is recommended by some but not all authorities. This consists of 2 g orally in four divided doses for 7 days [14,16,17,78,84,95]. Zidampidine, a derivative of zidovudine, is a new agent that seems effective in treating the CD-1 mouse model of Lassa VHF [96].

Control of rodents in or near dwellings and strict isolation of hospitalized patients are important [97]. In one survey in Ekpom, Nigeria, of 218 captured *M natalensis* rodents, 46.8% were positive for complement fixing antibody to Lassa virus [98].

New vaccines, including a DNA mini-gene vaccine that encodes for Lassa virus proteins (full-length Lassa nucleoprotein) has been found to induce $CD8^+$ T-cell responses in mice that can protect against lymphocytic choriomeningitis virus and Pichinde virus. A DNA vaccine that encodes for a nine amino acid sequence from Lassa nucleoprotein has also induced $CD8^+$ T cells and has been protective in the mouse model against viral challenges [99].

Another candidate vaccine has been produced from an attenuated recombinant vesicular stomatitis virus that expresses Lassa viral glycoprotein. The vaccine protected nonhuman primates against a lethal viral challenge, and none of the test animals was found to shed the virus. Both protective humoral and cellular responses occurred. Despite a documented Lassa fever virus viremia 7 days after the challenge, none of the vaccinated animals displayed evidence of clinical disease [100].

A live attenuated vaccine produced from the reassortment of genomic segments from Lassa virus and Mopeia virus encodes for major viral antigens (nucleocapsid and glycoprotein of Lassa virus and RNA polymerase and zinc-binding protein of Mopeia virus). Immunity against Lassa virus has been demonstrated in guinea pigs, mice, and Rhesus macaques. Two of the monkeys were examined and revealed no histologic lesions or signs of disease [101]. The nonpathogen, Uukuniemi virus (a Bunyaviridae), has been used as a model for more than 30 years to study the molecular and cell biology of the highly pathogenic members of this family [102,103].

Approximately 20 cases of Lassa fever imported into western countries have resulted in no secondary clinical cases. The contacts of an imported case from the Ivory Coast by way of Lisbon to Germany were studied. The patient was diagnosed by PCR and died of hemorrhagic fever by Day 14. Of 232 contacts, 149 (with 30 close contacts) were tested serologically. No clinical illness was reported, and only a physician who examined the patient on Day 9 was IgG antibody positive. Ribavirin (10 mg/kg orally four times daily for 5–8 days) prophylaxis was started by 16 of the high-risk and close contacts after the index case's diagnosis was confirmed. Eleven of these patients had reversible increases in bilirubin (one person with jaundice on Day 4 of therapy), and nine had decreases in hemoglobin [104].

Recommendations for the management of Lassa fever in Europe [105] include the following. Management of patients has varied. Negative pressure rooms and universal precautions (The Netherlands), completely enclosed "plastic bubble units" (Trexler Units, United Kingdom), and staff isolation suits (Germany) have all been used. The Trexler Units made it impossible to provide intensive care to the sickest patients, and the isolation suits made it difficult for staff to care for patients more than 3 hours at a time. One publication concluded that all patients should be hospitalized; mildly ill patients may be managed with negative pressure rooms and strict isolation. Patients more severely ill should be managed in high-security isolation facilities [105].

Low-risk contact monitoring should consist of self-monitoring of temperatures without reporting regularly to health authorities. Persons directly in contact with patients' body fluids, blood, or secretions should self-monitor temperatures and report regularly to the health departments [105].

Evidence of the efficacy of ribavirin prophylaxis is limited. Ideal dose is 1 g by mouth per day in two divided doses. In Germany and the United Kingdom, prophylaxis is offered to high-risk contacts only. It is recommended that contacts be informed of the adverse reactions and be offered the medication [105].

Guanarito virus: Venezuelan hemorrhagic fever

The virus for Venezuelan hemorrhagic fever was first described in 1990. The natural host is the cane mouse, *Zygodontomys brevicaudia*. The clinical presentation is similar to Argentine hemorrhagic fever (fever, thrombocytopenia, bleeding, and in some patients neurologic complications), with 7- to 14-day incubation and 10% to 16% mortality [16,17]. Treatment and prophylaxis are the same as for Lassa fever [16,17]. Convalescent serum therapy may also be effective [97]. Diagnosis is made by isolating the virus in a biosafety level 4 laboratory. Real-time PCR assays are under development [106].

Sabia virus: Sabia virus hemorrhagic fever

Sabia virus hemorrhagic fever is characterized by marked liver necrosis and may be mistaken for yellow fever [107]. A case has been successfully treated with ribavirin. Treatment and prophylaxis are the same as for Lassa fever [16,17,95]. Rodent control in or near dwellings is important [97]. Diagnosis is made by isolating the virus in a biosafety level 4 laboratory. Real-time PCR assays are under development [106].

Junin virus: Argentine hemorrhagic fever

As with Lassa fever, patients with Argentine hemorrhagic fever present with a nonspecific illness. In 3 to 4 days, they become extremely ill with hypotension, petechiae in the soft palate, axilla, and gingiva.

Neurologic findings are more common than in Lassa fever. They begin on the fourth day of the illness with the onset of hemorrhage. Patients are more irritable, lethargic, and display muscular hypotonia, hyporeflexia, areflexia, proprioceptive disturbances, inability to ambulate, tremor of the tongue and hands, and fluctuations in level of consciousness. Severely ill patients bleed from the mucous membranes and develop shock, anuria, seizures, and coma. Untreated, 15% to 30% die [16,108].

Diagnosis is made in the first few days of the illness by isolating the virus from blood, throat swabs, or urine in biosafety level 4 laboratory. Junin virus antigen and IgM and IgG antibodies may be detected by ELISA testing [16]. Real-time PCR assays are under development [106].

Treatment and prophylaxis are the same as for Lassa fever [14,16,17,84,95]. Convalescent serum therapy may also be effective [97]. Cationic peptides (cecropin A, melittin, and indolicidin) are newer agents that seem to have activity against Junin virus and herpes simplex I and II. Indolicidin inactivated cell-free Junin virus and cecropin A are active against the arenaviruses Tacaribe and Pichinde [109].

Rodent control in or near dwellings is important. A live-attenuated vaccine is available with increasing human safety data, animal efficacy data, but insufficient human efficacy and safety data to support Food and Drug Administration licensure. Unfortunately, the vaccine is only available in Argentina [14,15,110]. Candid #1 vaccine is manufactured in Argentina and in the United States. A 1998 study found vaccine manufactured in the United States to be safe and efficacious [110]. The Argentinean vaccine has been found to be equally safe, immunogenic, and protective in guinea pigs as the vaccine manufactured in the United States [111]. Oils from aromatic plants native to San Luis Province, Argentina, exhibited antiviral activity. *Lippia junelliana* and *L turbinata* were the most potent [112].

Machupo virus: Bolivian hemorrhagic fever

Bolivian hemorrhagic fever is only naturally endemic in the Beni region of northeast Bolivia. The natural host is the rodent *C callosus*. Incubation period is 7 to 14 days and mortality is 10% to 16% [16,17,95]. Treatment and prophylaxis are the same as for Lassa fever [16,17,95]. Convalescent serum therapy may also be effective [97]. Diagnosis is made by isolating the virus in a biosafety level 4 laboratory. Real-time PCR assays are under development [106]. Rodent control in or near dwellings is important. There is evidence of cross-protection by Junin virus vaccine [84,97].

Whitewater Arroyo virus: Whitewater Arroyo virus hemorrhagic fever

The virus for Whitewater Arroyo virus hemorrhagic fever was first isolated from the white-throated wood rat *Neotoma albigula* in northwestern New Mexico. Infection (in mice) results in lymphocytic meningitis and perivascular lymphocytic cuffing. Neonatal infection in the mouse results in chronic (lifelong) infection and viral shedding [113,114]. There have been only a handful of cases.

New therapeutic modalities for Arenaviridae and other RNA viruses

Because RNA viruses replicate with high error rates, they have the potential to rapidly develop drug-resistant mutants. Rather than "chase" the resistant strains with newer anti-infective agents, Grande-Perez and coworkers and others [115,116] attempted to increase the replication error rate to force viral extinction before resistance mutants arise. They did this in vitro (cell cultures) with lymphocytic choriomeningitis virus treated with fluorouracil. The phenomenon was seen at both high and low doses of the mutagen.

The Bunyaviridae

Bunyavirus genus

In California encephalitis, La Crosse virus, Jamestown Canyon virus, and Oropouche virus there is encephalitis and generalized febrile illnesses usually without hemorrhagic fever. Bunyamwera virus (previously referred to as Garissa virus) was isolated from two patients and serologically detected in 27% of the patients during a large outbreak of hemorrhagic fever (1997–1998) in Kenya, Tanzania, and Somalia [117]. Studies of the two isolates found that there was genetic reassortment that altered its potential for disease. The Ngari virus was responsible for this outbreak. The Garissa virus is an isolate of Ngari virus, which is a Bunyamwera virus reassortment species [117,118].

Phlebovirus genus: Rift Valley fever

Rift Valley fever virus is a zoonosis that commonly causes abortions in livestock herds. Mortality in ruminants is 10% to 30%, and 1% in humans [119]. Outbreaks are associated with heavy rainfall, sustained flooding, and the appearance of large numbers of mosquitoes [120]. Humans become infected by mosquito bite or handling infected animal blood or tissue. Although human-to-human transmission has not been reported, appropriate infection control procedures should be used. After a 2- to 6-day incubation period, most patients develop a self-limited nonspecific febrile illness [121]. Patients present with sudden onset of fever, headache, joint and muscle pains, conjunctivitis, and photophobia. In a few patients, after a brief initial illness and partial recovery, symptoms return followed by a protracted convalescence.

Five percent to 10% of patients develop retinal disease 1 to 3 weeks after the febrile illness. Patients experience macular exudates, retinal hemorrhages, and vasculitis. Half of these patients have permanent visual impairment. One percent to 5% develops central nervous system complications. One percent develops typical VHF [16,122].

Aggressive supportive care and ribavirin (in similar doses as for Lassa fever) are recommended therapies for complicated cases. Human immune serum is also recommended when available [16,17,121].

Virus may be isolated from the blood during the first week of illness by intracerebral injection into baby mice. Laboratory-acquired cases have been reported and viral isolation should be performed in a biosafety 4 level laboratory. RT-PCR detects virus in the blood and enzyme immunoassay detects IgG and IGM [121].

Treatment and prophylaxis are the same as for Lassa fever [14,16,17,49,84,95]. A live attenuated vaccine is available for livestock. A formalin-killed Rift Valley fever vaccine is available for humans, but requires an annual booster [122]. Mosquito and rodent control, insect repellants, and personal protective clothing are essential for preventing illness [49,79]. Attenuated mutagenised (by 5-fluorouracil) Rift Valley fever virus vaccine (RFV MP 12) has been tested in sheep, cattle, and Rhesus macaques [122–124]. The South African vaccine strain of lumpy skin disease virus (type SA-Neethling) is being tested for recombinant vaccines expressing the structural glycoprotein gene of bovine ephemeral fever virus or two glycoprotein genes of Rift Valley fever [125]. DNA vaccines for Rift Valley fever, CCHF, tick-borne encephalitis, and Hantaan virus were tested in mice. The Rift Valley fever and tick-borne encephalitis vaccines were protective, whereas the other two vaccines were less immunogenic [126].

Nairovirus genus: Congo-Crimean hemorrhagic fever

The first cases recognized in modern times were documented in 1944. The virus was isolated in 1967 from patients with the Crimean disease and was found to be identical with the virus isolated from a child from the Congo in 1956. Humans are infected by (*Hyalomma* sp) tick-bite, crushing infected ticks against their skin, contact with blood from infected livestock, or from infected patients blood and body fluids [16,17,127]. In some areas, the disease exhibits biannual peaks (March–May and August–October) [128].

The incubation following a tick bite is 1 to 3 days; the incubation following contact with contaminated blood is 5 to 6 days. Nosocomial transmission has been well documented [129]. Most infections are symptomatic. Patients present with sudden onset of fever, chills, headache, dizziness, neck pain, and myalgia. Lymphadenopathy and tender hepatomegaly is seen in most patients. Nausea, vomiting, neuropsychiatric symptoms, and cardiovascular signs and symptoms manifest themselves in some patients as the disease progresses [127]. Some patients develop nausea, vomiting, and diarrhea [130]. Patients later develop flushing and hemorrhage, especially profuse gastrointestinal bleeding. Severely ill patients develop DIC, and renal, hepatic, and respiratory failure [16]. There is a 30% overall mortality [127].

Laboratory studies reveal leucopenia, thrombocytopenia, and elevated transaminase levels. Mortality ranges from 15% to 30% [16,17].

Treatment consists of supportive therapy and ribavirin using the same regimen as outlined for Lassa fever or World Health Organization oral regimen: 30 mg/kg loading dose followed by 15 mg/kg every 6 hours for 4 days, followed by 7.5 mg/kg every 6 hours for 6 days [49,84,95]. This therapy is not approved by the Food and Drug Administration [127].

Although CCHF is transmissible by aerosol, technical difficulties stand in the way of mass production [14,131]. Control of the disease depends on tick control (spraying camp sites, clothing, and tick-infested areas with acaricide or repellents); ribavirin prophylaxis; effective disinfection; and decontamination. Patients must be cared for in strict isolation. Written procedures for the establishment of an isolation unit, barrier nursing, safety measures, handling of patient specimens, and laboratory protocols must be established and enforced [132,133]. Early recognition of disease is essential to limit spread and prevent mortality [134].

Hantavirus genus

Hemorrhagic fever with renal syndrome. During the Korean War (1950–1952), 3000 United Nations troops developed a symptom complex of fever, hemorrhage, acute renal failure, shock, and a mortality of 10% [16]. The etiologic agent (Hantaan virus) was isolated in 1978 from the field mouse, *A agrarius*. Related viruses are the Dobrava virus (the Balkans), which causes severe hemorrhagic fever; Seoul virus (the Far East), which causes a milder hemorrhagic fever; and Puumala virus (Scandinavia), which causes nephropathia epidemica. Puumala virus has also been implicated in cases of HFRS [16,135].

The usual incubation period is 2 to 3 weeks, but may range from 2 days to 2 months. Distinct clinical disease phases have been described [16,136].

1. Febrile phase: Patients present acutely with a flu-like illness with low back pain from retroperitoneal edema, flushing of the face, and conjunctival and pharyngeal injection secondary to vascular dilatation.
2. Hypotensive phase: The second phase consists of mild hypotension or shock and hemorrhage lasing for 1 to 2 days. Patients may only manifest petechiae or develop massive gastrointestinal bleeding or low-grade DIC.
3. Oliguric phase: The third phase is associated with hypertension and renal failure, and in some patients pulmonary edema and change in mental status. If untreated, 50% of the deaths occur at this time.
4. Diuretic phase: The diuretic phase may last for several months.
5. Convalescent phase

Laboratory findings include thrombocytopenia, leukocytosis, hemoconcentration, abnormal clotting profile, and proteinuria. Mortality is estimated at 1%, to 5% to 15% [16,17].

Puumala and Dobrava viruses principally attack the kidneys. All clinically ill patients had enlarged kidneys by sonography. The minority of patients manifest ascites (32% of Dobrava virus infections and 4% of Puumala virus infections) and pleural effusion (16% of Dobrava virus infections). Dobrava virus–infected patients tended to be more ill. They had higher serum creatinine and urea nitrogen levels, 28% required dialysis, and 4% died [137].

An 18-year survey in the Pomurje region of Slovenia found that most cases of HFRS occurred between May and August, and in patients with outdoor occupations. The median age was 39 years, and 19 of the 25 patients were male. Puumala virus caused many more cases than Dobrava virus (23 versus 2 cases). Oliguric renal failure was seen in 13 (57%) of 23 Puumala virus–infected patients. Six (26%) of the 23 patients with Puumala virus infection and one (50%) of the two patients with Dobrava virus infection were hypotensive with signs of shock. Seven (47%) of 15 patients had elevated cerebrospinal fluid protein (all patients), and 7 (41%) of 17 Puumala virus patients had sinus bradycardia [135].

Seoul virus produces milder disease with febrile, mild hemorrhagic manifestations, with hepatomegaly and mildly elevated liver enzymes. Puumala virus produces the mildest infection with fever, petechiae, and the onset of oliguria on Day 6 of disease. Ten percent of patients require dialysis, and 20% develop reversible central nervous system symptoms (confusion and dizziness) [16,17].

A recent outbreak of HFRS among Russian military personnel stationed in the Primorskii region reported the greatest number of cases within 2 weeks of the first case. There were 104 cases; 77.8% were 18 to 20 year olds; and there was 7.4% mortality [138].

A study of 1600 Korean War veterans who had contracted HFRS found no increase in long-term mortality and only a questionable increase in selective morbidities [139]. Hypopituitarism with an atrophic pituitary gland and an empty sella (on MRI) has been reported as a late complication of HFRS [140].

Aggressive supportive therapy and ribavirin has been shown significantly to improve survival. A killed vaccine is available with increasing human safety data, animal efficacy data, but insufficient human efficacy and safety data to support Food and Drug Administration licensure [84]. Formalin inactivated vaccines for Hantaan and Seoul viruses have been used in Asia [16,141]. Chinese monovalent vaccines are said to be 95% effective. The Chinese have data on a new bivalent vaccine that seroconverts 85% of patients with an adverse reaction rate of 0.5% [141].

Hepatitis B virus core particles with the amino-terminal 120 amino acids of the nucleocapsid of Dobrava, Hantaan, or Puumala viruses (chimeric core particles) were found to be highly immunogenic in BALB/c and C57BL/6 mice [142]. Another candidate vaccine is the recombinant *Peromyscus maniculatus* cytomegalovirus vaccine that contains Sin Nombre virus glycoprotein GI fused to enhanced green fluorescent protein gene [143].

Limiting human exposure to rodents and excreta is essential for prevention of this disease [16]. There are two studies that suggest that person-to-person spread of hantavirus of the type that causes HPS [144,145] is unlikely in the hospital setting and one study that demonstrates the possibility [22]. The differential diagnosis includes leptospirosis, typhus, pyelonephritis, poststreptococcal glomerulonephritis, acute surgical abdomen, and other hemorrhagic fevers [16,17]. Although HFRS is transmissible by aerosol, technical difficulties stand in the way of virus mass production [14].

Hanta virus pulmonary syndrome: Sin Nombre virus. HPS incubation period typically is 1 to 2 weeks but ranges from 1 to 4 weeks. Prodromal stage is usually 3 to 5 days (range: 1–10 days). Patients have an abrupt onset of symptoms: fever, myalgia, malaise, chills, anorexia, and headache. As the patient worsens, there is prostration and significant nausea, vomiting, abdominal pain, and diarrhea. Some patients present with only mild to moderate generalized discomfort. In the cardiorespiratory compromise stage, patients initially are short of breath and have evidence of pulmonary edema. They have a productive or nonproductive cough, tachypnea, fever, mild hypotension, and arterial oxygen desaturation.

Chest radiographs may be initially normal, but progressively worsen, displaying signs of pulmonary edema and acute respiratory distress syndrome. Other laboratory abnormalities include thrombocytopenia, leukocytosis, atypical lymphocytes, mildly elevated aspartate transaminase serum, prolonged partial thromboplastin time, increased serum lactate dehydrogenase, and lactic acidosis. Few patients develop DIC and bleeding.

Patients deteriorate at different rates, some dying rapidly, whereas others deteriorate and desaturate more slowly. Most deaths occur within 48 hours of admission. One third of the patients are managed successfully, and if patients survive the first 2 to 3 days, they will probably recover.

Independent of the pulmonary pathology, patients are found to have low cardiac outputs, elevated systemic vascular resistance, and normal to low pulmonary wedge pressures. Patients succumb to fatal shock and lactic acidosis. Those who survive without complications of therapy are often discharged in 2 weeks [18]. Renal failure requiring hemodialysis has accompanied acute infection [146]. Ribavirin is apparently ineffective. Intensive care decreased the mortality and a vigorous neutralizing antibody response seems to be predictive of survival [147]. Serologic testing for Sin Nombre virus may be accomplished by ELISA or Western blot assays [148].

The Filoviridae

Ebola virus: Ebola hemorrhagic fever

Following a 4- to 10-day (range: 2–21 days) incubation period, patients present with an abrupt onset of fever, severe headaches, myalgia, abdominal pain, diarrhea, and pharyngitis, with herpetic-like lesions on the mouth and pharynx. There is severe conjunctival injection and bleeding from the gums. Light-skinned patients often have a prominent maculopapular rash, which evolves into petechiae; ecchymosis; and bleeding from venepuncture sites and mucosa (with hematemesis, bloody diarrhea, and generalized mucosal hemorrhage). Neurologic complications (hemiplegia, psychosis, coma, and seizures) are common. Patients go on to develop shock, metabolic acidosis, and diffuse coagulopathy. Patients succumb by Day 10 with mortality rates from 60% to 90% for Ebola Zaire and 50% to 60% for Ebola Sudan. Mortality rates are higher for those infected by contaminated needles [16,17,65].

Initial leucopenia and lymphopenia is replaced by increases in the white blood cell counts and the appearance of viral-infected large abnormal lymphocytes with dark cytoplasm (virocytes) [16]. Although the clinical presentation for both viral infections seems to be severe disease, serosurveys in equatorial Africa in the mid-1990s found a 20% seropositivity rate for filoviruses in some populations. This suggests that the diseases maybe be widespread, and the most common infections are mild or asymptomatic [65].

Differential diagnosis is the same as for Lassa fever. Diagnosis is made in the first few days of the illness by isolating the virus in Vero cells in biosafety level 4 laboratory. Antigen may be detected by RT-PCR and antigen-capture ELISA. IgM and IgG antibodies may be detected by ELISA testing [16].

Strict isolation, safe burial practices, and an active surveillance system are described [149]. Presently, there is no vaccine or therapy available for Marburg or Ebola virus hemorrhagic fevers. Filovirus matrix protein VP40 drives spontaneous production and release of virus-like particles that resemble the infectious virions. Addition of other filovirus proteins (VP24, VP30, VP35, and filovirus glycoprotein) increases the virus-like particles production and particles that express multiple filovirus antigens. Injection of rodents with (Ebola or Marburg) virus-like particles containing glycoprotein and VP40 protects them from lethal challenges with Ebola and Marburg viruses [150–152].

Cytotoxic T lymphocytes are essential for survival during an Ebola virus infection. In C57BL/6 mice, vaccination with Venezuelan equine encephalitis virus replicons encoding for Ebola virus nucleoprotein survived a normally lethal Ebola virus infection. Polyclonal antiserum against Ebola virus nucleoprotein was not protective, whereas transfer of cytotoxic T lymphocytes specific for Ebola virus nucleoprotein was protective against Ebola virus infection [153].

Vaccines against Ebola virus are particularly difficult to develop because the disease observed in primates differs from the disease in rodents. Work with the unsuccessful vaccine candidates (attenuated Venezuelan equine encephalitis virus expressing Ebola glycoprotein and nucleoprotein; recombinant vaccinia virus expressing Ebola glycoprotein; liposomes containing lipid A and inactivated Ebola virus; and concentrated inactivated whole-virion preparation) demonstrated protection against Ebola for mice and guinea pigs, but failed in nonhuman primates [154]. Vaccine against Ebola and Marburg viruses based on recombinant vesicular stomatitis virus has been shown to protect macaques from lethal doses of the corresponding filovirus [155,156].

Prediction of epidemic spread of Ebola has been attempted by monitoring the spread of disease in nonhuman primates. Ebola outbreaks in the forest zone between Gabon and the Republic of Congo (2001–2003) were the result of handling wild animals (carcasses) that had died of infection. A monitoring system collected 98 carcasses of which analysis of 21 found that 10 gorillas, 3 chimpanzees, and 1 duiker were seropositive for Ebola virus. Between 2001 and 2003, there were five human Ebola outbreaks, each preceded by an animal zootic. The surveillance method was able to alert the health departments of two of the outbreaks weeks in advance [157].

Marburg virus: Marburg hemorrhagic fever

The clinical presentation of Marburg virus infection is similar to that of Ebola virus. The incubation period is 3 to 10 days after which there is a sudden onset of fever, chills, headache, and myalgia. After 6 to 8 days the illness may progress to severe hemorrhagic fever. On the fifth day of illness, some patients develop a maculopapular rash followed by nausea, vomiting, chest pain, sore throat, abdominal pain, and diarrhea. As patients become worse, jaundice, pancreatitis, weight loss, delirium, shock, liver failure, massive bleeding, and multiorgan failure develops [158].

Although the mortality has been recorded as 25% to 90%, it is closer to 25% to 30%. Virus may be isolated from survivors' semen as long as 3 months after recovery. Uveitis with viral isolation from the anterior chamber has been reported [16,17].

Diagnosis is made by isolating the virus in biosafety level 4 laboratory. Antigen may be detected by PCR and antigen-capture ELISA. IgM and IgG antibodies may persist for long periods [16].

An effective public health response (as seen during the outbreak in Angola, 2005) involves (1) accurate diagnosis, (2) isolation of patients and contacts, and (3) proper infection control procedures at health care facilities. Strict isolation precautions for patients are absolutely necessary. There is no vaccine or specific antiviral therapy presently available [158,159].

The Flaviviridae

Dengue and dengue hemorrhagic fever

This is the most common VHF with some estimates of over 100 million cases per year worldwide. The disease is found in every tropical country and is principally spread by *A aegypti*. There are four serotypes that produce three clinical syndromes: (1) nonspecific febrile illness; (2) dengue fever (fever, arthralgia, and rash); and (3) dengue hemorrhagic fever.

Classical dengue. The incubation period for dengue is 2 to 7 days. Patients develop "break bone fever," a sudden onset of high fevers, severe muscle pains, headache, and prostration with facial flushing, retro-orbital pain, and conjunctival injection. Half the patients have an early transient erythematous rash. Patients remain febrile, anorexic, and restless for 4 to 6 days and display mild hemorrhagic signs (positive tourniquet test, epistaxis, petechiae, or purpura). Platelet counts are usually above 100,000/mm^3, but may drop to low levels with the white blood cell count. The fever then rapidly resolves and a morbilliform or scarlatiniform rash appears, first on the extremities (with petechiae on the legs) along with generalized lymphadenopathy. Liver enzymes are abnormal but usually there is no hepatomegaly. There is a second febrile phase lasting 2 to 3 days followed by a desquamation of the rash. Convalescence is long, and patients remain debilitated and depressed during this period [16,17,121].

Dengue hemorrhagic fever. Dengue hemorrhagic fever begins on Day 2 to 5 of the classical illness. At this time, the patient goes into shock and exhibits restlessness; diaphoresis; hypotension; and hemorrhagic manifestations (positive tourniquet test, petechiae, purpura, spontaneous bleeding from the gums and gastrointestinal tract). The liver becomes enlarged and tender and some patients develop hypoproteinemia, hyponatremia, and mild elevations of the liver enzymes. Thrombocytopenia, sometimes below 10,000, develops. There is increased capillary permeability with hemoconcentration (hematocrit increasing $\leq$20%), DIC, and leucopenia, and patients develop hypotension (dengue shock syndrome). Respiratory failure ensues from alveolar hemorrhage and fluid accumulation. Renal failure secondary to hypotension and immune complex deposition, and rarely encephalopathy, follows. Mortality is 10% for dengue hemorrhagic fever and may be reduced to $<$1% with adequate fluid resuscitation [16,121].

Virus may be detected early in the disease by growth on cell culture or RNA detected by PCR. Serologic tests are also available (hemagglutination inhibition test, enzyme immunoassay, or immunofluorescence assay) on acute and convalescent serum samples [16,121].

There is no specific antiviral therapy. Aggressive supportive therapy is necessary. Candidate vaccines and chemotherapeutic agents have been discussed (see Yellow fever next). Strict isolation except for the exclusion of mosquitoes is not necessary [16,121].

Ampligen (polyI:polyC12U) is a mismatched double-stranded RNA that induces interferon production. It is being investigated for therapy of chronic fatigue syndrome; HIV infection; Epstein-Barr virus–positive Hodgkin's lymphoma; severe acute respiratory syndrome; hepatitis C; renal cell carcinoma; invasive or metastatic malignant melanoma; immune dysfunction syndrome; and flaviviruses (West Nile virus, equine encephalitis virus, dengue fever virus, and Japanese encephalitis virus). Hemispherx Biopharma has an oral Ampligen-like (polyI-polyC126) compound available, that could possibly be of great value in a mass-casualty setting [160].

A live-attenuated vaccine is available with increasing human safety data, animal efficacy data, but insufficient human efficacy and safety data to support Food and Drug Administration licensure [84]. Some authorities do not consider dengue a bioterrorism risk because primary dengue rarely causes hemorrhagic fever, and it does not seem to be transmissible by small particle inhalation [14,131]. Others, however, think otherwise. As an example, Dr. Kamal Datta, director of the National Institute of Communicable Diseases (India), referred to the outbreak of dengue in Delhi in 1996 (10,252 cases; 423 deaths) as "suspicious" [161].

Yellow fever

Yellow fever is found in tropical Africa and South and Central America. In the nineteenth and early twentieth century, it was also endemic in temperate areas as far north as Philadelphia. The virus is maintained in *Haemagogus* and *Sabethes* mosquitoes in forests, and *A aegypti* are usually responsible for outbreaks in population centers. In Africa, there are monkey-mosquito-monkey cycles involving other *Aedes* species. In Brazil, the *Amblyomma variegatum* tick transmits the virus transstadially and passes the virus to uninfected monkeys.

The incubation period is 3 to 6 days. In endemic areas, many have unapparent infections with significant immunity. Most symptomatic infections are mild with patients recovering within 48 hours or less. The minority of patients has severe headache, myalgia, low back pain, and proteinuria. Patients exhibit a relative bradycardia for the degree of fever (Faget's sign).

Patients with severe illness have abrupt onset of high fever; severe headache; nausea, vomiting; and abdominal, back, loins, and limb pain. Patients become dehydrated, jaundiced, and develop bleeding from the nose and gums. This "period of infection" (viremia) last for 3 days. Patients may enter a recovery phase or temporarily improve over the next 24 hours and then rapidly deteriorate (jaundice deepens and patients develop epigastric pain, vomiting, and gastrointestinal bleeding). Patients become hypotensive and develop heart failure and prolongation of the PR and QT intervals on EKG. Patients may recover over 3 to 4 days to 2 weeks, or death may occur on the seventh to tenth day.

Complications include parotitis and pneumonia. Increasing proteinuria, bleeding, tachycardia, oliguria, renal insufficiency, and hypotension are all bad prognostic signs. Mortality is 20% to 50% [16,121].

Virus may be isolated from the blood in the first 3 days. Other methods of diagnosis are antigen-capture enzyme immunoassay; RT-PCR; or on liver biopsy specimen by immunofluorescence assay, probe hybridization, or RT-PCR [121]. A licensed live-attenuated vaccine is available [85].

Kyasanur Forest disease virus and hemorrhagic fever

Kyasanur Forest disease is a tick-borne (*Haemaphysalis* ticks) flavivirus of southwestern India. There is a 3- to 8-day incubation period. It produces a febrile or hemorrhagic disease. A vaccine is available and infection control methods include treatment of cows for tick infestations and the use of insect repellents. Mortality is 3% to 10% [16,17]. Asymptomatic infection probably occurs because serology studies (2401 samples from six locations on the Andaman and Nocobar Islands of India) found 22.4% antibody prevalence [162].

Because of its potential use as a bioterrorist weapon, this virus requires a biosafety level 4 laboratory for isolation [15].

Omsk hemorrhagic fever virus and disease

Dermacentor ticks are the principle reservoir, and the infection is found in many small mammals in Siberia including the muskrat. Human infection is acquired by either handling dead carcasses or by tick bites. Infected muskrat hunters are often asymptomatic. There is a 3- to 8-day incubation period for symptomatic disease. Some develop papulovesicular lesions on the soft palate, and mucosal and gastrointestinal bleeding. There is a 0.5% to 10% mortality in symptomatic cases [16,17].

BALB/c mouse model has been used for Omsk hemorrhagic fever and the neurotropic flavivirus, Powassan virus. Pathologic differences (cerebellar involvement with Powassan virus infection and different splenic pathology) were demonstrated. Omsk viral antigen was seen in the spleen, brain, and endothelial cells of the liver but was absent from the kidneys. Powassan virus was detected in the brain but was absent from the spleen and kidneys. The distribution of the viral particles in the brain differed [163].

Because of its potential use as a bioterrorist weapon, this virus requires a biosafety level 4 laboratory for isolation [15].

Alkhumra virus and hemorrhagic fever

Four pilgrims from the 2001 Hajj to the holy city of Mecca, Saudi Arabia, were identified in February of that year as having typical VHF. A new flavivirus, a close relative to the tick-borne Kyasanur forest disease virus, was the same virus isolated in 1995 from six patients with dengue-like hemorrhagic fever from the Alkhumra district, south of Jeddah, Saudi Arabia [164–167]. Further investigation found two additional cases in 1994, both in butchers and both organisms recovered from wounds [166]. Sources of infection identified in the original cases included contaminated wounds (butchers, six); tick bites (student and engineer, two); and consumption of raw camel milk (soldier, driver, and poultry worker, three) [166]. The investigation identified 37 patients (20 laboratory confirmed). All presented with an acute febrile flu-like illness and hepatitis; half displayed hemorrhagic findings (55%); and 20% had encephalitis. It was concluded that the disease was transmitted by mosquito bite or direct contact with infected sheep, goats, and rodents. How the virus is maintained in nature is under investigation. Of 11 cases identified between 1994 and 1999, four died [166]. Overall, there was 25% mortality with this outbreak [164,165].

Because of its potential use as a bioterrorist weapon, this virus requires a biosafety level 4 laboratory for isolation [15,167].

Summary

Specific pharmacologic therapy (ribavirin) for VHF is recommended for Lassa fever and the other arenavirus hemorrhagic fevers, Rift Valley fever,

CCHF, HFRS, and related viruses. There is no specific antiviral therapy available for flavivirus or filovirus hemorrhagic fevers. The lack of an approved vaccine or proved prophylaxis and survival of many of the most severely ill patients with inpatient intensive care make this group of viruses potential bioterrorism agents with the intention of overwhelming society's resources.

Mobilization is immediately needed for:

1. Vaccine development
2. Specific prophylactic and therapeutic interventions
3. Strengthened public health response including an efficient system to monitor contacts and populations at risk
4. Invigorated hospital infection control practices
5. Effective regional or national triage systems
6. Expansion of inpatient isolation facilities to accommodate intensive levels of care
7. Regionalization of inpatient intensive care facilities to maximize the care that may be delivered to the sickest victims
8. Development of effective and acceptable outpatient therapeutic care

A unique suggestion has been the development of immune response modifiers that stimulate the immune system's antiviral and antineoplastic activity. Coley Pharmaceutical Group, 3M Pharmaceuticals, Hybridon, SciClone, Hemispherx Biopharma, Corixa Corporation, and AFG Biosolutions have products in various stages of development. Hybridon's second-generation immunomodulatory oligonucleotide may be potentially useful for prophylaxis or therapeutically for variola, dengue, and Ebola in addition to other pathogens [168].

Toll-like receptors on immune cells recognize pathogen macromolecules with wide specificity. 3M Pharmaceuticals' Aldara (imiquimod) has been shown to be active against human papillomavirus, molluscum contagiosum, and leishmaniasis, and is approved for the treatment of actinic keratoses, basal cell carcinoma, and genital warts. The drug stimulates toll-like receptor–7 and toll-like receptor–8, which have activity (in the mouse and primate models) against herpes simplex 1 and 2, cytomegalovirus, influenza, Banzivirus, Rift Valley fever, and West Nile virus. Coley Pharmaceutical Group's GPG 7909 is a toll-like receptor–9 agonist [168].

With the best defense being prevention, a worldwide inventory of existing viral stocks must be both accurately recorded and secured. Aggressive international profiling and tracking of individuals who acquire or seek to acquire specialized viral laboratory equipment, viral cultures, viral hosts or vectors, and visit viral habitats, or have contact with their natural victims, needs to be undertaken. Such programs deter all but the most determined, resourceful, and elaborately sponsored malefactors. Denying resources to a determined and well-financed enemy protected by a foreign government and its international boundaries is difficult if not impossible. Only intelligence agencies' clandestine targeting of state and "stateless" organizations is able to address threats from the remainder.

A valuable and frequently updated resource that tabulates the etiologic agents, their characteristics, a resource list, and clinical pathways may be found at the Infectious Diseases Society of America website (http://www.idsociety.org/) under "Resources" and "Bioterrorism."

References

[1] Sidwell RW, Smee DF. Viruses of the Bunya- and Togaviridae families: potential as bioterrorism agents and means of control. Antiviral Res 2003;57:101–11.
[2] Kortepeter M, Christopher G, Cieslak T, et al. Viral hemorrhagic fevers. In: USAMRIID's medical management of biological casualties handbook. 4th edition. Fort Detrick (MD): Operational Medicine Department, US Army Medical Research Institute of Infectious Diseases; 2001. p. 61–8.
[3] Salvato MS, Lukashevich IS. Arenavirus: Arenaviridae. In: Tidona CA, Darai G, editors. The Springer index of viruses. Berlin: Springer-Verlag; 2002. p. 36–42.
[4] Gonzalez-Scarano F. Bunyavirus: Bunyaviridae. In: Tidona CA, Darai G, editors. The Springer index of viruses. Berlin: Springer-Verlag; 2002. p. 142–9.
[5] Hooper J, Schmalhohn CS. Hantavirus: Bunyaviridae. In: Tidona CA, Darai G, editors. The Springer index of viruses. Berlin: Springer-Verlag; 2002. p. 150–6.
[6] Nuttall PA. Nairovirus: Bunyaviridae. In: Tidona CA, Darai G, editors. The Springer index of viruses. Berlin: Springer-Verlag; 2002. p. 157–62.
[7] Bouloy M. Phlebovirus: Bunyaviridae. In: Tidona CA, Darai G, editors. The Springer index of viruses. Berlin: Springer-Verlag; 2002. p. 163–8.
[8] Goldbach R, Kormelink R. Tospovirus: Bunyaviridae. In: Tidona CA, Darai G, editors. The Springer index of viruses. Berlin: Springer-Verlag; 2002. p. 169–74.
[9] Sanchez A. Ebola-like viruses: Filoviridae. In: Tidona CA, Darai G, editors. The Springer index of viruses. Berlin: Springer-Verlag; 2002. p. 296–9.
[10] Klenk H-D, Feldmann H. Marburg-like viruses: Filoviridae. In: Tidona CA, Darai G, editors. The Springer index of viruses. Berlin: Springer-Verlag; 2002. p. 300–3.
[11] Westaway EG. Flavivirus: Flaviviridae. In: Tidona CA, Darai G, editors. The Springer index of viruses. Berlin: Springer-Verlag; 2002. p. 306–19.
[12] Spaeth GB, Rice CM. Hepacivirus: Flaviviridae. In: Tidona CA, Darai G, editors. The Springer index of viruses. Berlin: Springer-Verlag; 2002. p. 320–6.
[13] Becher P, Thiel H-J. Pestivirus: Flaviviridae. In: Tidona CA, Darai G, editors. The Springer index of viruses. Berlin: Springer-Verlag; 2002. p. 327–31.
[14] Borio L, Inglesby TV, Peters CJ, et al. Hemorrhagic fever viruses as biological weapons. In: Henderson DA, Inglesby TV, O'Toole T, editors. Bioterrorism: guidelines for medical and public health management. Chicago: AMA Press; 2002. p. 191–220.
[15] Peters CJ. Bioterrorism: viral hemorrhagic fever. In: Mandell GL, Bennett JE, Dolin R, editors. Mandell, Douglas, and Bennett's principles and practice of infectious diseases, vol 2. 6th edition. Philadelphia: Elsevier Churchill Livingston; 2005. p. 3626–9.
[16] Solomon T. Viral haemorrhagic fevers. In: Cook GC, Sumla AI, editors. Manson's tropical diseases. 21st edition. Philadelphia: Saunders, an imprint of Elsevier Science Limited; 2003. p. 773–93.
[17] Bossi P, Tegnell A, Baka A, et al. Bichat guidelines for the clinical management of haemorrhagic fever viruses and bioterrorism-related haemorrhagic fever viruses. Euro Surveill 2004;9:E11–2.
[18] Peters CJ, Mills JN, Spiropoulou C, et al. Hantavirus infections. In: Guerrant RL, Walker DH, Weller PF, editors. Tropical infectious diseases: principles, pathogens, and practice, vol 2. Philadelphia: Churchill Livingston; 1999. p. 1217–35.

[19] Pigott DC. Hemorrhagic fever viruses. Crit Care Clin 2005;21:765–83.
[20] Salvaggio MR, Baddley JW. Other viral bioweapons: Ebola and Marburg hemorrhagic fever. Dermatol Clin 2004;22:291–302.
[21] Bossi P, Guihot A, Bricaire F. Emerging or re-emerging infections that can be used for bioterrorism. Presse Med 2005;34(2 Pt 2):149–55.
[22] Martinez VP, Bellomo C, San Juan J, et al. Person-to person transmission of Andes virus. Emerg Infect Dis 2005;11:1848–53.
[23] Buchmeier M, Bowen MD, Peters CJ. Arenaviruses. In: Fields BN, Knipe DM, Howley PM, editors. Fields virology, vol 2. 4th edition. Philadelphia: Lippincott Williams & Wilkins; 2001. p. 1635–69.
[24] Southern PJ. Arenaviridae: the viruses and their replication. In: Fields BN, Knipe DM, Howley PM, editors. Fields virology, vol 2. 3rd edition. Philadelphia: Lippincott Williams & Wilkins; 1996. p. 1505–19.
[25] Bowen MD, Peters CJ, Mills JN, et al. Oliveros virus: a novel arenavirus from Argentina. Virology 1996;217:362–6.
[26] Mills JN, Barrera Oro JG, Bressler DS, et al. Characterization of Oliveros virus, a new member of the Tacaribe complex (Arenaviridae: Arenavirus). Am J Trop Med Hg 1996; 54:399–404.
[27] Suarez OV, Cueto GR, Cavia R, et al. Prevalence of infection with hantavirus in rodent populations of central Argentina. Mem Inst Oswaldo Cruz 2003;98:727–32.
[28] Cordo SM, Cesio y Acuna M, Candurra NA. Polarized entry and release of Junin virus, a New World arenavirus. J Gen Virol 2005;86(pt 5):1475–9.
[29] Kunz S, Rojek JM, Perez M, et al. Characterization of the interaction of Lassa fever virus with its cellular receptor alpha-dystroglycan. J Virol 2005;79:5979–87.
[30] Murphy FA, Winn WC Jr, Walker DH, et al. Early lymphoreticular viral tropism and antigen persistence: Tamiami virus infection in the cotton rat. Lab Invest 1976;34: 125–40.
[31] Asper M, Sternsdorf T, Hass M, et al. Inhibition of different Lassa virus strains by alpha and gamma interferons and comparison with a less pathogenic arenavirus. J Virol 2004; 78:3162–9.
[32] Wright KE, Ahmed R, Buchmeier MJ. Persistent infection of mice with Pichinde virus associated with failure to thrive. Microb Pathog 1995;19:73–82.
[33] Cajimat MN, Fulhorst CF. Phylogeny of the Venezuelan arenaviruses. Virus Res 2004;102: 199–206.
[34] Xiao SY, Zhang H, Yang Y, et al. Pirital virus (Arenaviridae) infection in the Syrian golden hamster, *Mesocricetus auratus*: a new animal model for arenaviral hemorrhagic fever. Am J Trop Med Hyg 2001;64:111–8.
[35] Schmaljohn CS, Hooper JW. Bunyaviridae: the viruses and their replication. In: Fields BN, Knipe DM, Howley PM, editors. Fields virology, vol 2. 4th edition. Philadelphia: Lippincott Williams & Wilkins; 2001. p. 1581–602.
[36] Nichol ST. Bunyaviruses. In: Fields BN, Knipe DM, Howley PM, editors. Fields virology, vol 2. 4th edition. Philadelphia: Lippincott Williams & Wilkins; 2001. p. 1603–33.
[37] Studdert MJ. Restriction endonuclease DNA fingerprinting of respiratory, foetal and perinatal foal isolates of equine herpesvirus type 1. Arch Virol 1983;77:249–58.
[38] Sanford SE, Josephson GK, MacDonald A. *Coxiella burnetii* (Q fever) abortion storms in goat herds after attendance at an annual fair. Can Vet J 1994;35:376–8.
[39] Davies FG. Tick virus diseases of sheep and goats. Parassitologia 1997;39:91–4.
[40] Hornyak A, Bakonyi T, Tekes G, et al. A novel subgroup among genotypes of equine arteritis virus: genetic comparison of 40 strains. J Vet Med B Infect Dis Vet Public Health 2005;52:112–8.
[41] Wouda W, Bartels CJ, Moen AR. Characteristics of *Neospora caninum*-associated abortion storms in dairy herds in The Netherlands (1995–1997). Theriogenology 1999;52: 233–45.

[42] Bartels CJ, Wouda W, Schukken YH. Risk factors for *Neospora caninum*-associated abortion storms in dairy herds in The Netherlands (1995–1997). Theriogenology 1999;52:247–57.
[43] Reichel MP. *Neospora caninum* infections in Australia and New Zealand. Aust Vet J 2000; 78:258–61.
[44] Daly P, Doyle S. The development of a competitive PCR-ELISA for the detection of equine herpesvirus-1. J Virol Methods 2003;107:237–44.
[45] Kradel DC. Abortion storms: projection for the future. Cornell Vet 1978;68(Suppl 7): 195–9.
[46] Ding X, Xu F, Chen H, et al. Apoptosis of hepatocytes caused by Punta toro virus (Bunyaviridae: Phlebovirus) and its implications for Phlebovirus pathogenesis. Am J Pathol 2005; 167:1043–9.
[47] Gharrel RN, Attoui H, Butenko AM, et al. Tick-borne virus diseases of human interest in Europe. Clin Microbiol Infect 2004;10:1040–55.
[48] Sironen T, Vaheri A, Plyusnin A. Phylogenetic evidence for the distinction of Saaremaa and Dobrava hantaviruses. Virol J 2005;2:90.
[49] Peters CJ. California encephalitis, hantavirus pulmonary syndrome, and Bunyavirid hemorrhagic fevers. In: Mandell GL, Bennett JE, Dolin R, editors. Mandell, Douglas, and Bennett's principles and practice of infectious diseases, vol 1. 6th edition. Philadelphia: Elsevier Churchill Livingston; 2005. p. 2086–9.
[50] Bayard V, Kitsutani PT, Barria EO, et al. Outbreak of hantavirus pulmonary syndrome, Los Santos, Panama, 1999–2000. Emerg Infect Dis 2004;10:1635–42.
[51] Fulhorst CF, Cajimat MN, Utrera A, et al. Maporal virus, a hantavirus associated with the fulvous pygmy rice rat (*Oligoryzomys fulvescens*) in western Venezuela. Virus Res 2004;104: 139–44.
[52] McIntyre NE, Chu YK, Owen RD, et al. A longitudinal study of Bayou virus, hosts and habitat. Am J Trop Med Hyg 2005;73:1043–9.
[53] Rosa ES, Mills JN, Padula PJ, et al. Newly recognized hantaviruses associated with hantavirus pulmonary syndrome in northern Brazil: partial genetic characterization of viruses and serologic implication of likely reservoirs. Vector Borne Zoonotic Dis 2005;5:11–9.
[54] Mendes WS, da Silva AA, Aragao LF. Hantavirus infection in Anajatuba, Maranhao, Brazil. . Emerg Infect Dis 2004;10:1496–8.
[55] Carroll DS, Mills JN, Montgomery JM, et al. Hantavirus pulmonary syndrome in central Bolivia: relationships between reservoir hosts, habitats, and viral genotypes. Am J Trop Med Hyg 2005;72:42–6.
[56] Bi P, Cameron S, Higgins G, et al. Are humans infected by Hantavviruses in Australia? Intern Med J 2005;35:672–4.
[57] Chow L, Shu P-Y, Huang J-H, et al. A retrospective study of hantavirus infection in Kinmen, Taiwan. J Microbiol Immunol Infect 2005;38:343–9.
[58] Chandy S, Mitra S, Sathish N, et al. A pilot study for serological evidence of hantavirus infection in human population in south India. Indian J Med Res 2005;122:211–5.
[59] Xu FL, Lee YL, Tsai WY, et al. Effect of cordycepin on Hantaan virus 76–118 infection of primary human embryonic pulmonary fibroblasts: characterization of apoptotic effects. Acta Virol 2005;49:183–93.
[60] Lim SI, Kweon CH, Yang DK, et al. Apoptosis in Vero cells infected with Akabane, Aino and Chuzan virus. J Vet Sci 2005;6:251–4.
[61] Fritz CL, Fulhorst CF, Enge B, et al. Exposure to rodents and rodent-borne viruses among persons with elevated occupational risk. J Occup Environ Med 2002;44:962–7.
[62] Plekhova NG, Somova LM, Slonova RA, et al. Metabolic activity of macrophages infected with hantavirus, an agent of hemorrhagic fever with renal syndrome. Biochemistry (Mosc) 2005;70:990–7.
[63] Peters CJ. Marburg and Ebola virus hemorrhagic fevers. In: Mandell GL, Bennett JE, Dolin R, editors. Mandell, Douglas, and Bennett's principles and practice of infectious diseases, vol 1. 6th edition. Philadelphia: Elsevier Churchill Livingston; 2005. p. 2057–9.

[64] Sanchez A, Khan AS, Zaki SR, et al. Filoviridae: Marburg and Ebola viruses. In: Fields BN, Knipe DM, Howley PM, editors. Fields virology, vol 1. 4th edition. Philadelphia: Lippincott Williams & Wilkins; 2001. p. 1279–304.
[65] Mahanty S, Bray M. Pathogenesis of filoviral haemorrhagic fevers. Lancet 2004;4: 487–98.
[66] Peters CJ, Sanchez A, Rollin PE, et al. Filoviridae: Marburg and Ebola viruses. In: Fields BN, Knipe DM, Howley PM, editors. Fields virology, vol 1. 3rd edition. Philadelphia: Lippincott Williams & Wilkins; 1996. p. 1161–76.
[67] Peters CJ. Marburg and Ebola: arming ourselves against the deadly filoviruses. N Engl J Med 2005;352:2571–3.
[68] Leroy EM, Kumulungui B, Pourrut X, et al. Fruit bats as reservoirs of Ebola virus. Nature 2005;438:575–6.
[69] Lindenbach BD, Rice CM. Flaviviridae: the viruses and their replication. In: Fields BN, Knipe DM, Howley PM, editors. Fields virology, vol 1. 4th edition. Philadelphia: Lippincott Williams & Wilkins; 2001. p. 991–1041.
[70] Burke DS, Monath TP. Flaviviruses. In: Fields BN, Knipe DM, Howley PM, editors. Fields virology, vol 1. 4th edition. Philadelphia: Lippincott Williams & Wilkins; 2001. p. 1043–125.
[71] Rice CM. Flaviviridae: the viruses and their replication. In: Fields BN, Knipe DM, Howley PM, editors. Fields virology, vol 1. 3rd edition. Philadelphia: Lippincott Williams & Wilkins; 1996. p. 931–60.
[72] Monath TP, Heinz FX. Flaviviruses. In: Fields BN, Knipe DM, Howley PM, editors. Fields virology, vol 1. 3rd edition. Philadelphia: Lippincott Williams & Wilkins; 1996. p. 961–1035.
[73] Shope RE. Other flavivirus infections. In: Fields BN, Knipe DM, Howley PM, editors. Fields virology, vol 2. 4th edition. Philadelphia: Lippincott Williams & Wilkins; 2001. p. 1275–9.
[74] Gubler DJ. Dengue and dengue hemorrhagic fever. In: Guerrant RL, Walker DH, Weller PF, editors. Tropical infectious diseases: principles, pathogens, & practice, vol 2. Philadelphia: Churchill Livingstone; 1999. p. 1265–79.
[75] Pugachev KV, Guirakhoo F, Monath TP. New developments in flavivirus vaccines with special attention to yellow fever. Curr Opin Infect Dis 2005;18:387–94.
[76] Estevva L, Mo Yang H. Mathematical model to assess the control of *Aedes aegypti* mosquitoes by the sterile insect technique. Math Biosci 2005;198:132–47.
[77] Quaresma JA, Barros VL, Pagliari C, et al. Revisiting the liver in human yellow fever: virus-induced apoptosis in haptocytes associated with TGF-beta, TNF-alpha, and NK cells activity. Virology 2006;345:22–30.
[78] Monath TP. Yellow fever. In: Guerrant RL, Walker DH, Weller PF, editors. Tropical infectious diseases: principles, pathogens, and practice, vol 2. Philadelphia: Churchill Livingstone; 1999. p. 1253–64.
[79] Tsai TF, Vaughn DW, Solomon T. Flaviviruses (yellow fever, dengue, dengue hemorrhagic fever, Japanese encephalitis, West Nile encephalitis, St. Louis encephalitis, tick-borne encephalitis). In: Mandell GL, Bennett JE, Dolin R, editors. Mandell, Douglas, and Bennett's principles and practice of infectious diseases, vol 2. 6th edition. Philadelphia: Elsevier Churchill Livingston; 2005. p. 1926–50.
[80] Monath TP. Yellow fever. In: Plotkin SA, Orenstein WA, editors. Vaccines. 3rd edition. Philadelphia: WB Saunders; 1999. p. 815–80.
[81] Ojwang JO, Ali S, Smee DF, et al. Broad-spectrum inhibitor of viruses in the Flaviviridae family. Antiviral Res 2005;68:49–55.
[82] Saxena VK. Ixodid ticks infesting rodents and sheep in diverse biotopes of southern India. J Parasitol 1997;83:766–7.
[83] Crowcroft NS, Meltzer M, Evans M, et al. The public health response to a case of Lassa fever in London in 2000. J Infect 2004;48:221–8.

[84] Schmaljohn A, Hevey M. Medical countermeasures for filoviruses and other viral agents. In: Lindler LE, Lebeda FJ, Korch GW, editors. Biological weapons defense: infectious diseases and counterbioterrorism. Totowa (NJ): Humana Press; 2005. p. 239–54.
[85] Donoso Mantke O, Schmitz H, Schmitz H, et al. Quality assurance for the diagnostics of viral diseases to enhance the emergency preparedness in Europe. Euro Surveill 2005;10: 102–6.
[86] Ippolito G, Nicastri E, Capobianchi M, et al. Hospital preparedness and management of patients affected by viral haemorrhagic fever or smallpox at the Lazzaro Spallanzani Institute, Italy. Euro Surveill 2005;10:36–9.
[87] Karwa M, Bronzert P, Kvetan V. Bioterrorism and critical care. Crit Care Clin 2003;19: 279–313.
[88] Enria D, Bowen MD, Mills JN, et al. Arenavirus infections. In: Guerrant RL, Walker DH, Weller PF, editors. Tropical infectious diseases: principles, pathogens, & practice, vol 2. Philadelphia: Churchill Livingston; 1999. p. 1191–212.
[89] Richmond JK, Baglole DJ. Lassa fever: epidemiology, clinical features, and social consequences. BMJ 2003;327:1271–5.
[90] Demby AH, Inapogui A, Kargbo K, et al. Lassa fever in Guinea: II. Distribution and prevalence of Lassa virus infection in small mammals. Vector Borne Zoonotic Dis 2001;1: 283–97.
[91] McCormick JB, Webb PA, Krebs JW, et al. A prospective study of the epidemiology and ecology of Lassa fever. J Infect Dis 1987;155:437–44.
[92] Gunther S, Lenz O. Lassa virus. Crit Rev Clin Lab Sci 2004;41:339–90.
[93] Centers for Disease Control and Prevention. Imported Lassa fever—New Jersey, 2004. MMWR Morb Mortal Wkly Rep 2004;53:894–7.
[94] Webb PA, McCormick JB, King IJ, et al. Lassa fever in children in Sierra Leone, West Africa. Trans R Soc Trop Med Hyg 1986;80:577–82.
[95] Gilbert DN, Moellering RC, Eliopoulos GM, et al. Antiviral therapy (non HIV). In: Gilbert DN, Moellering RC, Eliopoulos GM, et al, editors. The Sanford guide to antimicrobial therapy 2005. 35th revision. Hyde Park (VT): Antimicrobial Therapy; 2005. p. 104–12.
[96] Uckun FM, Venkatachalam TK, Erbeck D, et al. Zidampidine, an aryl phosphate derivative of AZT: in vivo pharmacokinetics, metabolism, toxicity, and anti-viral efficacy against hemorrhagic fever caused by Lassa virus. Bioorg Med Chem 2005;13:3279–88.
[97] Peters CJ. Lymphocytic chroiomeningitis virus, Lassa virus, and the South American Hemorrhagic fevers. In: Mandell GL, Bennett JE, Dolin R, editors. Mandell, Douglas, and Bennett's principles and practice of infectious diseases, vol 1. 6th edition. Philadelphia: Elsevier Churchill Livingston; 2005. p. 2090–7.
[98] Okoror LE, Esumeh FI, Agbonlahor DE, et al. Lassa virus: seroepidemiological survey of rodents caught in Ekpoma and environs. Trop Doct 2005;35:16–7.
[99] Rodriguez-Carreno MP, Nelson MS, Botten J, et al. Evaluating the immunogenicity and protective efficacy of a DNA vaccine encoding Lassa virus nucleoprotein. Virology 2005; 335:87–98.
[100] Geisbert TW, Jones S, Fritz EA, et al. Development of a new vaccine for the prevention of Lassa fever. PloS Med 2005;2:e183.
[101] Lukashevich IS, Patterson J, Carrion R, et al. A live attenuated vaccine for Lassa fever made by reassortment of Lassa and Mopeia viruses. J Virol 2005;79:13934–42.
[102] Flick R, Elgh F, Pettersson RF. Mutational analysis of the Uukuniemi virus (Bunyaviridae family) promoter reveals two elements of functional importance. J Virol 2002; 76:10849–60.
[103] Flick K, Katz A, Overby A, et al. Functional analysis of the noncoding regions of the Uukuniemi virus (Bunyaviridae) RNA segments. J Virol 2004;78:11726–38.
[104] Haas WH, Breuer T, Pfaff G, et al. Imported Lassa fever in Germany: surveillance and management of contact persons. Clin Infect Dis 2003;36:1254–8.

[105] Crowcroft NS. Management of Lassa fever in European countries. Euro Surveill 2002;7: 50–3.
[106] Vieth S, Drosten C, Charrel R, et al. Establishment of conventional and fluorescence resonance energy transfer-based real-time PCR assays for detection of pathogenic New World arenaviruses. J Clin Virol 2005;32:229–35.
[107] Lisieux T, Coimbra M, Nassar ES, et al. New arenavirus isolated in Brazil. Lancet 1994; 343:391–2.
[108] Alvarez FA, Biquard C, Figini HA, et al. Neurological complications of Argentinean hemorrhagic fever. Neurol Neurocir Psiquiatr 1977;18(2–3 Suppl):357–73.
[109] Albiol Matanic VC, Castilla V. Antiviral activity of antimicrobial cationic peptides against Junin virus and herpes simplex virus. Int J Antimicrob Agents 2004;23:382–9.
[110] Maiztegui JI, McKee KT Jr, Barrera Oro JG, et al. Protective efficacy of live attenuated vaccine against Argentine hemorrhagic fever. AHF Study Group. J Infect Dis 1998;177:277–83.
[111] Ambrosio AM, Riera LM, Saavedra Mdel C, et al. Preclinical assay of candid #1 vaccine against Argentine hemorrhagic fever made in Argentina. Medicina (B Aires) 2005;65: 329–32.
[112] Garcia CC, Talarico L, Almeida N, et al. Virucidal activity of essential oils from aromatic plants of San Luis, Argentina. Phytother Res 2003;17:1073–5.
[113] Fulhorst CF, Milazzo ML, Bradley RD, et al. Experimental infection of *Neotoma albigula* (Muridae) with Whitewater Arroyo virus (Arenaviridae). Am J Trop Med Hyg 2001;65: 147–51.
[114] Lele SM, Milazzo ML, Graves K, et al. Pathology of Whitewater Arroyo viral infection in the white-throated woodrat (*Neotoa albigula*). J Comp Pathol 2003;128:289–92.
[115] Grande-Perez A, Lazaro E, Lowenstein P, et al. Suppression of viral infectivity through lethal defection. Proc Natl Acad Sci U S A 2005;102:4448–52.
[116] de la Torre JC. Arenavirus extinction through lethal mutagenesis. Virus Res 2005;107: 207–14.
[117] Gerrard SR, Li L, Barrett AD, et al. Ngari virus is a Bunyamwera virus reassortant that can be associated with large outbreaks of hemorrhagic fever in Africa. J Virol 2004;78:8922–6.
[118] Bowen MD, Trappier SG, Sanchez AJ, et al. A reassortant bunyavirus isolated from acute hemorrhagic fever cases in Kenya and Somalia. Virology 2001;29:185–90.
[119] Ikegami T, Makino S. Rift Valley fever virus. Uirusu 2004;54:229–35.
[120] Gerdes GH. Rift Valley fever. Rev Sci Tech 2004;23:613–23.
[121] Broom AK, Smith DW, Hall RA, et al. Arbovirus infections. In: Cook GC, Sumla AI, editors. Manson's tropical diseases. 21st edition. Philadelphia: WB Saunders, an imprint of Elsevier Science Limited; 2003. p. 725–64.
[122] Morrill JC, Peters CJ. Pathogenicity and neurovirulence of a mutagen-attenuated Rift-Valley fever vaccine in rhesus monkeys. Vaccine 2003;21:2994–3002.
[123] Morrill JC, Mebus CA, Peters CJ. Safety of a mutagen-attenuated Rift Valley fever virus vaccine in fetal and neonatal bovids. Am J Vet Res 1997;58:1110–4.
[124] Hunter P, Erasmus BJ, Vorster JH. Teratogenicity of a mutagenised Rift Valley fever virus (MVP 12) in sheep. Onderstepoort J Vet Res 2002;69:95–8.
[125] Wallace DB, Viljoen GJ. Immune responses to recombinants of the South African vaccine strain of lumpy skin disease virus generated by using thymidine kinase gene insertion. Vaccine 2005;23:3061–7.
[126] Spik K, Shurtleff A, McElroy AK, et al. Immunogenicity of combination DNA vaccines for Rift Valley fever virus, tick-borne encephalitis virus, Hantaan virus, and Crimean Congo hemorrhagic fever virus. Vaccine 2005;Sept:17.
[127] Whitehouse CA. Crimean-Congo hemorrhagic fever. Antiviral Res 2004;64:145–60.
[128] Sheikh AS, Sheikh AA, Sheikh NS, et al. Bi-annual surge of Crimean-Congo haemorrhagic fever (CCHF): a five-year experience. Int J Infect Dis 2005;9:37–42.
[129] Harxhi A, Pilaca A, Delia Z, et al. Crimean-Congo hemorrhagic fever: a case of nosocomial transmission. Infection 2005;33:295–6.

[130] Flick R, Whitehouse CA. Crimean-Congo hemorrhagic fever virus. Curr Mol Med 2005;5: 753–60.
[131] Rigaudeau S, Bricaire F, Bossi P. Haemorrhagic fever viruses, possible bioterrorist use. Presse Med 2005;34(2 Pt 2):169–76.
[132] Kuljic-Kapulica N. Emerging diseases: Crimean-Congo hemorrhagic fever. Med Pregl 2004;57:453–6.
[133] Frangoulidis D, Meyer H. Measures undertaken in the German Armed forces Field Hospital deployed in Kosovo to contain a potential outbreak of Crimean-Congo hemorrhagic fever. Mil Med 2005;170:366–9.
[134] Jamil B, Hasan RS, Sarwari AR, et al. Crimean-Congo hemorrhagic fever: experience at a tertiary care hospital in Karachi, Pakistan. Trans R Soc Trop Med Hyg 2005;99:577–84.
[135] Pal E, Strle F, Avsic-Zupanc T. Hemorrhagic fever with renal syndrome in the Pomurje region of Slovenia: an 18-year survey. Wien Klin Wochenschr 2005;117:398–405.
[136] Tai PW, Chen LC, Huang CH. Hanta hemorrhagic fever with renal syndrome: a case report and review. J Microbiol Immunol Infect 2005;38:221–3.
[137] Hukic M, Tulumovic D, Calkic L. The renal failure and capillary leak during the acute stage of (Dobrava) DOB and PUU (Puumala infection). Med Arh 2005;59:227–30.
[138] Slonova RA, Kompanets GG, Obraztosov IUG. Hemorrhagic fever with renal syndrome among servicement in Primorskii Region of Russia. Voen Med Zh 2005;326:20–5.
[139] Mathes RW, Page WF, Crawford HM, et al. Long-term sequelae of hemorrhagic fever with renal syndrome attributable to hantaan virus in Korean War veterans. Mil Med 2005;170: 315–9.
[140] Pekic S, Cvijovic G, Stojanovic M, et al. Hypopituitarism as a late complication of hemorrhagic fever. Endocrine 2005;26:79–82.
[141] Dong G-M, Han L, An Q, et al. Immunization effect of purified bivalent vaccine to haemorrhagic fever with renal syndrome manufactured from primary cultured hamster kidney cells. Chin Med J (Engl) 2005;118:766–8.
[142] Geldmacher A, Skrastina D, Borisova G, et al. A hantavirus nucleocapsid protein segment exposed on hepatitis B virus core particles is highly immunogenic in mice when applied without adjuvants or in the presence of preexisting anti-core antibodies. Vaccine 2005;23: 3973–83.
[143] Rizvanov AA, van Geelen AG, Morzunov S, et al. Generation of a recombinant cytomegalovirus for expression of hantavirus glycoprotein. J Virol 2003;77:12203–10.
[144] Chaparro J, Vega J, Terry W, et al. Assessment of person-to-person transmission of hantavirus pulmonary syndrome in a Chilean hospital setting. J Hosp Infect 1998;40:281–5.
[145] Vitek CR, Breiman RF, Ksiazek TG, et al. Evidence against person-to-person transmission of hantavirus to health care workers. Clin Infect Dis 1996;22:824–6.
[146] Dara SI, Albright RC, Peters SG. Acute Sin Nombre hantavirus infection complicated by renal failure requiring hemodialysis. Mayo Clin Proc 2005;80:703–4.
[147] Ferres M, Vial P. Hantavirus infection in children. Curr Opin Pediatr 2004;16:70–5.
[148] Schmidt J, Meisel H, Hjelle B, et al. Development and evaluation of serological assays for detection of human hantavirus infections caused by Sin Nombre virus. J Clin Virol 2005;33: 247–53.
[149] Boumandouki P, Formenty P, Epelboin A, et al. clinical management of patients and deceased during the Ebola outbreak from October to December 2003 in Republic of Congo. Bull Soc Pathol Exot 2005;98:218–23.
[150] Warfield KL, Swenson DL, Demmin G, et al. Filovirus-like particles as vaccines and discovery tools. Expert Rev Vaccines 2005;4:429–40.
[151] Warfield KL, Olinger G, Deal EM, et al. Induction of humoral and CD8 + T cell responses are required for protection against lethal Ebola virus infection. J Immunol 2005;175: 1184–91.
[152] Warfield KL, Swenson DL, Negley DL, et al. Marburg virus-like particles protect guinea pigs from lethal Marburg virus infection. Vaccine 2004;22:3495–502.

[153] Wilson JA, Hart MK. Protection from Ebola virus mediated by cytotoxic T lymphocytes specific for the viral nucleoprotein. J Virol 2001;75:2660–4.
[154] Geisbert TW, Pushko P, Anderson K, et al. Evaluation of nonhuman primates of vaccines against Ebola virus. Emerg Infect Dis 2002;8:503–7.
[155] Hampton T. Vaccines against Ebola and Marburg viruses show promise in primate studies. JAMA 2005;294:163–4.
[156] Jones SM, Feldmann H, Stroher U, et al. Live attenuated recombinant vaccine protects nonhuman primates against Ebola and Marburg viruses. Nat Med 2005;11:720–1.
[157] Rouquet P, Froment JM, Bermejo M, et al. Wild animal mortality monitoring and human Ebola outbreaks, Gabon and Republic of Congo, 2001–2003. Emerg Infect Dis 2005;11: 283–90.
[158] Centers for Disease Control and Prevention. Brief report: outbreak of Marburg virus hemorrhagic fever—Angola, October 1, 2004—March 29, 2005. MMWR Morb Mortal Wkly Rep 2005;54:308–9.
[159] Harboe ZB, Qureshi KM, Skinhoj P, et al. Marburg haemorrhagic fever in Angola, 2005. Ugeskr Laeger 2005;167:4087–90.
[160] Mismatched double-stranded RNA:polyI:polyC12U. Drugs R D 2004;5:297–304.
[161] Sharma R. India wakes up to threat of bioterrorism. BMJ 2001;323:714.
[162] Padbidri VS, Wairagkar NS, Joshi GD, et al. A serological survey of arboviral diseases among the human population of the Andaman and Nicobar Islands, India. Southeast Asian J Trop Med Public Health 2002;33:794–800.
[163] Holbrook MR, Aronson JF, Campbell GA, et al. An animal model for the tickborne flavivirus—Omsk hemorrhagic fever virus. J Infect Dis 2005;191:100–8.
[164] Madani TA. Alkhumra virus infection, a new viral hemorrhagic fever in Saudi Arabia. J Infect 2005;51:91–7.
[165] Memish ZA, Balkhy HH, Francis C, et al. Alkhumra haemorrhagic fever: case report and infection control details. Br J Biomed Sci 2005;62:37–9.
[166] Charrel RN, Zaki AM, Fakeeh M, et al. Low diversity of Alkhurma hemorrhagic fever virus: Saudi Arabia, 1994–1999. Emerg Infect Dis 2005;11:683–8.
[167] Charrel RN, de Lamballierie X. The Alkhurma virus (family Flaviviridae, genus Flavivirus): an emerging pathogen responsible for hemorrhagic fever in the Middle East. Med Trop (Mars) 2003;63:296–9.
[168] Amlie-Lefond C, Paz DA, Connelly MP, et al. Innate immunity for biodefense: a strategy whose time has come. J Allergy Clin Immunol 2005;116:1334–42.

ELSEVIER
SAUNDERS

Infect Dis Clin N Am
20 (2006) 395–421

INFECTIOUS
DISEASE CLINICS
OF NORTH AMERICA

Category B Potential Bioterrorism Agents: Bacteria, Viruses, Toxins, and Foodborne and Waterborne Pathogens

Georgios Pappas, MD[a,*],
Paraskevi Panagopoulou, MD, MPH[a],
Leonidas Christou, MD[b], Nikolaos Akritidis, MD[c]

[a]*Institute for Continuing Medical Education of Ioannina, Velissariou 15-19, 45221, Ioannina, Greece*
[b]*Internal Medicine Department, University Hospital, 45110, Ioannina, Greece*
[c]*Internal Medicine Department, General Hospital "G. Hatzikosta," Makrygianni Avenue, 45500, Ioannina, Greece*

Category B of potential weapons of bioterrorism is by far the broadest, because it includes a wide variety of bacteria, viruses, protozoa, and toxins. Category B agents have been listed both by the Centers for Disease Control and Prevention [1] and the National Institute of Allergy and Infectious Diseases (NIAID) Biodefense Research [2]. The NIAID list is practically an expanded, detailed Centers for Disease Control and Prevention list, and it is used as the basis of this article (Box 1). Inclusion of a certain pathogen in this list implicates either its attractive nature as a potential bioweapon that is accompanied by a low ability to cause massively destructive (and socially deconstructive) consequences, or an ability to induce major public health consequences that is accompanied by certain difficulties in the development and execution of a potential attack (and low probability). Basic aspects of the pathogens included in category B, along with important parameters related to their potential as biological weapons, are discussed.

* Corresponding author.
E-mail address: gpele@otenet.gr (G. Pappas).

doi:10.1016/j.idc.2006.02.002

Box 1. Category B potential bioterrorism agents

Bacteria
Brucella species (brucellosis)
Burkholderia pseudomallei (melioidosis) and *B mallei* (glanders)
Chlamydia psittaci (psittacosis)[a]
Coxiella burnetii (Q fever)
Rickettsia prowazekii (typhus fever)

Viruses
Alphaviruses
- Venezuelan equine encephalitis
- Eastern equine encephalitis
- Western equine encephalitis

Bunyaviruses
- LaCrosse
- California encephalitis

Flaviviruses
- West Nile virus
- Japanese encephalitis virus
- Kyasanur Forest virus

Foodborne and waterborne pathogens
Bacteria
- *Escherichia coli*
- Pathogenic vibrios
- *Shigella* species
- *Salmonella*
- *Listeria monocytogenes*
- *Campylobacter jejuni*
- *Yersinia enterocolitica*

Viruses
- Noroviruses
- Hepatitis A virus

Protozoa
- *Cryptosporidium parvum*
- *Cyclospora cayatanensis*
- *Giardia lamblia*
- *Entamoeba histolytica*
- *Toxoplasma*
- Microsporidia

Toxins
Epsilon toxin of *Clostridium perfringens*

Ricin toxin (from *Ricinus communis*)
Staphylococcus enterotoxin B

[a] Psittacosis is not included in this list, but is included in the Centers for Disease Control and Prevention list [1].

From the National Institute of Allergy and Infectious Diseases Biodefense Research. NIAID biodefense agenda for CDC category B and C priority pathogens. Available at: http://www3.niaid.nih.gov/Biodefense/Research/categorybandc.pdf. Accessed January 10, 2006.

Brucella

The pathogen

Brucella is a gram-negative zoonotic bacterium, certain species of which are pathogenic to humans [3]. Brucellosis is possibly the commonest zoonosis worldwide, with an increasing number of new disease loci emerging in recent years in various underdeveloped countries [4], and reacquaintance of the developed world with the disease as a result of travel-related infections and through international food trading [5]. Most disease is called by *Brucella melitensis*, whereas other species, such as *Brucella suis*, *Brucella abortus*, and *Brucella canis*, are considered less virulent. The pathogenesis of the disease is unique, as exhibited by the complex immune response evoked by the pathogen and the fact that the bacteria practically hide inside the macrophages, in unique compartments of acidic environment, replicating without affecting cellular viability [6]. The disease is transmitted by direct contact with infected animals (sheep and goats for *B melitensis*, bovine for *B abortus*); consumption of contaminated dairy products or undercooked meat from infected animals; and by inhalation of infective aerosol particles. Person-to-person transmission does not generally occur. Brucellosis in humans causes a febrile disease with nonspecific manifestations. A wide variety of complications have been described in the literature [7], of which spondylitis, central nervous system involvement of various presentations, and endocarditis are the most troublesome. Chronic brucellosis has not been adequately defined. Diagnosis requires isolation of the organism from blood or bone marrow specimens [8], but the reported sensitivity varies significantly in the literature, ranging from 10% to more than 70%. Serodiagnosis (serum agglutination test and similar tests) is widely used, whereas ELISA exhibits better sensitivity and specificity [9]. Polymerase chain reaction (PCR) assays have been developed [10], and real-time PCR assays allow for rapid diagnosis [11]. The traditional treatment options include a combination of doxycycline and rifampin for 6 weeks, or doxycycline for 6 weeks and streptomycin for 2 to 3 weeks [12]. Alternative regimens use other aminoglycosides [13], co-trimoxazole, and quinolones [12]. Relapse rates with accepted regimens are at the level of 10%, and relapse usually presents in the first year posttreatment, related to well-recognized parameters.

Bioterrorism potential

Brucella was one of the first agents to be used in the development of biological weapons, in particular *B suis*, which had been weaponized in the shape of particle-filled bombs, allegedly by the United States, and possibly by other countries more than 50 years ago [14]. The attractiveness of the pathogen lies in its exquisite ability to be transmitted as an inhalational pathogen; laboratory-acquired brucellosis [15] is a common event in nonspecialized laboratories dealing with the agent. The rare respiratory complications of the disease have not been related to inhalational exposure [16]. Reports on attack rates vary, and the mortality of the disease is minimal. The relatively protracted incubation period (varying from 10 days to 3 months) further compromises its potential as a biological weapon to disrupt social structures. Existence of adequate antibiotic options further compromises this pathogen's potential, although development of resistant strains could not be excluded. Moreover, in a situation of deliberate exposure, the use of prophylactic antibiotic administration has not been clarified [17], and universally acceptable human vaccines are not at present available [18]. A final important implication of brucellosis if used as a biological weapon is the effect on animal population of the targeted area, which might be significant for the overall economy of the region, if largely based on animal husbandry.

Burkholderia mallei* and *pseudomallei

The pathogens

Burkholderia mallei and *Burkholderia pseudomallei* are closely related species of the genus *Burkholderia*, until recently [19] categorized as *Pseudomonas mallei* and *Pseudomonas pseudomallei*, respectively. They are both small, gram-negative, strictly aerobic pathogens that cause zoonoses of varying severity in humans, known as "glanders" and "melioidosis," respectively. Their joint discussion is warranted, although criticized in past efforts [20], because of the paucity of current clinical knowledge about the former of the pathogens, which is in part compensated by application of experience with the latter.

Burkholderia mallei is an ancient pathogen, described by Aristotle [21] as an equine disease, and termed in Greek as "malis/melis," a term further used in nomenclature, also naming the clinical syndrome of melioidosis (melis-like). Glanders is even present in the works of Shakespeare (in The Taming of the Shrew [21]). *B pseudomallei* and *B mallei* are morphologically similar, although the latter exhibits motility because of polar flagella [22]. Glanders is an extremely rare disease nowadays, with extremely few human cases reported in the literature in the second half of the twentieth century, most in laboratory workers working with the pathogen [23]. Melioidosis is an important infectious disease of selected areas, especially Northeast Thailand (but also neighboring countries, including China) and North Australia; recently, however, the disease has been reported in Brazil.

The disease usually presents during the rainy seasons, in people who are in direct contact with soil and surface water, and the usual mode of transmission is percutaneous contact through small skin abrasions. Inhalation of infected aerosol particles is another means of transmission. Person-to-person transmission does not generally occur. *B pseudomallei* exhibit ability to survive intracellularly in phagocytes, forming small colony units.

Most patients exhibit underlying illnesses, diabetes mellitus being the commonest (but also renal and hepatic disease, thalassemia, alcohol consumption, and chronic lung disease including cystic fibrosis). Incubation period ranges from 1 to 14 days, 1 to 5 days in cases of septicemia, and possibly even hours in cases of inhalatory exposure [24]. The disease usually presents dramatically as a rapidly fatal septicemia, mortality rates ranging from 19% to 50%, even with adequate antibiotic treatment. Respiratory failure caused by acute necrotizing pneumonia or acute respiratory distress syndrome may develop. Profound weight loss accompanies the clinical picture. Pulmonary disease often exhibits a chronic form resulting in cavitation, causing misdiagnoses of tuberculosis. Neurologic manifestations are rare but important in terms of morbidity. *B pseudomallei* have a tendency for abscess formation, with a particular tropism for the spleen, but also prostate, liver, and soft tissues. In children in Thailand the disease often presents as unilateral suppurative parotitis. A localized form of the infection with ulceration, subcutaneous nodules, and regional lymphadenopathy is more benign (a similar form of *B mallei* infection is called "farcy").

Despite adequate treatment, the disease can relapse, even after a period of decades. Isolation of the organism in cases of septicemia is feasible, and even throat swabs have been useful in certain clinical settings. The use of selective media, such as Ashdown's medium, enhances diagnostic sensitivity, but misidentifications may occur with automated systems [25]. Serologic diagnosis by means of ELISA is useful in nonendemic areas (in endemic areas, nonprotective seroconversion ensues early in life), but no commercial kits are available. Treatment is prolonged and biphasic: intravenous therapy with ceftazidime or carbapenems has proved superior to traditional regimens [26] in recent years, and should be continued until definite clinical improvement ensues. Amoxicillin-clavulanate has been used as a less efficient, but cheaper, alternative. A second oral antibiotic phase for at least 20 weeks uses doxycycline and co-trimoxazole, with the addition of chloramphenicol for 8 weeks. Monotherapy with co-trimoxazole in the second phase in a recent study showed excellent results. For glanders, the experience on treatment is largely based on in vitro data [27] demonstrating a similar antibiotic susceptibility profile to that of *B pseudomallei*, apart from the additional sensitivity to gentamicin for *B mallei*.

Bioterrorism potential

B mallei have been used as biological weapons in World War I, albeit targeting the enemy's cavalry. It has also been reported that during World

War II Japan carried on experiments in humans at the Pinfang Institute in China [28].

The high infectivity of both diseases in their aerosolized form (attack rates in laboratory exposure being up to 46%), and the possible severe pulmonary or septicemic form of pathology exhibited after such an exposure [29], makes them possible biological weapons. Furthermore, both agents are practically unknown, even to specialists, in the Western World, and a prompt diagnosis and response might not be feasible, especially when taking into account the need for specialized, early, and costly, antibiotic administration. Prophylaxis is another issue because of the absence of adequate data, and co-trimoxazole might be an attractive option, although further issues would ensue over who should receive such a prophylactic regimen. There are no vaccines available (natural immunity does not offer protection). As for brucellosis, animal disease in the setting of a biological weapon incident is also a factor to consider: the notorious outbreak in animals of Paris zoos in 1973, ensuing after a Panda suffering from melioidosis was imported as a gift from Mao ZeDong to the French president, is a characteristic incident of unintentional international bioterrorism at the highest level [30].

Chlamydia psittaci

The pathogen

Chlamydia psittaci (alternatively called *Chlamydophila psittaci*) is the etiologic agent of psittacosis (alternatively called ornithosis), a rare cause of atypical pneumonia that mainly presents as an occupational disease in persons exposed to domestic (and rarely free-ranging) birds. The disease is transmitted through the inhalational route, after exposure to contaminated bird droppings or dust generated in environments contaminated by infected bird droppings. *C psittaci* is an environmentally stable pathogen. Incubation period is 1 to 2 weeks, and the disease produced ranges in severity from asymptomatic to severe pneumonia. Case fatality rate is 15% to 20% in untreated patients, but <1% posttreatment. Prominent headache is reported as characteristic in the clinical presentation. During convalescence, cases of thrombophlebitis and subsequent pulmonary embolism have been reported. Diagnosis is based on serology (complement-fixing antibody, cross-reacts with other *Chlamydia* species). PCR assays have been developed, whereas culture is laborious and hazardous. Treatment with doxycycline (alternatively macrolides) results in prompt response [31].

Bioterrorism potential

Psittacosis is included in the Centers for Disease Control and Prevention list [1] but not in the NIAID list [2]. Undoubtedly, as an inhalational disease, it is far less potent than other pathogens of this group in creating major public health consequences. Moreover, psittacosis is a largely forgotten disease, which implies that knowledge of its pathogenetic properties is limited (a fact that may prove problematic both for weaponization and improvement of response policies). The one intriguing characteristic of the disease in terms of bioterrorism is the ability to be transferred wide distances through infected free-ranging birds. Limited data exist, however, about the ecology of the disease outside captive settings.

Coxiella burnetii

The pathogen

Coxiella burnetii is a gram-negative coccobacillus, usually described in parallel with Rickettsiae, although their phylogenetic differences have been largely outlined in recent years [32]. The disease is a global zoonosis that often runs undetected because of its low mortality. It is an intracellular pathogen, which after infection can survive for prolonged periods in the autophagosomes, leading to chronic infections [33]. It is usually transmitted by inhalation, and the inoculum needed to induce human infection is extremely low, often mentioned as even a sole organism. The disease produced, Q fever, is largely an occupational disease in people in close contact with animal hosts of the pathogen, such as sheep. *C burnetii* exhibits a remarkable environmental stability, and generation of aerosols (dustborne disease) from previously infected areas does not require current presence or contact with infected animal hosts. Person-to-person transmission does not occur.

The clinical syndrome induced 10 to 21 days after exposure is usually mild, in the form of a flulike illness or an atypical pneumonia, with varying radiologic appearances. Mild elevations of serum aminotransferases, indicating hepatitis, are also common. Serious complications are rare, and mortality is minimal, but the disease exhibits a tendency for chronicity, which can manifest in various forms, the most important of which is chronic endocarditis [34]. A chronic fatigue–like syndrome has also been recognized. The diagnosis is usually based on serologic tests, such as ELISA and indirect immunofluorescence assays. PCR detection has gradually become the diagnostic gold standard [35], although its use is still limited to reference laboratories. Q fever is often asymptomatic and self-limited. In detected clinical cases, a short course of doxycycline (7–10 days) is the choice regimen, although alternatives, such as quinolones, erythromycin, and in special populations co-trimoxazole and rifampin, exist [36]. Chronic endocarditis requires protracted administration of doxycycline in combination with hydroxychloroquine, although valve replacement may not be avoided [37].

Bioterrorism potential

The historical military significance of Q fever is characteristically outlined in the large number of outbreaks in military personnel stationed in

Mediterranean countries during World War II [38], although none of these outbreaks was attributed to deliberate release. Q fever exhibits most characteristics of a potential biological weapon, excluding mortality [39]. It is extremely stable in the environment, easily found and aerosolized in large quantities, and has further significance for the animal population and the economy and subsequent living in a targeted area. Various countries have experimented with weaponizing the pathogen in the past, including the United States [40]. In a recent attack scenario [41] targeting a 100,000-person city, massive disruption of societal and health structure was predicted despite an extremely low mortality rate, even without further interventions. Similar results were yielded from historical attack scenarios [42]. Questions regarding response were further raised: doxycycline is an acceptable prophylactic regimen, but whether it should be administered to everyone exposed or only to special populations at risk has not been clarified. Furthermore, the issue of vaccination for *C burnetii* remains underdiscussed: A formalin-activated whole-cell vaccine is extensively used in Australia, and candidate vaccines are under investigation.

Rickettsia prowazekii

The pathogen

Rickettsia prowazekii is the only *Rickettsia* listed as a potential biological weapon, although appeals for the inclusion of other rickettsial species, most notably *R rickettsi*, the causative agent of Rocky Mountain spotted fever, have emerged [43]. Epidemic typhus, a major determinant of significant historical turning points [44], is transmitted to humans by the human body louse, and is related to conditions of poor hygiene and social disruption, as outlined by the characteristics of recent epidemics in Burundi [45] and Russia. Head lice [46] and flying squirrels [47] have been also recently implicated as *R prowazekii* reservoirs. Human-to-human transmission does not occur. Self-inoculation by scratching the bite-site is the usual mode of transmission, although exposure to aerosol particles containing infected lice feces also leads to disease. The typical disease induced by *R prowazekii* 8 to 12 days after exposure is characterized by fever; severe headache; and a subsequent generalized maculopapular, sometimes finally purpuric, rash spreading centrifugally. Mortality is 20% when untreated, significantly higher in older adults and related to gangrene, central nervous system complications, diffuse intravascular coagulation, or severe hypovolemia. Adequate treatment leads to a decline in mortality rates to about 2% to 4%. Establishment of chronic infection can lead to recrudescence (Brill-Zinsser disease) in 15% of the patients, which is usually mild and may appear decades after the typhus episode, often related to external or internal stress. Diagnosis is based on serology (immunofluorescence assays and ELISA), although cross-reactions with other rickettsiae from the typhus group are extensive and their avoidance subject to newer techniques [48]. Moreover, the need for convalescent samples allows for a retrospective-only diagnosis. When epidemiologic situations related to the disease have been already recognized, the diagnosis is anticipated and can be achieved clinically [45]. Specific PCR techniques for this pathogen have been developed [49], including real-time PCR [50]. Treatment, apart from supportive measures in critically ill patients, relies on the administration of doxycycline, a single dose of which can be life saving [51]. Chloramphenicol is an acceptable alternative regimen.

Bioterrorism potential

An older attack scenario developed by the World Health Organization [42] outlined the grave sequences of an attack with an aerosolized form of *R prowazekii*, with an estimated number of 19,000 deaths. The process of weaponization with *R prowazekii* is not as easy, however, as with *C burnetii*, for example, and one can suppose that such a task could be abandoned in favor of weaponizing a category A pathogen. An alternative approach would use extended spread of infected lice, but in this case, the emerging epidemiologic situation would lead to anticipation of epidemic typhus and rapid response [41]. There are currently no vaccines available for epidemic typhus. The whole-cell vaccine that was successful during World War II in minimizing epidemic typhus among allied troops is not being produced anymore, but projects for new vaccine products are currently under way [52].

Epsilon toxin of *Clostridium perfringens*

The toxin

Epsilon toxin (ETX) is a major toxin produced by the type B and D strains of *Clostridium perfringens*, an anaerobic bacterium the other types of which cause various human diseases as gas gangrene and necrotizing enteritis. There is a paucity of knowledge over the effect of ETX on humans, because the types of *C perfringens* carrying it are not human pathogens [53] and data are largely based on experience from animal disease and mice models. It is known that ETX exhibits an exquisite neurotropism, indicated by the severe neurologic sequelae of certain *C perfringens* type D infections in sheep [54], and the rapid accumulation of ETX in mice brain, resulting in death, after intravenous administration of minimal quantities [55]. This neurotropism may be related to recognition of specific receptors on brain cells. ETX seems to act through alteration of the permeability of the cellular membrane, with formation of a heptameric pore [56]. Increasing knowledge about protective humoral immunity in infected animals may allow further understanding of the pathophysiology of ETX and further extrapolation on human risk.

Bioterrorism potential

ETX is an aberration in category B pathogen list, because practically nothing is known about its possible consequences in humans. To deliver a large-scale biological attack, it has to be used in the form of an aerosol, or through poisoning of water or food supplies. Yet, because nothing is known about ETX's interaction with human gastrointestinal and respiratory mucosa, no safe projections could be made over its lethality and its consequences [56]. For example, it is known that goats infected by *C perfringens* type D develop enterocolitis and a wasting syndrome that is compatible with the mechanism of action of ETX, yet apart from expecting that the cleavage of the protoxin secreted by *C* perfringens by trypsin and chymotrypsin definitely ensues in human gastrointestinal tract as well, no other projections can be made. Attempts to develop a recombinant vaccine against ETX are currently under way [57], although a formalin-inactivated vaccine exists for susceptible animals. Given these facts, one can support that ETX is more suitably placed in category C pathogens, because its potential for biological weapon use is still largely unexplored and unproved.

Ricin

The toxin

Ricin is a toxin derived from the bean of castor plant *Ricinus communis*, and has drawn medical interest since the nineteenth century, Ehrlich being among the scientists experimenting with it [53], but still attractive in the field of oncologic pharmacology. Its importance lies in its ability to act on the ribosomes and halt the procedure of protein synthesis, leading to cellular death. Its crystal structure has been outlined: it is a heterodimer, consisting of two glycoprotein chains, chain B facilitating anchoring to the targeted cell, allowing for chain A to intrude and attack the 28S ribosomal subunit. There are limited data over its effects on human subjects: workers exposed to castor dusts exhibited allergic symptoms [58], but the inhalational dose was presumably low. Mice and monkeys exposed to infected aerosols, however, developed rapidly fatal necrotizing airway pathology and alveolar flooding [59,60]. The inverse relationship between particle diameter and clinical severity has also been experimentally proved. When administered orally, based on the experience drawn from isolated cases of involuntary ingestion of castor beans [61] or from experimental data [62], gastrointestinal symptoms, including bloody diarrhea, predominated and significant histologic pathology was exhibited. There are currently no available methods of diagnosing ricin poisoning: detection of ricin from blood and other fluids is difficult because of its propensity for rapid and subtotal protein binding. Various immunologic methods have been described, but none has been field-tested. Treatment is largely supportive, and although numerous agents have been screened in vitro, none is currently advocated in the treatment of ricin poisoning. Antitoxins are currently also being evaluated [63]. In cases of gastrointestinal exposure, activated charcoal is recommended, although its interaction with ricin has not been ascertained.

Bioterrorism potential

Ricin exhibits various properties that suit a potential biological weapon: it is abundant worldwide, it is relatively environmentally stable in its aerosolized form, and it is susceptible to mass-production without the need of specialized technology. The toxin has been tested as a biological weapon by various countries in the past and it has been implicated in the murder of a Bulgarian dissident, Georgi Markov, in Great Britain in 1978 [64]. Furthermore, its recent isolation from White House mail facilities, a US senator's office [61], and after a London police raid [65] renewed interest in its potential. It could be distributed either through aerosolization, or through contamination of food or water sources, the former means of distribution being potentially more threatening to public health. In such a situation, preparedness is an issue, because a huge burden of patients with severe respiratory pathology should be handled by health authorities, the suitability of the various existing vaccines (including the ones in production) is a significant issue, and the absence of a definite diagnostic method and the difficulty in differential diagnosis from other respiratory pathogens would further slow the response. Its use through food or water poisoning seems more difficult, taking into account the rather large (compared with other toxins) lethal dose extrapolated for humans, in the range of 5 to 10 mg/kg.

A number of vaccines have been tested, and others are under evaluation: a formalin-treated toxoid was successful in protecting mice in a subsequent aerosol challenge, yet the golden equilibrium between attenuation and immunogenicity is hard to achieve [66], and postexposure prophylaxis has not been ascertained. A deglycosylated ricin chain A vaccine enhanced the toxicity, presumably through delayed clearance [53]. A number of recombinant vaccines have been developed or are under development, excellently summarized by Mantis [53], including mucosal vaccines that take advantage of the protective role of secretory IgA against the toxin, and the first recombinant vaccine to enter phase I trials was recently reported [67]. On the basis of all these factors, one could advocate the inclusion of ricin in category A pathogens in the future.

Staphylococcal enterotoxin B

The toxin

Staphylococcal enterotoxin B is the most widely studied of the enterotoxins produced by *Staphylococcus aureus*, and belongs to the family of superantigens, acting after transcytosis through the epithelium by binding to T lymphocytes and major histocompatibility complex class II molecules and triggering a cytokine storm, predominantly through the release of interferon-γ, tumor necrosis factor-α, and interleukin-1, leading to toxic shock syndrome [68]. Staphylococcal enterotoxin B is a prevalent cause of acute diarrheal illness when ingested, causing a self-limited syndrome of undetermined pathogenesis that starts hours after exposure and gradually wanes during the next 72 hours. Its inclusion, however, in category B pathogen list is warranted because of its possible effects when administered in aerosol form, based on limited human data (involving accidental military exposure) and various experimental animal models. Sixteen cases of inhalational exposure have been documented, resulting rapidly ($<$24 hours) in evolution of a clinical syndrome characterized by fever, malaise, cough, dyspnea, nausea, and vomiting. Ocular exposure in humans can result in purulent conjunctivitis [69]. In animal models exposed to aerosolized form of staphylococcal enterotoxin B initial gastrointestinal symptoms were followed by death caused by pulmonary edema by Day 3 [70]. The estimated minimum dose for evoking an emetic response in human volunteers is 5 μg [71], whereas in aerosolized exposure, the estimated 50% lethal dose (LD_{50}) is 0.02 μg/kg [72]. Immune protection through anti–staphylococcal enterotoxin B antibodies, even with passive administration, has been outlined [73]. Diagnosis is based on sophisticated toxin assays performed at reference laboratories. Treatment is largely supportive, although experimental therapeutic procedures are currently under investigation, aiming at halting the cytokine domino at various points of its activation [68].

Bioterrorism potential

Certain aspects of a potential deliberate release of staphylococcal enterotoxin B in inhalational form should be addressed, one of the most important being the difficulties posed in differential diagnosis, especially in the context of the absence of widely available diagnostic procedures. A wide variety of both formalin-inactivated and recombinant vaccines have been tested, but none has been approved for human use, although new candidates emerge [53].

Alphaviruses

The viruses

Venezuelan equine encephalitis (VEE), Eastern equine encephalitis (EEE), and Western equine encephalitis (WEE) belong to this category. All are mosquito-borne RNA viruses that rarely cause disease in humans but are significant causes of equine morbidity [74]. VEE is the commonest and the most extensively studied pathogen, with a geographic distribution encompassing Latin America and in certain outbreaks reaching the United States. The virus uses equine species as amplifiers, because equine disease is related to significant viremia (although this is not the case for newer strains implicated in recent epidemics in Mexico, where strains with particular neurotropism might be implicated) [75,76]. Human disease is rare, usually in the form of a self-remitting flulike syndrome. Progression to encephalitis occurs in 1% of the adults and 4% of the pediatric population, with 20% mortality.

EEE is principally located in the United States, east of the Mississippi River, but principally animal disease has also been reported from the Caribbean and Latin America. An average of 4.9 cases is reported annually in the United States, and the attack rates calculated from clusters of cases is 1 per 1000 population, and most detected cases occur in children and older adults. Incubation period is 5 to 7 days. The ratio of self-remitting or nonapparent to severe infections is 40:1 for adults, and 17:1 for the pediatric population [74]. The clinical syndrome is similar to VEE, but mortality is much higher (>50%), with an additional number of survivors exhibiting severe neurologic sequelae.

WEE is distributed in various western territories of the Untied States and Canada, but also in regions of Latin America. Human attack rates in past outbreaks reached up to 1.7 per 1000 population, and mortality is generally estimated at 3% to 4%. The ratio of self-remitting or nonapparent to severe infections is 1150:1 for adults, but only 1:1 for infants. As with EEE, the disease has a seasonal distribution, probably related to the increased outdoor activities during the summer period. The clinical syndrome induced, after an incubation period of 5 to 10 days, is particularly severe in infants, with common neurologic sequelae present in survivors of this age group.

The diagnosis is based on PCR detection of the viruses in cerebrospinal fluid samples (VEE and EEE) [77]; serum and cerebrospinal fluid serology might also be helpful in diagnosis. Treatment is supportive for all agents, although experimental data suggest a role for interferon-γ for VEE [78]. Human-to-human transmission does not occur for any of the agents.

Bioterrorism potential

The attractiveness of VEE as a biological weapon is based on its potential for widespread infection through aerosolization or release of infected mosquitoes, its relatively low infective dose for humans, its ease of production, and its implications for animal populations of the targeted area [79]. Studies on weaponization of VEE have allegedly taken place in the past [80]. A particular disturbing scenario regarding VEE's low attack rates (at least in the form of severe disease) might include genetic manipulation and evolution of highly neurotropic (inducing more severe disease) strains. Prophylaxis through vaccination is not available for civilians: an inactivated vaccine is available as an investigational new drug, and live attenuated vaccines are in development [81]. The weapon potential of EEE is roughly equal to that of VEE, its higher infective dose being compensated by the relative severity of the clinical syndrome. Pre-exposure prophylaxis through vaccination is not available for the public, but only through the US Army. On the contrary, the pathogenetic characteristics of WEE make it a pediatric biological weapon (and a wide deliberate release would have the same impact as Herod the Great in the targeted area: if WEE was not exclusively located in the Western Hemisphere, the notorious Massacre of the Innocents by Herod the Great could be viewed as an epidemic of WEE). Various experimental recombinant WEE vaccines are under development [82].

Bunyaviruses

The viruses

LaCrosse virus and California encephalitis viruses are the representatives of the Bunyaviridae family in category B, whereas Crimean-Congo hemorrhagic fever is listed in category C. LaCrosse virus remains the most important cause of pediatric encephalitis in the United States [74], with annual cases reported averaging 70, mostly from states from the middle-north, possibly reflecting the natural host (squirrels and chipmunks) residing in areas rich in forests [74]. The ratio of unapparent to apparent infection is huge, and mortality is extremely low (0.3%), whereas long-term neurologic sequelae are also rare (2%), despite LaCrosse virus's epileptogenic properties and initial clinical resemblance to herpetic encephalitis. Hyponatremia is a common finding, related to adverse prognosis [83]. Incubation period is 1 to 6 days. Distinct histologic findings have been described in the rare fatalities (focusing, in contrast to other viral encephalitis lesions, in the cortical gray matter). Diagnosis is based on serology and various PCR assays recently described [84]. Treatment is largely supportive. Other California encephalitis viruses are extremely rare human pathogens.

Bioterrorism potential

The weapon potential of LaCrosse virus is certainly lower than that of alphaviruses, because of the lower morbidity and mortality rates exhibited. One may assume that an episode involving deliberate release of a virus would preferentially use an alphavirus as VEE. There are no vaccines available, and development is still at preliminary stages [85].

Flaviviruses

The viruses

Japanese encephalitis virus, West Nile virus (WNV), and Kyasanur Forest virus are included in this genus and listed in category B. Other members of the genus, such as St. Louis encephalitis virus, could theoretically be included, yet much of what applies for the included viruses could be extrapolated to it. Japanese encephalitis virus is the cause of the most prevalent pediatric viral encephalitis worldwide, with an estimated 50,000 cases diagnosed annually in countries of East and Southeast Asia, although the virus has recently spread to Australia [86]. Pigs and birds serve as the amplifying hosts of this mosquito-borne virus, which causes a similar syndrome to the alphaviruses, with an unapparent to apparent case ratio of 50 to 400:1 and a case fatality rate above 20% (much of which is accredited to the pediatric population, because in adults this rate is 10%). The disease exhibits a peak during summer and the incubation period is 5 to 14 days. Low antibody levels at diagnosis are correlated to an adverse prognosis. The diagnosis is achieved through serology (ELISA) [87] and PCR [88]. Treatment is largely supportive.

WNV is a pathogen at the epicenter of medical interest since its introduction in the New World since 1999 and its subsequent spread to the West and South [89,90] and the evolution of a disease spectrum that encompasses severe neurologic sequelae in the last decade. Birds serve as the amplifying hosts for this virus, and a wide array of arthropods and animals can carry WNV or exhibit pathology [91]. Important issues were raised regarding its transmission through transfusion and transplantation [92], and public health policies had to be adapted quickly to rapidly emerging facts. Unlike other encephalitis viruses, WNV poses a significant risk for older adults, and possibly patients with various forms of immune compromise, especially diabetics [93] (other predisposing factors have been discussed, including hypertension, but are not universally accepted [91]). WNV spreads through the reticuloendothelial system after its entrance to the body by a mosquito bite inoculation, and the ensuing viremia facilitates entrance to the central nervous system (WNV is particularly neurotropic). Incubation period is 5 to 14 days. The clinical syndrome produced may have some characteristic aspects, such as hyponatremia, poliolike acute flaccid paralysis related to poor outcome, and increased dyskinesias in encephalitis cases [94]. Overall mortality reaches 10%, but neurologic sequelae may be observed in more than half of the survivors. Diagnosis can be achieved by real-time PCR [95] or ELISA, although the latter's increased percentage of cross-reactions with other flaviviruses has augmented the development of immunofluorescence assays. Regarding ELISA, persistence of IgM has been reported that may further hamper its diagnostic potential [96]. Experimental data on therapeutic options have offered few hopes until now, with a controversial role for human immunoglobulin [97], and preliminary reports with antisense gene–targeted compounds [98].

The inclusion of Kyasanur Forest virus in this category also seems like an aberration, because most other hemorrhagic fever viruses belong to category A, and Crimean-Congo hemorrhagic fever and Yellow fever belong to category C. Furthermore, the rationale of this classification is not explained in

NIAID documents [2]. Presumably, the propensity for neurologic complications during the second phase of the disease accounts for this joint with viral encephalitides classification. Kyasanur Forest virus is a tick-borne hemorrhagic fever virus found exclusively in Northern India. Incubation period is 3 to 8 days. Case fatality rate is 3% to 5%, and clinical presentation is characterized by a first febrile period during which hemorrhagic manifestations may appear, with bradycardia and hypotension being common findings, and a second febrile period 10 to 21 days after defervescence, which is accompanied by various neurologic symptoms. Diagnosis is based on serology, although the protracted viremia allows for laboratory isolation of the virus. Treatment is supportive [99].

Bioterrorism potential

One important aspect in regard to Japanese encephalitis virus and its bioweapon potential is the current status of vaccine availability: the development of a Food and Drug Administration–approved formalin-inactivated mouse brain vaccine for Japanese encephalitis virus and its wide application in endemic countries in the second half of the twentieth century was a significant weapon against the disease and an important prophylactic component of travel medicine. Its efficacy reached 91% [100]. The vaccine eventually will be replaced by an inactivated cell culture vaccine, or by an attenuated live vaccine similar to the current Chinese approach [101,102].

Regarding WNV, its introduction into the New World raised fears of a bioterrorism act, and such an approach (evolution of a long-term epidemic or endemic has been considered an alternative important aspect of bioterrorism [103]) has been discussed. At present WNV is the subject of significant and rapid scientific progress, which could be used in less benign ways, but still the scientific community remains one step ahead. Development of a vaccine is in process with preliminary reports and phase I trials for DNA vaccines and live attenuated chimeric vaccines [104]. Still, as the complete spectrum of WNV is clarified, its importance as a possible biological weapon may increase, and its inclusion in category A pathogens could be supported.

A formalin-inactivated vaccine for Kyasanur Forest virus has been used in endemic regions [105], but its efficacy is diminished in patients exposed to other flaviviruses.

Foodborne and waterborne pathogens

The bacteria

Most of the known bacterial causes of infectious diarrhea are included in category B pathogen list. Most of them are universally widespread, and responsible for millions of annual cases worldwide [106].

Salmonella species can induce acute infectious diarrhea (usually *Salmonella enterica* serovars *enteritidis* and *typhimurium*) that manifests usually within 1 day after exposure, demand a low inoculum of almost 100 colony-forming units, and can be treated only with supportive measures. More severe cases may demand the use of co-trimoxazole, quinolones, or ceftriaxone. *Salmonella typhi* is the causative agent of typhoid fever, a protracted systematic illness that, at least in experimental studies, demands a high inoculum [107]. The incubation period ranges from 7 to 14 days, and achlorhydria is one important risk factor. Characteristic (but inconsistently seen) clinical findings include relative bradycardia and truncal rose spots. The disease causes complications in the gastrointestinal tract or the central nervous system in 10% of patients, but the overall case-fatality rate is less than 2%. Blood and bone marrow cultures are the preferential diagnostic methods, the latter reaching a sensitivity of 95%. Quinolones are the treatment of choice, and alternative options include azithromycin (in cases of quinolone resistance); co-trimoxazole; amoxicillin; or ceftriaxone [108].

Shigella species may be the most fearsome foodborne and waterborne pathogen, because it can induce bloody diarrhea with a very low inoculum (on average 200 colony-forming units); can further be transmitted from person to person through the fecal-oral route; and is related to the late development of hemolytic uremic syndrome. Its incubation period is 1 to 7 days, and achlorhydria also predisposes to clinical disease. The importance of Shiga's toxin as a prototype toxin cannot be overemphasized. Treatment is based on co-trimoxazole or quinolones. Azithromycin and ceftriaxone may also be used [109].

Escherichia coli strains can be implicated in acute watery diarrhea (enteropathogenic *E coli*) [110], but also in a low-inoculum-induced, often afebrile (50%), bloody (in 90% of the patients) diarrhea by Shiga's toxin–producing strains [111], the importance of which is paramount, because the disease is also related to the development of hemolytic uremic syndrome in a significant percentage of children. Rapid diagnosis is imperative, because antibiotics may further predispose to hemolytic uremic syndrome development, although other reports suggest the opposite [112], and antimotility drugs are contraindicated. Attack rates for Shiga's toxin–producing strains are estimated at 20%.

Campylobacter jejuni is the most prevalent bacterial cause of infectious diarrhea in adults, with an incubation period of 1 to 7 days, and a very high ratio of subclinical to clinical cases, possibly because of its exquisite susceptibility to hydrochloric acid. It is also related to certain sequelae, as Guillain-Barré syndrome [113]; *Campylobacter* is the syndrome's most common identified cause. Macrolides and azithromycin are first-line therapeutic choices, especially because quinolone resistance to the pathogen has been continuously on the rise [114].

Of the Vibrios, *V cholerae* has been historically responsible for a huge number of epidemics worldwide [115], inducing through an exotoxin a severe watery diarrhea that leads to hypovolemia and death in certain clinical settings. Achlorhydria is also a risk factor for symptomatic disease. The attack rates are high, however, and treatment, beyond aggressive fluid and electrolyte resuscitation, may be achieved with a single dose of doxycycline or ciprofloxacin (or erythromycin in pregnancy). *V parahemolyticus* is the commonest pathogen implicated in vibrio-related diarrhea in the Western world, causing in less than 24 hours after exposure a usually benign gastroenteritis, although septicemia might develop in immunocompromised patients and patients with underlying liver disease. It requires a high inoculum (> 10,000 colony-forming units). Treatment is largely supportive, and in severe cases doxycycline and quinolones can be used [116].

Listeria monocytogenes, the gram-positive pathogen of the group, a facultative anaerobe, is known to induce significant disease in immunocompromised patients, with a spectrum including septicemia and meningitis [117]. Listeriosis is also important for pregnant women, but foremost for the safety of the fetus [118]. In the United States 2500 cases occur annually, with 500 deaths recorded on average (case-fatality ratio 20%). Most cases are noted in newborns, pregnant women, and immunosuppressed patients. Incubation period is 1 day in uncomplicated cases, but may be prolonged in invasive disease. High-dose ampicillin therapy is warranted.

Yersinia enterocolitica is a zoonotic pathogen largely localized to Northern Europe [119], which usually causes acute enteritis, especially in young children. The severity of infection (including septicemia, which even if treated is associated with 50% mortality) is related to host factors, namely iron overload as in thalassemia, underlying liver disease, diabetes mellitus, and old age; the disease may be more common in African Americans and infants in the United States [120]. Isolation of the organism suggests the diagnosis, although serology might be helpful. Treatment is usually suggested for immunocompromised patients and severe infections, using combinations of doxycycline, co-trimoxazole, aminoglycosides, or quinolones.

The viruses

Noroviruses are the commonest cause of acute infectious diarrhea worldwide, responsible for 90% of the outbreaks and 52% of total cases in the United States [121]. The inoculum is low (< 100 viral particles), and attack rates exquisitely high, reaching 100% in contained situations. Further human-to-human transmission is feasible, especially in the presence of severe symptoms. Incubation period is hours to 2 days, and supportive measures are usually the only indicated treatment. Diagnosis is based on real-time PCR, although ELISA may also be helpful. One important aspect of Noroviruses is their ability to exist in aerosolized form, and their relative environmental stability, because they are resistant to common disinfectants.

Hepatitis A virus has been related to massive epidemics because of consumption of infected seafood and can be relatively resistant to chlorination, surviving from common hygiene measures of potable water supplies. The inoculum for induction of infection is low (< 100 viral particles), and the incubation period is 3 to 6 weeks. The resulting acute hepatitis is benign (0.2% mortality in patients who developed jaundice) and does not exhibit chronicity. Reported attack rates vary widely. Serology is usually enough in terms for diagnosis [122].

The protozoa

Cryptosporidium parvum is an intracellular waterborne pathogen that has caused few significant epidemics [123], but is of main importance in the pathology of AIDS. Its cysts are environmentally stable, and a small number of cysts (even one to two) are required to induce infection. Incubation period is 1 to 14 days. Immunocompetent patients are usually symptom-free or exhibit limited symptoms, but the disease is more severe in immunocompromised patients, and can be related to significant weight loss. Human-to-human secondary transmission is feasible. Treatment is advocated for severe cases and paromomycin is the agent of choice, although new treatment options are emerging [124].

Cyclospora cayetanensis is a recently recognized coccidian parasite of unknown ecology, which can cause protracted, relapsing diarrheic syndromes, accompanied by fatigue and weight loss, and in 50% of the cases fever. Incubation period is 1 week, and infection has been related to contaminated basil and lettuce, and most notoriously Guatemalan raspberries [125]. Immunologically naive populations may be more susceptible to severe disease. Attack rates are estimated high, but experimental studies failed to induce disease even with high inocula [126]. Diagnosis can be achieved by staining or PCR, or by ultraviolet fluorescent microscopy, using the oocyst's autofluorescence. Co-trimoxazole is used for treatment. No human-to-human transmission occurs [127].

Entamoeba histolytica is a parasite with worldwide distribution, usually producing no symptoms (cyst passers), but also able to induce a usually afebrile colitis with ulcer formation, after an incubation period of 3 weeks. Amebomas and hepatic abscesses are known complications. Alternative diagnostic procedures, apart from microscopy of feces, include duodenal biopsy and serology (ELISA). Treatment uses a combination of metronidazole with either iodoquinol or paromomycin [128].

Giardia lamblia is also an intestinal parasite with worldwide distribution correlating with poor hygiene. It can induce a protracted diarrheic syndrome after an incubation period of 12 to 20 days, attack rates varying from 17% to 47%. Severe disease is almost exclusively seen in children and young women. Person-to-person transmission is feasible through the fecal-oral route. Treatment with metronidazole (or alternatively quinacrine or furazolidone) is advocated: 20% of treated patients experience treatment failure or relapse and are usually retreated [129].

Microsporidia have been recently recognized as human pathogens. They are unicellular, obligate intracellular eukaryotes with a characteristic polar tube [130].

Enterocytozoon bieneusi is the commonest human pathogen causing chronic intestinal inflammation in patients with AIDS (but also in other immunocompromised populations). Less than 20 cases have been described in immunocompetent adults, as benign cases of traveler's diarrhea. Diagnosis is based on light microscopy (to the genus level) and PCR. Treatment options are limited, and in general only fumagillin can be suggested [131]. Immune reconstitution through antiretroviral therapy augments clearing of the infection. The pathogen exhibits potential for transmission in aerosolized form, and can be transmitted from person-to-person through the fecal-oral route. *Encephalitozoon intestinalis* has caused similar symptoms in <200 immunocompromised patients reported in the literature, and two immunocompetent travelers. *E intestinalis* is usually sensitive to albendazole. Human infection with *Encephalitozoon hellem* and *Encephalitozoon cuniculi* is very rare.

Finally, *Toxoplasma gondii* is an intracellular foodborne pathogen, which poses significant risks for patients with AIDS, while also adversely affecting the outcome of the fetus when nonimmune pregnant mothers are infected. Rare cases of chorioretinitis are the most significant presentations in immunocompetent adults. The evolution of PCR has augmented accurate diagnosis. Treatment, when needed, is based on combinations of pyrimethamine and sulfadiazine (or clindamycin) [132].

Bioterrorism potential

Foodborne and waterborne bacteria can be implicated in potential bioterrorism events because, besides air, food and water supplies are the other options for accessing massive numbers of candidate patients [133]. Two characteristic episodes of deliberate release have outlined this potential. In 1984, a religious group used *S typhimurium* to contaminate salad bars to influence the outcome of a regional election [134], and an attempt of poisoning using Shiga's toxin was later reported [135]. Category A pathogens can also be implicated in poisoning of the food and water chain [136]. One critical aspect of a potential episode is recognition of intent, because many epidemics occur annually worldwide, often caused by inadvertent contamination of the same sources that are implicated in a voluntary release. For category B pathogens, however, the huge experience gained from naturally occurring outbreaks, the evolution of extended networks for surveillance, and the ability to cooperate in international epidemiologic studies (witness the example of the Guatemalan raspberries [125]), definitely facilitates a prompt, well-organized, and successful response. One problem that may emerge is that, as with naturally occurring outbreaks, a definite diagnosis should be reached quickly to exclude other toxic compounds, and to ensure that empirical decisions are not being made: for example, an outbreak that is ultimately attributed to Shiga's toxin–producing strains should be followed by a guideline for avoidance of antibiotics and antimotility drugs as much as possible (see above). The scale of danger posed by category B foodborne and waterborne pathogens is not similar: certain pathogens induce secondary medical problems, such as hemolytic uremic syndrome and Guillain-Barré syndrome (or even reactive arthritis), potentiating their overall effect on public health. Certain pathogens have the potential of the creation of a second wave of infection, caused by human-to-human transmission. Other pathogens can facilitate further transmission because of their shedding from nonsymptomatic carriers (Typhoid Mary–like). Certain of these pathogens, such as *V cholerae*, are related to a possibly more extreme public response, because of intrinsic fear of the pathogen [137]. Furthermore, it is obvious that if bioterrorists had the option to choose, they would choose a pathogen with low inoculum and high attack rates. One cannot exclude that certain populations at risk (ie, AIDS patients) might also become the specific target of extremist groups. Certain agents are not that well known, so it is difficult for extremist groups to develop them for dispersion: category B includes both *Shigella*, which might be a primary extremist choice, and cyclospora, scientific knowledge on which is still extremely limited.

Vaccine availability for foodborne and waterborne pathogens is limited at present. Commercially available vaccines exist for typhoid (a polysaccharide vaccine and an oral live attenuated vaccine) [108]; cholera (a killed whole cell vaccine and a live attenuated vaccine, both are not available in the United States) [138]; and hepatitis A virus. Other vaccine candidates for typhoid are emerging [139]. In development (or trials) are also vaccines for enteropathogenic *E coli* [140], *Shigella* [141], *C jejuni*, [142], *Y enterocolitica*, *Entamoeba histolytica* [143], and *Toxoplasma gondii*. Monoclonal antibodies directed against Shiga's toxin are also being studied [144].

Summary

Category B of potential bioterrorism agents is a vast pool of pathogens and toxins, with varying clinical characteristics, ranging from hard to develop as weapons viruses with significant mortality to easily weaponized bacteria that induce clinical syndromes with minimal mortality, to vaguely studied pathogens with unproved risk as weapons. Further stratification of this category is warranted, one that may bring certain agents as ricin, *Shigella*, and West Nile virus closer to category A agents, while simultaneously administering category C status to agents as Kyasanur Forest virus, cyclospora and microsporidia, and epsilon toxin of *C perfringens*. Further stratification of the existing classifications will result in more appropriate definitions of priorities.

References

[1] Centers for Disease Control and Prevention. Emergency preparedness and response: bioterrorism agents/ diseases. Available at: http://www.bt.cdc.gov/agent/agentlist-category.asp. Accessed January 10, 2006.

[2] National Institute of Allergy and Infectious Diseases Biodefense Research. NIAID biodefense agenda for CDC category B and C priority pathogens. Available at: http://www3.niaid.nih.gov/Biodefense/Research/categorybandc.pdf. Accessed January 10, 2006.
[3] Pappas G, Akritidis N, Bosilkovski M, et al. Brucellosis. N Engl J Med 2005;352:2325–36.
[4] Pappas G, Papadimitriou P, Akritidis N, et al. The new global map of human brucellosis. Lancet Infect Dis 2006;6:91–9.
[5] Memish ZA, Balkhy HH. Brucellosis and international travel. J Travel Med 2004;11:49–55.
[6] Gorvel JP, Moreno E. Brucella intracellular life: from invasion to intracellular replication. Vet Microbiol 2002;90:281–97.
[7] Colmenero JD, Reguera JM, Martos F, et al. Complications associated with Brucella melitensis infection: a study of 530 cases. Medicine (Baltimore) 1996;75:195–211 [Erratum: Medicine (Baltimore) 1997;76:139].
[8] Al Dahouk S, Tomaso H, Nockler K, et al. Laboratory-based diagnosis of brucellosis–a review of the literature. Part I: Techniques for direct detection and identification of Brucella spp. Clin Lab 2003;49:487–505.
[9] Al Dahouk S, Tomaso H, Nockler K, et al. Laboratory-based diagnosis of brucellosis–a review of the literature. Part II: serological tests for brucellosis. Clin Lab 2003;49:577–89.
[10] Navarro E, Casao MA, Solera J. Diagnosis of human brucellosis using PCR. Expert Rev Mol Diagn 2004;4:115–23.
[11] Queipo-Ortuno MI, Colmenero JD, Baeza G, et al. Comparison between LightCycler real-time polymerase chain reaction (PCR) assay with serum and PCR-enzyme-linked immunosorbent assay with whole blood samples for the diagnosis of human brucellosis. Clin Infect Dis 2005;40:260–4.
[12] Pappas G, Akritidis N, Tsianos E. Effective treatments in the management of brucellosis. Expert Opin Pharmacother 2005;6:201–9.
[13] Solera J, Martinez-Alfaro E, Espinoza A. Recognition and optimum treatment of brucellosis. Drugs 1997;53:245–56.
[14] Christopher GW, Agan MB, Cieslak TJ, et al. History of US military contributions to the study of bacterial zoonoses. Mil Med 2005;170(4 Suppl):39–48.
[15] Yagupsky P, Baron EJ. Laboratory exposures to brucellae and implications for bioterrorism. Emerg Infect Dis 2005;11:1180–5.
[16] Pappas G, Bosilkovski M, Akritidis N, et al. Brucellosis and the respiratory system. Clin Infect Dis 2003;37:e95–9.
[17] Bossi P, Tegnell A, Baka A, et al. Bichat guidelines for the clinical management of brucellosis and bioterrorism-related brucellosis. Euro Surveill 2004;9:E15–6.
[18] Schurig GG, Sriranganathan N, Corbel MJ. Brucellosis vaccines: past, present and future. Vet Microbiol 2002;90:479–96.
[19] Yabuuchi E, Kosako Y, Oyaizu H, et al. Proposal of *Burkholderia* gen. nov. and transfer of seven species of the genus *Pseudomonas* homology group II to the new genus, with the type species *Burkholderia cepacia* (Palleroni and Holmes 1981) comb. nov. Microbiol Immunol 1992;36:1251–75 [Erratum: Microbiol Immunol 1993;37:335].
[20] Cheng AC, Dance DA, Currie BJ. Bioterrorism, glanders, and melioidosis. Euro Surveill 2005;10:E1–2.
[21] Wilkinson L. Glanders: medicine and veterinary medicine in common pursuit of a contagious disease. Med Hist 1981;25:363–84.
[22] Currie BJ. Melioidosis: an important cause of pneumonia in residents of and travellers returned from endemic regions. Eur Respir J 2003;22:542–50.
[23] Srinivasan A, Kraus CN, DeShazer D, et al. Glanders in a military research microbiologist. N Engl J Med 2001;345:256–8.
[24] White NJ. Melioidosis. Lancet 2003;361:1715–22.
[25] Inglis TJ, Merritt A, Chidlow G, et al. Comparison of diagnostic laboratory methods for identification of *Burkholderia pseudomallei*. J Clin Microbiol 2005;43:2201–6.

[26] Currie BJ, Fisher DA, Howard DM, et al. Endemic melioidosis in tropical northern Australia: a 10-year prospective study and review of the literature. Clin Infect Dis 2000;31: 981–6.
[27] Kenny DJ, Russell P, Rogers D, et al. In vitro susceptibilities of *Burkholderia mallei* in comparison to those of other pathogenic *Burkholderia* spp. Antimicrob Agents Chemother 1999;43:2773–5.
[28] Bossi P, Tegnell A, Baka A, et al. Bichat guidelines for the clinical management of glanders and melioidosis and bioterrorism-related glanders and melioidosis. Euro Surveill 2004;9: E17–8.
[29] Lever SM, Nelson M, Ireland PI, et al. Experimental aerogenic *Burkholderia mallei* (glanders) infection in the BALB/c mouse. J Med Microbiol 2003;52(Pt 12):1109–15.
[30] Dance DA. Melioidosis: the tip of the iceberg? Clin Microbiol Rev 1991;4:52–60.
[31] Gregory DW, Schaffner W. Psittacosis. Semin Respir Infect 1997;12:7–11.
[32] Maurin M, Raoult D. Q fever. Clin Microbiol Rev 1999;12:518–53.
[33] Raoult D, Marrie T, Mege J. Natural history and pathophysiology of Q fever. Lancet Infect Dis 2005;5:219–26.
[34] Fenollar F, Fournier PE, Carrieri MP, et al. Risks factors and prevention of Q fever endocarditis. Clin Infect Dis 2001;33:312–6.
[35] Scola BL. Current laboratory diagnosis of Q fever. Semin Pediatr Infect Dis 2002;13: 257–62.
[36] Choi E. Tularemia and Q fever. Med Clin North Am 2002;86:393–416.
[37] Marrie TJ, Raoult D. Update on Q fever, including Q fever endocarditis. Curr Clin Top Infect Dis 2002;22:97–124.
[38] Kelly DJ, Richards AL, Temenak J, et al. The past and present threat of rickettsial diseases to military medicine and international public health. Clin Infect Dis 2002;34(Suppl 4): S145–69.
[39] Madariaga MG, Rezai K, Trenholme GM, et al. Q fever: a biological weapon in your backyard. Lancet Infect Dis 2003;3:709–21.
[40] Kagawa FT, Wehner JH, Mohindra V. Q fever as a biological weapon. Semin Respir Infect 2003;18:183–95.
[41] Pappas G, Akritidis N, Tsianos EV. Attack scenarios with rickettsial species: implications for response and management. Ann NY Acad Sci 2005;163:451–8.
[42] World Health Organization. Health aspects of chemical and biological weapons: report of a WHO group of consultants. Geneva, Switzerland: World Health Organization; 1970.
[43] Azad A, Radulovic S. Pathogenic rickettsiae as bioterrorism agents. Ann N Y Acad Sci 2003;990:734–8.
[44] Raoult D, Woodward T, Dumler JS. The history of epidemic typhus. Infect Dis Clin North Am 2004;18:127–40.
[45] Raoult D, Ndihokubwayo JB, Tissot-Dupont H, et al. Outbreak of epidemic typhus associated with trench fever in Burundi. Lancet 1998;352:353–8.
[46] Robinson D, Leo N, Prociv P, et al. Potential role of head lice, *Pediculus humanus capitis*, as vectors of *Rickettsia prowazekii*. Parasitol Res 2003;90:209–11.
[47] Duma RJ, Sonenshine DE, Bozeman FM, et al. Epidemic typhus in the United States associated with flying squirrels. JAMA 1981;245:2318–23.
[48] La Scola B, Raoult D. Laboratory diagnosis of rickettsioses: current approaches to diagnosis of old and new rickettsial diseases. J Clin Microbiol 1997;35:2715–27.
[49] Carl M, Tibbs CW, Dobson ME, et al. Diagnosis of acute typhus infection using the polymerase chain reaction. J Infect Dis 1990;161:791–3.
[50] Jiang J, Temenak JJ, Richards AL. Real-time PCR duplex assay for *Rickettsia prowazekii* and *Borrelia recurrentis*. Ann N Y Acad Sci 2003;990:302–10.
[51] Perine PL, Chandler BP, Krause DK, et al. A clinico-epidemiological study of epidemic typhus in Africa. Clin Infect Dis 1992;14:1149–58.

[52] Coker C, Majid M, Radulovic S. Development of *Rickettsia prowazekii* DNA vaccine: cloning strategies. Ann N Y Acad Sci 2003;990:757–64.
[53] Mantis NJ. Vaccines against the category B toxins: staphylococcal enterotoxin B, epsilon toxin and ricin. Adv Drug Deliv Rev 2005;57:1424–39.
[54] Finnie JW. Pathogenesis of brain damage produced in sheep by *Clostridium perfringens* type D epsilon toxin: a review. Aust Vet J 2003;81:219–21.
[55] Nagahama M, Sakurai J. High-affinity binding of *Clostridium perfringens* epsilon-toxin to rat brain. Infect Immun 1992;60:1237–40.
[56] Nagahama M, Ochi S, Sakurai J. Assembly of *Clostridium perfringens* epsilon-toxin on MDCK cell membrane. J Nat Toxins 1998;7:291–302.
[57] Oyston PC, Payne DW, Havard HL, et al. Production of a non-toxic site-directed mutant of *Clostridium perfringens* epsilon-toxin which induces protective immunity in mice. Microbiology 1998;144(Pt 2):333–41.
[58] Bradberry SM, Dickers KJ, Rice P, et al. Ricin poisoning. Toxicol Rev 2003;22:65–70.
[59] Roy CJ, Hale M, Hartings JM, et al. Impact of inhalation exposure modality and particle size on the respiratory deposition of ricin in BALB/c mice. Inhal Toxicol 2003;15:619–38.
[60] Wilhelmsen CL, Pitt ML. Lesions of acute inhaled lethal ricin intoxication in rhesus monkeys. Vet Pathol 1996;33:296–302.
[61] Audi J, Belson M, Patel M, et al. Ricin poisoning: a comprehensive review. JAMA 2005;294:2342–51.
[62] Sekine I, Kawase Y, Nishimori I, et al. Pathological study on mucosal changes in small intestine of rat by oral administration of ricin. I. Microscopical observation. Acta Pathol Jpn 1986;36:1205–12.
[63] Rainey GJ, Young JA. Antitoxins: novel strategies to target agents of bioterrorism. Nat Rev Microbiol 2004;2:721–6.
[64] Crompton R, Gall D. Georgi Markov: death in a pellet. Med Leg J 1980;48:51–62.
[65] Mayor S. UK doctors warned after ricin poison found in police raid. BMJ 2003;326:126.
[66] Griffiths GD, Phillips GJ, Bailey SC. Comparison of the quality of protection elicited by toxoid and peptide liposomal vaccine formulations against ricin as assessed by markers of inflammation. Vaccine 1999;17:2562–8.
[67] Smallshaw JE, Richardson JA, Pincus S, et al. Preclinical toxicity and efficacy testing of RiVax, a recombinant protein vaccine against ricin. Vaccine 2005;23:4775–84.
[68] Krakauer T. Chemotherapeutics targeting immune activation by staphylococcal superantigens. Med Sci Monit 2005;11:RA290–5.
[69] Rusnak JM, Kortepeter M, Ulrich R, et al. Laboratory exposures to staphylococcal enterotoxin B. Emerg Infect Dis 2004;10:1544–9.
[70] Mattix ME, Hunt RE, Wilhelmsen CL, et al. Aerosolized staphylococcal enterotoxin B-induced pulmonary lesions in rhesus monkeys (*Macaca mulatta*). Toxicol Pathol 1995;23:262–8.
[71] Balaban N, Rasooly A. Staphylococcal enterotoxins. Int J Food Microbiol 2000;61:1–10.
[72] Gill DM. Bacterial toxins: a table of lethal amounts. Microbiol Rev 1982;46:86–94.
[73] Boles JW, Pitt ML, LeClaire RD, et al. Generation of protective immunity by inactivated recombinant staphylococcal enterotoxin B vaccine in nonhuman primates and identification of correlates of immunity. Clin Immunol 2003;108:51–9.
[74] Calisher CH. Medically important arboviruses of the United States and Canada. Clin Microbiol Rev 1994;7:89–116.
[75] Weaver SC, Barrett AD. Transmission cycles, host range, evolution and emergence of arboviral disease. Nat Rev Microbiol 2004;2:789–801.
[76] Charles PC, Walters E, Margolis F, et al. Mechanism of neuroinvasion of Venezuelan equine encephalitis virus in the mouse. Virology 1995;208:662–71.
[77] Linssen B, Kinney RM, Aguilar P, et al. Development of reverse transcription-PCR assays specific for detection of equine encephalitis viruses. J Clin Microbiol 2000;38:1527–35.

[78] Grieder FB, Vogel SN. Role of interferon and interferon regulatory factors in early protection against Venezuelan equine encephalitis virus infection. Virology 1999;257:106–18.
[79] Bronze MS, Huycke MM, Machado LJ, et al. Viral agents as biological weapons and agents of bioterrorism. Am J Med Sci 2002;323:316–25.
[80] Smith JF, Davis K, Hart MK, et al. Viral encephalitides. In: Zajtchuk R, Bellamy RF, editors. Textbook of military medicine: medical aspects of chemical and biological warfare. Washington: Office of the Surgeon General, Department of the Army, United States of America; 1997. p. 561–91.
[81] Lee JS, Hadjipanayis AG, Parker MD. Viral vectors for use in the development of biodefense vaccines. Adv Drug Deliv Rev 2005;57:1293–314.
[82] Schoepp RJ, Smith JF, Parker MD. Recombinant chimeric western and eastern equine encephalitis viruses as potential vaccine candidates. Virology 2002;302:299–309.
[83] McJunkin JE, de los Reyes EC, Irazuzta JE, et al. La Crosse encephalitis in children. N Engl J Med 2001;344:801–7.
[84] Lambert AJ, Nasci RS, Cropp BC, et al. Nucleic acid amplification assays for detection of La Crosse virus RNA. J Clin Microbiol 2005;43:1885–9.
[85] Blakqori G, Weber F. Efficient cDNA-based rescue of La Crosse bunyaviruses expressing or lacking the nonstructural protein NSs. J Virol 2005;79:10420–8.
[86] Mackenzie JS. Emerging zoonotic encephalitis viruses: lessons from Southeast Asia and Oceania. J Neurovirol 2005;11:434–40.
[87] Solomon T, Thao LT, Dung NM, et al. Rapid diagnosis of Japanese encephalitis by using an immunoglobulin M dot enzyme immunoassay. J Clin Microbiol 1998;36:2030–4.
[88] Huang JL, Lin HT, Wang YM, et al. Sensitive and specific detection of strains of Japanese encephalitis virus using a one-step TaqMan RT-PCR technique. J Med Virol 2004;74: 589–96.
[89] Hayes EB, Komar N, Nasci RS, et al. Epidemiology and transmission dynamics of West Nile virus disease. Emerg Infect Dis 2005;11:1167–73.
[90] Campbell GL, Marfin AA, Lanciotti RS, et al. West Nile virus. Lancet Infect Dis 2002;2: 519–29.
[91] Granwehr BP, Lillibridge KM, Higgs S, et al. West Nile virus: where are we now? Lancet Infect Dis 2004;4:547–56.
[92] Busch MP, Caglioti S, Robertson EF, et al. Screening the blood supply for West Nile virus RNA by nucleic acid amplification testing. N Engl J Med 2005;353:460–7.
[93] Iwamoto M, Jernigan DB, Guasch A, et al. Transmission of West Nile virus from an organ donor to four transplant recipients. N Engl J Med 2003;348:2196–203.
[94] Sejvar JJ, Haddad MB, Tierney BC, et al. Neurologic manifestations and outcome of West Nile virus infection. JAMA 2003;290:511–5 [Erratum: JAMA 2003;290:1318].
[95] Lanciotti RS, Kerst AJ, Nasci RS, et al. Rapid detection of West Nile virus from human clinical specimens, field-collected mosquitoes, and avian samples by a TaqMan reverse transcriptase-PCR assay. J Clin Microbiol 2000;38:4066–71.
[96] Roehrig JT, Nash D, Maldin B, et al. Persistence of virus-reactive serum immunoglobulin m antibody in confirmed West Nile virus encephalitis cases. Emerg Infect Dis 2003;9:376–9.
[97] Ben-Nathan D, Lustig S, Tam G, et al. Prophylactic and therapeutic efficacy of human intravenous immunoglobulin in treating West Nile virus infection in mice. J Infect Dis 2003; 188:5–12.
[98] Shi PY. Strategies for the identification of inhibitors of West Nile virus and other flaviviruses. Curr Opin Investig Drugs 2002;3:1567–73.
[99] Pavri K. Clinical, clinicopathologic, and hematologic features of Kyasanur Forest disease. Rev Infect Dis 1989;11(Suppl 4):S854–9.
[100] Marfin AA, Eidex RS, Kozarsky PE, et al. Yellow fever and Japanese encephalitis vaccines: indications and complications. Infect Dis Clin North Am 2005;19:151–68.
[101] Monath TP, Guirakhoo F, Nichols R, et al. Chimeric live, attenuated vaccine against Japanese encephalitis (ChimeriVax-JE): phase 2 clinical trials for safety and immunogenicity,

effect of vaccine dose and schedule, and memory response to challenge with inactivated Japanese encephalitis antigen. J Infect Dis 2003;188:1213–30.
[102] Ohrr H, Tandan JB, Sohn YM, et al. Effect of single dose of SA 14–14–2 vaccine 1 year after immunisation in Nepalese children with Japanese encephalitis: a case-control study. Lancet 2005;366:1375–8.
[103] Casadevall A, Pirofski LA. The weapon potential of a microbe. Trends Microbiol 2004;12: 259–63.
[104] Hall RA, Khromykh AA. West Nile virus vaccines. Expert Opin Biol Ther 2004;4: 1295–305.
[105] Dandawate CN, Desai GB, Achar TR, et al. Field evaluation of formalin inactivated Kyasanur forest disease virus tissue culture vaccine in three districts of Karnataka state. Indian J Med Res 1994;99:152–8.
[106] Allos BM, Moore MR, Griffin PM, et al. Surveillance for sporadic foodborne disease in the 21st century: the FoodNet perspective. Clin Infect Dis 2004;38(Suppl 3):S115–20.
[107] Glynn JR, Hornick RB, Levine MM, et al. Infecting dose and severity of typhoid: analysis of volunteer data and examination of the influence of the definition of illness used. Epidemiol Infect 1995;115:23–30.
[108] Parry CM, Hien TT, Dougan G, et al. Typhoid fever. N Engl J Med 2002;347:1770–82.
[109] Niyogi SK. Shigellosis. J Microbiol 2005;43:133–43.
[110] Qadri F, Svennerholm AM, Faruque AS, et al. Enterotoxigenic *Escherichia coli* in developing countries: epidemiology, microbiology, clinical features, treatment, and prevention. Clin Microbiol Rev 2005;18:465–83.
[111] Paton JC, Paton AW. Pathogenesis and diagnosis of Shiga toxin-producing *Escherichia coli* infections. Clin Microbiol Rev 1998;11:450–79.
[112] Boyce TG, Swerdlow DL, Griffin PM. *Escherichia coli* O157:H7 and the hemolytic-uremic syndrome. N Engl J Med 1995;333:364–8.
[113] Nachamkin E, Allos BM, Ho T. *Campylobacter* species and Guillain-Barré syndrome. Clin Microbiol Rev 1998;11:555–67.
[114] Butzler JP. Campylobacter, from obscurity to celebrity. Clin Microbiol Infect 2004;10: 868–76.
[115] Kaper JB, Morris JG Jr, Levine MM. Cholera. Clin Microbiol Rev 1995;8:48–86 [Erratum: Clin Microbiol Rev 1995;8:316].
[116] Butt AA, Aldridge KE, Sanders CV. Infections related to the ingestion of seafood Part I: Viral and bacterial infections. Lancet Infect Dis 2004;4:201–12.
[117] Schlech WF III. Foodborne listeriosis. Clin Infect Dis 2000;31:770–5.
[118] Mylonakis E, Paliou M, Hohmann EL, et al. Listeriosis during pregnancy: a case series and review of 222 cases. Medicine (Baltimore) 2002;81:260–9.
[119] Bottone EJ. *Yersinia enterocolitica*: overview and epidemiologic correlates. Microbes Infect 1999;1:323–33.
[120] Ray SM, Ahuja SD, Blake PA, et al. Population-based surveillance for *Yersinia enterocolitica* infections in FoodNet sites, 1996–1999: higher risk of disease in infants and minority populations. Clin Infect Dis 2004;38(Suppl 3):S181–9.
[121] Musher DM, Musher BL. Contagious acute gastrointestinal infections. N Engl J Med 2004; 351:2417–27.
[122] Cuthbert JA. Hepatitis A: old and new. Clin Microbiol Rev 2001;14:38–58 [Erratum: Clin Microbiol Rev 2001;14:642].
[123] Mac Kenzie WR, Hoxie NJ, Proctor ME, et al. A massive outbreak in Milwaukee of cryptosporidium infection transmitted through the public water supply. N Engl J Med 1994;331: 161–7 [Erratum: N Engl J Med 1994;331:1035].
[124] Smith HV, Corcoran GD. New drugs and treatment for cryptosporidiosis. Curr Opin Infect Dis 2004;17:557–64.
[125] Herwaldt BL, Ackers ML. An outbreak in 1996 of cyclosporiasis associated with imported raspberries. The Cyclospora Working Group. N Engl J Med 1997;336:1548–56.

[126] Alfano-Sobsey EM, Eberhard ML, Seed JR, et al. Human challenge pilot study with *Cyclospora cayetanensis*. Emerg Infect Dis 2004;10:726–8.
[127] Herwaldt BL. *Cyclospora cayetanensis*: a review, focusing on the outbreaks of cyclosporiasis in the 1990s. Clin Infect Dis 2000;31:1040–57.
[128] Bruckner DA. Amebiasis. Clin Microbiol Rev 1992;5:356–69.
[129] Wolfe MS. Giardiasis. Clin Microbiol Rev 1992;5:93–100.
[130] Mathis A, Weber R, Deplazes P. Zoonotic potential of the microsporidia. Clin Microbiol Rev 2005;18:423–45.
[131] Molina JM, Tourneur M, Sarfati C, et al. Fumagillin treatment of intestinal microsporidiosis. N Engl J Med 2002;346:1963–9.
[132] Montoya JG, Liesenfeld O. Toxoplasmosis. Lancet 2004;363:1965–76.
[133] Elad D. Risk assessment of malicious biocontamination of food. J Food Prot 2005;68:1302–5.
[134] Torok TJ, Tauxe RV, Wise RP, et al. A large community outbreak of salmonellosis caused by intentional contamination of restaurant salad bars. JAMA 1997;278:389–95.
[135] Kolavic SA, Kimura A, Simons SL, et al. An outbreak of *Shigella dysenteriae* type 2 among laboratory workers due to intentional food contamination. JAMA 1997;278:396–8.
[136] Wein LM, Liu Y. Analyzing a bioterror attack on the food supply: the case of botulinum toxin in milk. Proc Natl Acad Sci U S A 2005;102:9984–9.
[137] Rotz LD, Khan AS, Lillibridge SR, et al. Public health assessment of potential biological terrorism agents. Emerg Infect Dis 2002;8:225–30.
[138] Lucas ME, Deen JL, von Seidlein L, et al. Effectiveness of mass oral cholera vaccination in Beira, Mozambique. N Engl J Med 2005;352:757–67.
[139] Von Seidlein L. The need for another typhoid fever vaccine. J Infect Dis 2005;192:357–9.
[140] Boedeker EC. Vaccines for enterotoxigenic *Escherichia coli*: current status. Curr Opin Gastroenterol 2005;21:15–9.
[141] Katz DE, Coster TS, Wolf MK, et al. Two studies evaluating the safety and immunogenicity of a live, attenuated *Shigella flexneri* 2a vaccine (SC602) and excretion of vaccine organisms in North American volunteers. Infect Immun 2004;72:923–30.
[142] Walker RI. Campylobacter vaccine development: a key to controlling enteric diseases. Expert Opin Investig Drugs 1999;8:107–13.
[143] Chaudhry OA, Petri WA Jr. Vaccine prospects for amebiasis. Expert Rev Vaccines 2005;4:657–68.
[144] Tzipori S, Sheoran A, Akiyoshi D, et al. Antibody therapy in the management of shiga toxin-induced hemolytic uremic syndrome. Clin Microbiol Rev 2004;17:926–41.

ELSEVIER
SAUNDERS

Infect Dis Clin N Am
20 (2006) 423–441

INFECTIOUS
DISEASE CLINICS
OF NORTH AMERICA

Category C Potential Bioterrorism Agents and Emerging Pathogens

Adnan Mushtaq, MD, Mohamed El-Azizi, PhD, Nancy Khardori, MD, PhD*

Department of Medicine, Division of Infectious Diseases, Southern Illinois University, School of Medicine, 701 North First Street, Room A 480, Springfield, IL 62702, USA

Category C bioterrorism agents

Infectious agents have been, and in the foreseeable future will remain, potential tools of mass casualties. The intentional use of living organisms or infected materials derived from them has occurred over centuries during war and peacetime by armies, states, groups, and individuals [1–5]. A wide range of microorganisms could be used as biological weapons. Few microorganisms can be used for production of weapons of mass destruction, however. Eligible agents should meet criteria such as availability, ease of dissemination, stability, and potential for high morbidity and mortality to qualify as a weapon of mass destruction [6].

The Centers for Disease Control and Prevention (CDC) has classified critical biologic agents into three major categories [7]. The agents classified as category C by the CDC currently are Nipah virus, Hantavirus, tick-borne hemorrhagic fever viruses, tick-borne encephalitis (TBE) virus complex, yellow fever, and multidrug-resistant tuberculosis (MDR-TB). These agents could be produced, disseminated, and engineered easily for mass exposure in the future. Preparedness for category C agents requires ongoing research to improve disease detection, diagnosis, treatment, and prevention.

Nipah virus

Nipah virus, a zoonotic virus, was discovered in 1999 [8]. The virus is named after the location where it was first detected in Malaysia. Nipah is

* Corresponding author.
E-mail address: nkhardori@siumed.edu (N. Khardori).

doi:10.1016/j.idc.2006.03.003

closely related to another zoonotic virus, Hendra virus. Nipah and Hendra are members of the virus family Paramyxoviridae [9]. Nipah virus has caused only a few focal outbreaks [10,11]; however, its capability of causing significant mortality in humans has made this emerging viral infection a public heath concern. In the Malaysian outbreak, a total of 265 people were infected, of whom 105 died. The Singapore outbreak led to 11 cases, with 1 death [12].

Transmission

The risk of transmission of Nipah virus from sick animals to humans is thought to be low, and person-to-person transmission has not been documented yet, even in the context of a large outbreak. In Malaysia and Singapore outbreaks, most of the patients had direct contact with pigs [13]. The mode of transmission from animal to animal and from animal to human is uncertain, but seems to require close contact with contaminated tissue or body fluids from infected animals [14]. It is believed that certain species of fruit bats are the natural hosts for Nipah virus [15]. The bats seem to be susceptible to infection with this virus, but they do not become ill. It is unknown how the virus is transmitted from bats to animals. The role of species other than pigs in transmitting infection to other animals has not yet been determined.

Clinical symptoms

The incubation period of the disease is 4 to 18 days. The infection may be mild or subclinical, and in symptomatic cases, the onset is usually with influenza-like symptoms with high fever and myalgia. The disease may progress to encephalitis with drowsiness, disorientation, convulsions, and coma.

Laboratory diagnosis

Procedures for the laboratory diagnosis of Nipah virus infection include serology, histopathology, immunohistochemistry, electron microscopy, polymerase chain reaction (PCR), and virus isolation [16,17].

Treatment

No drug therapies have been proved to be effective in treating Nipah infection. Treatment relies on providing intensive supportive care. There is some evidence that treatment with the antiviral drug ribavirin may reduce the mortality of acute Nipah encephalitis [18].

Disinfection

Phenolic disinfectants are not effective against Paramyxoviruses, but polar lipophilic solvents, such as chloroform, are effective.

Hantaviruses

Hantaviruses are serologically related members of the family Bunyaviridae [19]. The term *Hantavirus* is derived from the Hantaan River, where the prototype Old World hantavirus (Hantaan virus) was first isolated. The disease associated with the Old World hantaan virus is called Korean hemorrhagic fever or hemorrhagic fever with renal syndrome. Regions especially affected by hemorrhagic fever with renal syndrome include China, the Korean Peninsula, Russia (Hantaan and Seoul viruses), and northern and western Europe (Puumala and Dobrava viruses).

In 1993, a newly recognized species of hantavirus (New World hantavirus) was found to cause the hantavirus pulmonary syndrome in the southwestern United States [20–22]. Hantavirus pulmonary syndrome subsequently was recognized throughout the contiguous United States and the Americas. As of June 6, 2002, a total of 318 cases of hantavirus pulmonary syndrome had been identified in 31 states, with a case-fatality rate of 37% [23]. Several hantaviruses that are pathogenic for humans have been identified in the United States, including New York virus [24], Black Creek Canal virus [25], and Bayou virus [26].

Transmission

Hantaviruses are rodent-borne, and no arthropod vector has been implicated in the transmission of any of them. Hantaviruses do not cause overt illness in their reservoir hosts [27]. Transmission to humans is believed to be via aerosols of infected excreta of rodents [28]. No person-to-person transmission has been reported with the Old World hantavirus or in the United states [23]. All hantaviruses known to cause hantavirus pulmonary syndrome are carried by the New World rats and mice, family Muridae, subfamily Sigmodontinae [23].

Clinical features

Hemorrhagic fever with renal syndrome is characterized by fever and myalgia, which develop days or weeks (incubation period 5–42 days) after exposure to rodents. The disease progresses to hemorrhage and hemodynamic instability, occasionally progressing to shock. The disease enters a second phase affecting the kidneys characterized at first by oliguria then polyuria, hypertension, bleeding of the mucous membranes, and edema of the lungs. Mortality is usually from shock or hemorrhage. The fatality rate is 1% to 3% for Puumala virus, 7% for Hantaan virus, and 5% to 15% for Dobrava virus.

Hantavirus pulmonary syndrome is characterized by fever, chills, and severe myalgia, which progress to variably severe respiratory compromise and hemodynamic instability. Thrombocytopenia is common, and hemoconcentration and other hematologic abnormalities occur commonly in severe cases.

Laboratory diagnosis

The diagnosis of hantaviruses is based on history of any possible contact with rodents, the clinical findings, and serology results. In the early phase of the illness, the infection cannot be differentiated from other viral fevers. Direct detection of antigen, for early diagnosis of the disease, also has been used. The virus antigen can be shown in the blood or urine. Isolation of the virus from urine is successful early in the illness, whereas isolation of the virus from the blood is less consistent.

Treatment

Ribavirin is effective against Hantaan virus and was made available for postexposure prophylaxis to soldiers in Operation Desert Shield/Storm. Supportive care, such as dialysis support of the kidneys and maintenance of blood volume, also is important.

Decontamination

The viruses can be killed by sodium hypochlorite (1%), glutaraldehyde (2%), and ethanol (70%).

Yellow fever virus

Yellow fever is a viral hemorrhagic fever transmitted by infected mosquitoes. Infection causes a wide spectrum of disease, from mild symptoms to severe illness and death. The *yellow* in the name stands for the jaundice that affects some patients. Yellow fever occurs only in Africa and South America [29]. The World Health Organization has estimated that 200,000 cases of yellow fever occur each year [30].

Sylvatic (jungle), intermediate, and urban are the three cycles of infection of the yellow fever virus [31]. Jungle yellow fever is a disease of monkeys. It is a rare disease that occurs mainly in individuals who are exposed to tropical rain forests and are bitten by mosquitoes that have been infected by monkeys. The intermediate cycle of yellow fever occurs only in humid or semihumid savannahs of Africa and in small-scale epidemics in rural areas. Semidomestic mosquitoes infect monkey and human hosts. Urban yellow fever is a disease of humans. It is spread by *Aedes aegypti* mosquitoes that have been infected by other people. These mosquitoes have adapted to living among humans in cities, towns, and villages. Urban yellow fever is the cause of most yellow fever outbreaks and epidemics.

Transmission

The mosquito takes a blood meal from an infected monkey or human (urban), then bites a human. It injects saliva containing the virus into the bite to prevent blood clotting and infects the human.

Clinical features

The clinical spectrum of yellow fever ranges from subclinical infection to overwhelming multisystem disease [32]. Symptoms occur after 3 to 6 days of infection and usually include fever, prostration, headache, photophobia, lumbosacral pain, extremity pain (including knee joints), epigastric pain, anorexia, and vomiting. The second phase involves the liver and kidneys, and hemorrhagic symptoms and signs caused by thrombocytopenia and abnormal coagulation can occur. The fatality rate of severe yellow fever is approximately 20% [29].

Laboratory diagnosis

Definitive diagnosis is made by viral culture from blood or tissue specimens. It also is made by identification of yellow fever virus antigen or nucleic acid in tissues using immunohistochemistry, enzyme-linked immunosorbent assay (ELISA), or PCR tests [33]. Detection of IgM antibody by capture ELISA with confirmation of fourfold or greater increase in neutralizing antibody titers between acute-phase and convalescent-phase serum samples also is diagnostic [29].

Treatment

Live attenuated virus preparation made from the 17D yellow fever virus strain is available [34]. It is provides immunity for about 10 years. No effective specific antiviral therapy for yellow fever has been identified. Treatment consists of providing general supportive care and varies depending on which organs are involved.

Decontamination

The yellow fever virus is killed by 1% sodium hypochlorite, 2% glutaraldehyde, formaldehyde, and 70% ethanol. It also is killed by heating at 60°C for 10 minutes.

Tick-borne encephalitis complex

TBE is a human viral infectious disease involving predominantly the central nervous system. It is one of the most dangerous human infections occurring in Europe and many parts of Asia. TBE is caused by members of the TBE virus complex of the Flaviviridae [35]. TBE virus is believed to cause at least 14,000 human cases of encephalitis in Europe annually [36]. Other viruses within the same group, including louping ill virus, Langat virus, and Powassan virus, also are known to cause human encephalitis, but rarely on an epidemic scale [36].

Transmission

TBE virus is spread by the bite of ticks of the genus *Ixodes,* and it can be spread through consumption of contaminated raw milk [37]. Ticks act as the vector and reservoir for TBE virus, small rodents are the main host, and humans are accidental hosts [38]. TBE cases occur during the period of highest tick activity (April–November), when humans are infected in rural areas through tick bites [38].

Clinical features

After an incubation period of 4 to 14 days, patients develop typical flulike symptoms that resolve in about 1 week. After a remission of a few days to a few weeks, about a quarter of patients develop severe symptoms, including meningitis or meningoencephalitis [39]. In severe cases (no more than a quarter of cases), a partial paralysis may be seen. Although most patients recover from the disease, about a third are believed to have long-lasting neurologic problems, including problems with cognition, balance, and coordination [40].

Laboratory diagnosis

The diagnosis is based on confirmed exposure to ticks in a high-risk area, a tick bite within the previous 3 weeks, clinical symptoms, infected cerebrospinal fluid, and IgM and IgG antibodies in the serum [37].

Treatment

A vaccine of killed virus is available in Europe. No specific therapies are available, and supportive care is used to treat symptoms as necessary.

Decontamination

The virus is killed by 1% sodium hypochlorite, 2% glutaraldehyde, formaldehyde, and 70% ethanol. It also is killed by heating at 60°C for 10 minutes.

Tick-borne hemorrhagic fever viruses

Tick-borne hemorrhagic fever viruses include Crimean-Congo hemorrhagic fever (CCHF), Omsk hemorrhagic fever, Kyasanur Forest disease, and Alkhurma viruses [36]. CCHF virus is a tick-borne virus of the genus *Nairovirus* within the family Bunyaviridae [41]. The disease was first characterized in the Crimea in 1944, then later recognized in 1969 as the cause of illness in the Congo, resulting in the current name of the disease [42]. The virus is widespread and has been found in Africa, Asia, the Middle

East, and eastern Europe. The *Nairovirus* genus includes 32 members, all of which are transmitted by argasid or ixodid ticks, but only 3 have been implicated as causes of human disease: the Dugbe and Nairobi sheep viruses and CCHF, which is the most important human pathogen among them [43].

Transmission

The virus is transmitted by the bite of an infective adult tick of the genus *Hyalomma* [41]. Nosocomial outbreaks also have occurred as a result of exposure to blood and secretions [44,45]. Transmission also can occur by drinking raw milk or slaughtering infected animals [41,46].

Clinical features

The incubation period is about 2 to 7 days and has not been recorded as longer than 12 days. Illness begins abruptly with high fever, myalgia, headache, vomiting, and pain in the epigastrium, lower back, and thighs. Loose stools, dry cough, and relative bradycardia may be present. After 3 to 5 days, hemorrhage begins and is seen as a red or purple discoloration of the skin and the development of nosebleeds. In about half of all cases, the liver is enlarged. Blood is found in saliva, urine, black skin patches, and vomit. Bleeding leads to shock, vascular collapse, and death about 10 days after the onset of symptoms. Fatality rates in hospitalized patients range from 9% to 50% [42].

Laboratory diagnosis

Rapid diagnosis of CCHF virus is made by classic reverse transcriptase (RT)-PCR methods [47,48]. IgG and IgM antibodies can be detected with ELISA and indirect immunofluorescence tests from about day 7 of illness [41].

Treatment

No vaccine is available for CCHF. Intensive supportive management is required at an early stage and sometimes for prolonged periods. Convalescence is often slow, with debility lasting for some weeks after recovery. There is evidence that CCHF responds to treatment with ribavirin [49].

Decontamination

The virus is killed by common disinfectants and by dry heat at 56°C for 30 minutes.

Multidrug-resistant tuberculosis

MDR-TB is caused by *Mycobacterium tuberculosis,* which is resistant to at least isoniazide and rifampicin. MDR-TB has emerged as a serious problem in many areas of the world. The World Health Organization [50] estimates that one third of the world's population is infected with *M tuberculosis,* and that MDR-TB prevalence is greater than 4% among new tuberculosis cases in eastern Europe, Latin America, Africa, and Asia. In 2003, the CDC reported that 7.7% of tuberculosis cases in the United States were resistant to isoniazid, whereas 1.3% were resistant to isoniazid and rifampicin [51]. With the difficulty of treatment and its ability to disseminate by aerosol, MDR-TB might be used as a biological weapon in the future [6].

Emerging pathogens with potential for bioterrorism

In the early twenty-first century and with advances in technology, one may think that major infectious diseases threats would be conquered, but the world is connected through massive and easy international travel, politics, trade, economics, and culture, which makes possible the potential global spread of pathogens of the microbial world that previously might have been confined to a remote, local area. Novel infectious diseases agents keep getting discovered because they continue to emerge and re-emerge, have expanded their geographic range, have the potential of genetic manipulation and bioweaponization, and pose substantial threat throughout the world. Infectious diseases presenting significant challenges as emerging and re-emerging threats include severe acute respiratory syndrome (SARS), West Nile virus (WNV) infection, pandemic influenza, and monkey poxvirus infection.

Pandemic and avian influenza

Historically, the twentieth century saw three pandemics of influenza. The influenza pandemic of 1918 caused at least 500,000 US deaths and 50 million deaths worldwide. The 1957 influenza pandemic caused at least 70,000 US deaths and 1 to 2 million deaths worldwide. The 1968 influenza pandemic caused about 34,000 US deaths and about 700,000 deaths worldwide. The influenza virus responsible for the 1918 pandemic remains uncertain. In the 1957 and 1968 pandemics, the new virus contained components of previous human and avian influenza viruses.

A pandemic occurs when a mutant influenza virus emerges as a virus that exhibits more radical changes (antigenic shift) than the changes occurring continuously in influenza viruses (antigenic drift) and that is more virulent and pathogenic [52]. Although avian influenza viruses generally replicate inefficiently in humans, some subtypes of avian influenza can replicate within the respiratory tract of humans to cause disease. Since 2003, the highly pathogenic H5N1 strain of avian influenza A has spread to poultry in 17 countries in Asia and eastern Europe and now is considered endemic in some of these countries [53]. At the time of writing, this strain has caused about 160 human cases and 85 deaths so far in countries including Cambodia, China, Indonesia, Thailand, and Vietnam [54].

There is concern that the currently circulating H5N1 strain of avian influenza will evolve into a pandemic strain by adapting to humans through genetic mutation or reassortment with human influenza strains. It has been noted that pig's trachea contains receptors for avian and human influenza viruses and supports the growth of viruses of human and avian origin. Genetic reassortment between human and avian influenza viruses may occur in pigs leading to a novel strain against which there would be little or no population immunity and that would be highly pathogenic, capable of human-to-human transmission and having pandemic potential. The currently circulating strain of H5N1 avian influenza A also has potential as a bioterrorism agent because of the aforementioned properties and ease of propagation, lack of vaccine, environmental stability of the virus, and emerging resistance to the antiviral agent oseltamivir.

Transmission

For human influenza A (H5N1) infections, evidence is consistent with bird-to-human and possibly environment-to-human transmission. There is limited, nonsustained human-to-human transmission to date [55], although it has been suggested in several household clusters [56] and is apparent in one case of child-to-mother transmission [57].

The virus causing avian influenza in poultry has spread to humans as a result of contact with infected poultry by airborne spread from their secretions or by contamination during food preparation. Undercooked poultry also has been implicated. Human-to-human transmission of influenza virus occurs by inhalation of infectious droplets and droplet nuclei caused by coughing and sneezing, by direct contact, and by indirect (fomite) contact.

Clinical features

The incubation period of H5N1 ranges from 2 to 8 days (median 4 days). Initial symptoms of H5N1 influenza A in humans include fever, cough, sore throat, muscle aches, and pneumonia. Diarrhea, vomiting, abdominal pain, pleuritic pain, and bleeding from the nose and gums also have been reported early in the course of illness [58,59]. Progression to respiratory failure has been associated with acute respiratory distress syndrome. Other complications, such as renal dysfunction, cardiac failure, and multiorgan failure, have been reported [58–60].

Laboratory diagnosis

Rapid antigen testing kits cannot differentiate between various subtypes of influenza A virus. Diagnosis of H5N1 can be made by virus isolation through viral culture or by detection of H5-specific RNA by RT-PCR.

Treatment

Early initiation of antiviral agents seems to be beneficial. Avian influenza virus is susceptible in vitro to the neuraminidase inhibitors oseltamivir and zanamivir [61,62]. Oral oseltamivir and inhaled zanamivir are active in animal models of H5N1, but inhaled zanamivir has not been studied in cases of H5N1 in humans.

Mechanistically, neuraminidase molecular rearrangement occurs to create a pocket to which oseltamivir attaches. Viral resistance to oseltamivir results from the substitution of a single amino acid resulting in H274Y, R292K, or N294S mutation. Any of these mutations causes inhibition of neuraminidase molecule active site changes to create a pocket for oseltamivir [63]. None of these mutations prevents the binding of zanamivir, and that is why no virus resistant to zanamivir has yet been isolated [63]. There have been case reports of neuraminidase conferring high-level resistance to oseltamivir in two Vietnamese patients during oseltamivir treatment [64].

Prevention

At present, there is no licensed vaccine available against avian influenza for humans, but several candidate vaccines are under study. Chemoprophylaxis with 75 mg of oseltamivir by mouth every 24 hours for prevention for 7 to 10 days is recommended for individuals who have had a possible unprotected exposure and for household contacts [65,66].

Severe acute respiratory syndrome

SARS is a respiratory viral illness caused by the newly discovered coronavirus [67], SARS-associated coronavirus (SARS-CoV) [68]. SARS first appeared in southern China in November 2002. Over the next few months, the illness spread to more than 24 countries in North America, South America, Europe, and Asia, and it was recognized as a global threat in March 2003. This major outbreak was contained by July 2003. The most recent human cases of SARS were reported from China in April 2004 in an outbreak that was caused by laboratory-acquired infections [69]. At the time of this writing, there is no known SARS transmission in the world [70]. SARS is a potential agent for bioterrorism. Rapid and easy transmissibility of this agent by respiratory droplet and airborne spread and short incubation period add to its threat.

SARS-CoV-like viruses were isolated from Himalayan palm civets and a raccoon dog in an animal market in southern China, which suggests that SARS-CoV may have originated from these or other wild animals [71]. Considering the possibility that these wild animals or a human reservoir of SARS-CoV still may exist, there is a concern that SARS may return [72].

Transmission

SARS is transmitted from person to person by respiratory droplet and airborne spread [73,74]. SARS-CoV has been isolated from sputum, nasal secretions, serum, feces, and bronchial washing specimens, however, which suggests that alternate modes of transmission may exist. Strict adherence to contact and droplet precautions with added airborne precautions can prevent SARS transmission in most cases. Use of surgical or N95 masks significantly reduces the transmission [75].

Clinical features

The incubation period typically is 2 to 10 days, but it may be prolonged. Initial symptoms include a prodrome of fever usually accompanied by dry cough, headache, myalgias, and other nonspecific symptoms, which usually is followed by development of pneumonia with worsening of respiratory symptoms.

Laboratory diagnosis

Diagnosis of SARS should be confirmed by SARS-CoV-specific microbiologic and serologic studies, including viral culture and RT-PCR from clinical specimens and antibody testing using enzyme immunoassay. Sensitive and specific tests that can yield results within hours are needed, especially in the setting of an outbreak. Real-time nested PCR has the potential for increased sensitivity and early diagnosis of SARS [76].

Treatment

Several antiviral and anti-inflammatory agents have been evaluated for treatment of SARS, including ribavirin, oseltamivir, ritonavir-lopinavir, interferon alfa, and corticosteroids [77–81]. Sufficient evidence to recommend any specific therapy is lacking, and the mainstay of treatment remains supportive care.

West Nile virus

WNV, a single-stranded RNA arbovirus, is in the family Flaviviridae. WNV was first isolated from Uganda in 1937 and subsequently was reported from Africa, Europe, Asia, Israel, and Egypt. WNV represents a potential and effective biological weapon because of persistent animal reservoir, seasonal predilection, relatively short incubation period, broad spectrum of clinical illness, and lack of vaccination.

In August 1999, WNV was detected for the first time in North America by causing an outbreak in New York City [82–84]. The WNV strain from the United States is closely related genetically to a strain from Israel from 1998, which supports the hypothesis that the WNV outbreak in the United States originated from introduction of a strain circulating in Israel [85,86]. There is no evidence, however, that WNV was introduced in the United States deliberately. It is possible that the virus was imported to North America through infected birds, infected mosquitoes, or viremic humans [85,87]. WNV is now a seasonal epidemic in the United States lasting from summer through fall.

Transmission

WNV is maintained in nature by a cycle involving mosquitoes and birds. Birds usually develop high levels of prolonged viremia and serve as amplifying hosts. Humans, horses, and dogs serve as incidental hosts. Human WNV infection can result from a mosquito bite (usually of the *Culex* spp.), infected blood products [88,89], and transplanted organs from infected donors [90].

Pathogenesis

WNV initially replicates at the site of inoculation after a mosquito bite. Virus may infect fibroblasts and vascular endothelial cells and subsequently spread to lymph nodes and bloodstream [91]. Central nervous system infection may occur as a result of viremia.

Clinical features

The incubation period for infection ranges from 2 to 14 days, but it may be prolonged. Most human infections are asymptomatic. Individuals in whom symptoms develop present with a self-limited febrile illness characterized by fever, headache, fatigue, malaise, myalgias, and gastrointestinal symptoms.

Neuroinvasive disease occurs in less than 1% of infected patients as meningitis or encephalitis, which can be complicated by acute asymmetric flaccid paralysis. Paralysis also can occur without overt meningitis or encephalitis, however [92]. Flaccid paralysis results from involvement of anterior horn cells by WNV and is similar to that seen with poliomyelitis.

Laboratory diagnosis

The most commonly used method of diagnosis is detection of IgM antibody to WNV in serum or cerebrospinal fluid, which provides strong evidence of recent WNV infection. WNV also can be detected from cerebrospinal fluid, blood, or tissue by isolation or nucleic acid amplification tests. RT-PCR and nucleic acid sequence-based amplification techniques are more sensitive than culture to detect WNV infection [93].

Treatment

Treatment is mainly supportive care. Trials of interferon alfa and intravenous immunoglobulin for treatment of WNV infection are currently ongoing. Currently no human vaccine is available for WNV infection.

Monkeypox virus

Human monkeypox is caused by monkeypox virus, a member of the family Poxviridae and genus *Orthopoxvirus*. Other important viruses in this group include variola virus (virus that causes smallpox) and vaccinia virus (virus used in smallpox vaccine). The first human cases of monkeypox were reported in 1970 in the Democratic Republic of Congo (formerly the Republic of Zaire) [94,95]. Since then, the disease has been endemic in Congo basin countries of Africa.

Since the discontinuation of routine smallpox vaccination and resulting lack of immunity in the population, there are concerns about the potential use of monkeypox virus as a bioterrorism agent. The risk also includes recombination between various pox viruses and genetically engineered manipulation of monkeypox virus to exhibit greater virulence and transmissibility. In 2003, monkeypox virus emerged for the first time in the Western Hemisphere when an outbreak of human monkeypox occurred in the midwestern United States [96–98]. Most of the patients got sick by having direct contact with pet prairie dogs that became infected after being housed with rodents imported from Ghana in western Africa [96,97]. In contrast to African patients, most US patients with mild self-limited illness.

Transmission

Monkeypox is transmitted to humans by direct contact or during handling of infected animals. Human-to-human transmission can occur by large respiratory droplets during prolonged face-to-face contact [99] or by touching body fluids of a sick person.

Clinical features

The incubation period is 10 to 14 days. Prodromal symptoms include fever, malaise, and lymphadenopathy. Most clinical features of human monkeypox disease resemble those of ordinary smallpox, but lymphadenopathy is considered a distinguishing feature of human monkeypox. Rash is distributed mainly on the trunk, but it can spread in a peripheral fashion toward the palms and soles. The clinical course can be complicated by secondary skin and soft tissue infections, pneumonitis, encephalitis, and ocular complications [100].

Laboratory diagnosis

Various laboratory tests for diagnosis of monkeypox virus include PCR, electron microscopy, IgM and IgG ELISA, immunofluorescent antibody assay, and histopathology, but many of these tests cannot differentiate between different orthopoxviruses. Virus isolation using cell culture or chick chorioallantoic membrane in conjunction with DNA-based assay is considered to be a definitive test for identification of monkeypox virus [101].

Treatment and prevention

Cidofovir is a broad-spectrum antiviral drug that has in vitro activity against monkeypox virus [102], but because of its relative toxicity, it can be considered only in severe cases of human monkeypox virus infection. No data are currently available on effectiveness of vaccinia immunoglobulin for treating human monkeypox virus infection or its complications.

Vaccination with vaccinia virus is protective against infection with monkeypox virus [103,104].

Genetically engineered biological weapons

Biologic threats now are categorized as conventional or genetically modified agents. Traditional biological weapons include naturally occurring organisms or toxins characterized by their ease of production, toxicity, stability, and modes of transmission. The dangers associated with conventional agents can be enhanced by genetic modification. Examples of potential genetic modifications include increased virulence, antibiotic resistance, toxin production, enhanced aerosol stability, and improved survival of the biologic agents.

Continuous development and advances in biotechnology have tremendous potential to revolutionize present and future biologic threats by facilitating an entirely new class of fully engineered agents, referred to as advanced biological warfare agents. Advanced biological warfare agents are specifically engineered to target specific organ system (eg, cardiovascular, gastrointestinal, neurologic) or specific biologic processes (eg, incapacitation, neurologic impairment, death) [105].

Summary

The threat of using weaponized forms of certain biologic agents against civilian populations through bioterrorism attacks has emerged over the past few years. With advances in biotechnology, category C bioterrorism agents and emerging pathogens may become attractive weapons for bioterrorists. For bioterrorists, category C bioterrorism agents and emerging pathogens have many advantages over conventional weapons and other biologic agents listed under categories A and B, including their relatively low costs; their relative accessibility; and the relative ease with which they could be produced, be delivered, and avoid detection. Their use, or even threatened use, is potentially capable of producing widespread social disruption. Although biotechnology is a tool by which bioterrorists could develop weapons of mass destruction, it also should be used to improve the methods of fighting such weapons.

References

[1] Beeching NJ, Dance DA, Miller AR, et al. Biological warfare and bioterrorism. BMJ 2002; 324:336–9.

[2] Christopher GW, Cieslak TJ, Pavlin JA, et al. Biological warfare: a historical perspective. JAMA 1997;278:412–7.

[3] Eitzen EM, Takafuji ET. Historical overview of biological warfare. In: Sidell FR, Takafuji ET, Franz DR, editors. Medical aspects of chemical and biological warfare. Washington, DC: Borden Institute; 1997. p. 415–23.
[4] Relman DA, Olson JE. Bioterrorism preparedness: what practitioners need to know? Infect Med 2001;18:497–514.
[5] Tucker JB. Historical trends related to bioterrorism: an empirical analysis. Emerg Infect Dis 1999;5:498–504.
[6] Moran GJ. Threats in bioterrorism: II. CDC category B and C agents. Emerg Med Clin N Am 2002;20:311–30.
[7] Centers for Disease Control and Prevention (CDC). Bioterrorism agents/diseases. Available at: http://www.bt.cdc.gov/agent/agentlist-category.asp. Accessed January 5, 2006.
[8] Centers for Disease Control and Prevention (CDC). Update: outbreak of Nipah virus—Malaysia and Singapore. MMWR Morb Mortal Wkly Rep 1999;48:335–7.
[9] Lim CC, Sitoh YY, Lee KE, et al. Meningoencephalitis caused by a novel paramyxovirus: an advanced MRI case report in an emerging disease. Singapore Med J 1999;40:356–8.
[10] Paton NI, Leo YS, Zaki SR, et al. Outbreak of Nipah-virus infection among abattoir workers in Singapore. Lancet 1999;354:1253–6.
[11] Tambyah PA. The Nipah virus outbreak-a reminder. Singapore Med J 1999;40:329–30.
[12] Chua KB, Bellini WJ, Rota PA, et al. Nipah virus: a recently emergent deadly paramyxovirus. Science 2000;288:1432–5.
[13] Chua KB, Goh KJ, Wong KT, et al. Fatal encephalitis due to Nipah virus among pig farmers in Malaysia. Lancet 1999;354:1257–9.
[14] Amal NM, Lye MS, Ksiazek TG, et al. Risk factors for Nipah virus transmission, Port Dickson, Negeri Sembilan, Malaysia: results from a hospital-based case-control study. Southeast Asian J Trop Med Public Health 2000;31:301–6.
[15] Enserink M. Emerging diseases: Malaysian researchers trace Nipah virus outbreak to bats. Science 2000;289:518–9.
[16] Daniels P, Ksiazek T, Eaton BT. Laboratory diagnosis of Nipah and Hendra virus infections. Microbes Infect 2001;3:289–95.
[17] Food and Agriculture Organization of the United Nations Regional Office for Asia and the Pacific Animal Production and Health Commission for Asia and the Pacific (APHCA). Manual on the diagnosis of Nipah virus infection in animals. Thailand: Food and Agriculture Organization of the United Nations. RAP publication no. 2002/01. 2002; p. 29–37.
[18] Chong HT, Kamarulzaman A, Tan CT, et al. Treatment of acute Nipah encephalitis with ribavirin. Ann Neurol 2001;49:810–3.
[19] Elliott RM, Schmaljohn CS, Collett MS. Bunyavirus genome structure and gene expression. Curr Top Microbiol Immunol 1991;169:91–141.
[20] Nichol ST, Spiropoulou CF, Morzunov S, et al. Genetic identification of a Hantavirus associated with an outbreak of acute respiratory illness. Science 1993;262:914–7.
[21] Childs JE, Ksiazek TG, Spiropoulou CF, et al. Serologic and genetic identification of *Peromyscus maniculatus* as the primary rodent reservoir for a new Hantavirus in the southwestern United States. J Infect Dis 1994;169:1271–80.
[22] Duchin JS, Koster FT, Peters CJ, et al. Hantavirus pulmonary syndrome: a clinical description of 17 patients with a newly recognized disease. N Engl J Med 1994;330:949–55.
[23] Centers for Disease Control and Prevention (CDC). Hantavirus pulmonary syndrome—United States: updated recommendations for risk reduction. MMWR Morb Mortal Wkly Rep 2002;51(RR09):1–12.
[24] Song J-W, Baek L-J, Gajdusek DC, et al. Isolation of pathogenic hantavirus from white-footed mouse (*Peromyscus leucopus*). Lancet 1994;344:1637.
[25] Rollin PE, Ksiazek TG, Elliott LH, et al. Isolation of Black Creek Canal virus, a new Hantavirus from *Sigmodon hispidus* in Florida. J Med Virol 1995;46:35–9.
[26] Ksiazek TG, Nichol ST, Mills JN, et al. Isolation, genetic diversity, and geographic distribution of Bayou virus (Bunyaviridae: Hantavirus). Am J Trop Med Hyg 1997;57:445–8.

[27] Peters CJ, Mills JN, Spiropoulou C, et al. Hantavirus infections. In: Guerrant RL, Walker DH, Weller PF, editors. Tropical infectious diseases: principles, pathogens, and practice. Philadelphia: Churchill Livingstone; 1999. p. 1217–35.
[28] Tsai TF. Hemorrhagic fever with renal syndrome: mode of transmission to humans. Lab Anim Sci 1987;37:428–30.
[29] Centers for Diseases Control and Prevention (CDC). Yellow fever vaccine recommendations of the Advisory Committee on Immunization Practices (ACIP). MMWR Morb Mortal Wkly Rep 2002;51(RR17):1–10.
[30] World Health Organization. District guidelines for yellow fever surveillance. Publication no. (WHO/EPI/GEN) 98.09. Geneva: WHO; 1998. Available at:. http://www.who.int/emc-documents/yellow_fever/whoepigen9809c.html.
[31] World Health Organization (WHO). Endemic and pandemic alert response—yellow fever. Available at: http://www.who.int/mediacentre/factsheets/fs100/en/. Accessed January 12, 2006.
[32] Monath TP. Yellow fever. In: Plotkin SA, Orenstein WA, editors. Vaccines. 3rd edition. Philadelphia: Saunders; 1999. p. 815–79.
[33] Centers for Disease Control and Prevention (CDC). Fatal yellow fever in a traveler returning from Amazonas, Brazil. MMWR Morb Mortal Wkly Rep 2002;51:324–5.
[34] Smithburn KC, Durieux C, Koerber R, et al. Yellow fever vaccination. WHO monograph series no. 30. Geneva: World Health Organization; 1956.
[35] Dumpis U, Crook D, Oksi J. Tick-borne encephalitis. Clin Infect Dis 1999;28:882–90.
[36] Gritsun TS, Lashkevich VA, Gould EA. Tick-borne encephalitis. Antiviral Res 2003;57:129–46.
[37] Lademann M, Wild B, Reisinger EC. Tick-borne encephalitis (FSME)—how great is the danger really? MMW Fortschr Med 2003;145:47–9.
[38] Centers for Diseases Control and Prevention (CDC). Tick-borne encephalitis. Available at: http://www.cdc.gov/ncidod/dvrd/spb/mnpages/dispages/TBE.htm. Accessed December 20, 2005.
[39] Haglund M, Gunther G. Tick-borne encephalitis—pathogenesis, clinical course and long-term follow-up. Vaccine 2003;21(Suppl 1):S11–8.
[40] Kondrusik M, Hermanowska-Szpakowicz T. Tick-borne encephalitis: clinical, pathological aspects and sequelae. Neurol Neurochir Pol 2004;38(Suppl 1):S67–70.
[41] Charrel RN, Attoui H, Butenko AM, et al. Tick-borne virus diseases of human interest in Europe. Clin Microbiol Infect 2004;10:1040–55.
[42] Centers for Diseases Control and Prevention (CDC). Crimean-Congo hemorrhagic fever. Available at: http://www.cdc.gov/ncidod/dvrd/spb/mnpages/dispages/cchf.htm. Accessed January 24, 2006.
[43] World Health Organization (WHO). Crimean-Congo haemorrhagic fever. Available at: http://www.who.int/mediacentre/factsheets/fs208/en/. Accessed January 24, 2006.
[44] Burney MI, Ghafoor A, Saleen M, et al. Nosocomial outbreak of viral hemorrhagic fever caused by Crimean hemorrhagic fever-Congo virus in Pakistan, January 1976. Am J Trop Med Hyg 1980;29:941–7.
[45] Weber DJ, Rutala WA. Risks and prevention of nosocomial transmission of rare zoonotic diseases. Clin Infect Dis 2001;32:446–56.
[46] Swanepoel R, Shepherd AJ, Leman PA, et al. A common-source outbreak of Crimean-Congo haemorrhagic fever on a dairy farm. S Afr Med J 1985;68:635–7.
[47] Drosten C, Gottig S, Schilling S, et al. Rapid detection and quantification of RNA of Ebola and Marburg viruses, Lassa virus, Crimean-Congo hemorrhagic fever virus, Rift Valley fever virus, dengue virus, and yellow fever virus by real-time reverse transcription-PCR. J Clin Microbiol 2002;40:2323–30.
[48] Papa A, Bozovi B, Pavlidou V, et al. Genetic detection and isolation of Crimean-Congo hemorrhagic fever virus, Kosovo, Yugoslavia. Emerg Infect Dis 2002;8:852–4.
[49] Watts DM, Ussery MA, Nash D, et al. Inhibition of Crimean-Congo hemorrhagic fever viral infectivity yields in vitro by ribavirin. Am J Trop Med Hyg 1989;41:581–5.

[50] World Health Organization (WHO). Drug and multidrug-resistant tuberculosis. Available at: http://www.who.int/tb/dots/dotsplus/faq/en/. Accessed January 5, 2006.
[51] Centers for Disease Control and Prevention (CDC). Reported Tuberculosis in the US, 2003. Available at: http://www.cdc.gov/nchstp/tb/surv/surv2003/default.htm. Accessed January 5, 2006.
[52] Fleming D. Influenza pandemic and avian flu. BMJ 2005;331:1066–9.
[53] Macfarlane JT, Lim WS. Bird flu and pandemic flu. BMJ 2005;331:975–6.
[54] World Health Organization (WHO). Cumulative number of confirmed human cases of avian influenza A/(H5N1) reported to WHO. Available at: http://www.who.int/csr/disease/avian_influenza/country/cases_table_2006_01_30/en/index.html. Accessed January 7, 2006.
[55] Capua I, Alexander DJ. Avian influenza and human health. Acta Trop 2002;83:1–6.
[56] Hien TT, Liem NT, Dung NT, et al. Avian influenza A (H5N1) in 10 patients in Vietnam. N Engl J Med 2004;350:1179–88.
[57] Ungchusak K, Auewarakul P, Dowell SF, et al. Probable person-to-person transmission of avian influenza A (H5N1). N Engl J Med 2005;352:333–40.
[58] Chan PK. Outbreak of avian influenza A(H5N1) virus infection in Hong Kong in 1997. Clin Infect Dis 2002;34(Suppl 2):S58–64.
[59] Chotpitayasunondh T, Ungchusak K, Hanshaoworakul W, et al. Human disease from influenza A (H5N1), Thailand, 2004. Emerg Infect Dis 2005;11:201–9.
[60] Hien TT, Liem NT, Dung NT, et al. Avian influenza A (H5N1) in 10 patients in Vietnam. N Engl J Med 2004;350:1179–88.
[61] Leneva IA, Roberts N, Govorkova EA, et al. The neuraminidase inhibitor GS4104 (oseltamivir phosphate) is efficacious against A/Hong Kong/156/97 (H5N1) and A/Hong Kong/1074/99 (H9N2) influenza viruses. Antiviral Res 2000;48:101–15.
[62] Govorkova EA, Leneva IA, Goloubeva OG, et al. Comparison of efficacies of RWJ-270201, zanamivir, and oseltamivir against H5N1, H9N2, and other avian influenza viruses. Antimicrob Agents Chemother 2001;45:2723–32.
[63] Moscona A. Oseltamivir resistance—disabling our influenza defenses. N Engl J Med 2005; 353:2633–6.
[64] de Jong MD, Thanh TT, Khanh TH, et al. Oseltamivir resistance during treatment of influenza A (H5N1) infection. N Engl J Med 2005;353:2667–72.
[65] Hayden FG, Belshe R, Villanueva C, et al. Management of influenza in households: a prospective, randomized comparison of oseltamivir treatment with or without postexposure prophylaxis. J Infect Dis 2004;189:440–9.
[66] Welliver R, Monto AS, Carewicz O, et al. Effectiveness of oseltamivir in preventing influenza in household contacts: a randomized controlled trial. JAMA 2001;285:748–54.
[67] Ksiazek TG, Erdman D, Goldsmith CS, et al. A novel coronavirus associated with severe acute respiratory syndrome. N Engl J Med 2003;348:1953–66.
[68] Kuiken T, Fouchier RAM, Schutten M, et al. Newly discovered coronavirus as the primary cause of severe acute respiratory syndrome. Lancet 2003;362:263–70.
[69] World Health Organization (WHO). Available at: www.wpro.who.int/sars/docs/update/update_07022004.asp. Accessed January 7, 2006.
[70] Centers for Disease Control and Prevention (CDC). Available at: www.cdc.gov/ncidod/sars/situation.htm. Accessed January 7, 2006.
[71] Guan Y, Zheng BJ, He YQ, et al. Isolation and characterization of viruses related to the SARS coronavirus from animals in southern China. Science 2003;302:276–8.
[72] Christian MD, Poutanen SM, Loutfy MR, et al. Severe acute respiratory syndrome. Clin Infect Dis 2004;38:1420–7.
[73] Booth TF, Kournikakis B, Bastien N, et al. Detection of airborne severe acute respiratory syndrome (SARS) coronavirus and environmental contamination in SARS outbreak units. J Infect Dis 2005;191:1472–7.
[74] Yu ITS, Wong TW, Chiu YL, et al. Temporal-spatial analysis of severe acute respiratory syndrome among hospital inpatients. Clin Infect Dis 2005;40:1237–43.

[75] Seto WH, Tsang D, Yung RW, et al. Effectiveness of precautions against droplets and contact in prevention of nosocomial transmission of severe acute respiratory syndrome (SARS). Lancet 2003;361:1519–20.
[76] Jiang SS, Chen T, Yang J, et al. Sensitive and quantitative detection of severe acute respiratory syndrome coronavirus infection by real-time nested polymerase chain reaction. Clin Infect Dis 2004;38:293–6.
[77] Chu CM, Cheng VC, Hung IF, et al. Role of lopinavir/ritonavir in the treatment of SARS: initial virological and clinical findings. Thorax 2004;59:252–6.
[78] Groneberg DA, Poutanen SM, Low DE, et al. Treatment and vaccines for severe acute respiratory syndrome. Lancet Infect Dis 2005;5:147–55.
[79] Tsang KW, Ho PL, Ooi GC, et al. A cluster of cases of severe acute respiratory syndrome in Hong Kong. N Engl J Med 2003;348:1977–85.
[80] Ho JC, Ooi GC, Mok TY, et al. High-dose pulse versus nonpulse corticosteroid regimens in severe acute respiratory syndrome. Am J Respir Crit Care Med 2003;168:1449–56.
[81] Stroher U, DiCaro A, Li Y, et al. Severe acute respiratory syndrome-related coronavirus is inhibited by interferon-alpha. J Infect Dis 2004;189:1164–7.
[82] Outbreak of West Nile-like viral encephalitis New York, 1999. MMWR Morb Mortal Wkly Rep 1999;48:845–9.
[83] Update: West Nile-like viral encephalitis—New York, 1999. MMWR Morb Mortal Wkly Rep 1999;48:890–2.
[84] Asnis DS, Conetta R, Teixeira AA, et al. The West Nile Virus outbreak of 1999 in New York: the Flushing Hospital experience. Clin Infect Dis 2000;30:413–8.
[85] Lanciotti RS, Roehrig JT, Deubel V, et al. Origin of the West Nile virus responsible for an outbreak of encephalitis in the northeastern United States. Science 1999;286:2333–7.
[86] Giladi M, Metzkor-Cotter E, Martin DA, et al. West Nile encephalitis in Israel, 1999: the New York connection. Emerg Infect Dis 2001;7:659–61.
[87] Jia XY, Briese T, Jordan I, et al. Genetic analysis of West Nile New York 1999 encephalitis virus. Lancet 354;1971–2.
[88] Pealer LN, Marfin AA, Petersen LR, et al. Transmission of West Nile virus through blood transfusion in the United States in 2002. N Engl J Med 2003;349:1236–45.
[89] Detection of West Nile virus in blood donations—United States, 2003. MMWR Morb Mortal Wkly Rep 2003;52:769–72.
[90] Iwamoto M, Jernigan DB, Guasch A, et al. Transmission of West Nile virus from an organ donor to four transplant recipients. N Engl J Med 2003;348:2196–203.
[91] Diamond MS, Shrestha B, Mehlhop E, et al. Innate and adaptive immune responses determine protection against disseminated infection by West Nile encephalitis virus. Viral Immunol 2003;16:259–78.
[92] Sejvar JJ, Haddad MB, Tierney BC, et al. Neurologic manifestations and outcome of West Nile virus infection. JAMA 2003;290:511–5.
[93] Parida M, Posadas G, Inoue S, et al. Real-time reverse transcription loop-mediated isothermal amplification for rapid detection of West Nile virus. J Clin Microbiol 2004;42: 257–63.
[94] Centers for Diseases Control and Prevention (CDC). Human monkeypox—Kasai Oriental, Democratic Republic of Congo, February 1996-October 1997. MMWR Morb Mortal Wkly Rep 1997;46:1168–71.
[95] Breman JG, Henderson DA. Poxvirus dilemmas—monkeypox, smallpox. N Engl J Med 1998;339:556–9.
[96] Centers for Disease Control and Prevention. Multistate outbreak of monkeypox—Illinois, Indiana, and Wisconsin, 2003. MMWR Morb Mortal Wkly Rep 2003;52:537–40.
[97] Centers for Disease Control and Prevention. Update: multistate outbreak of monkeypox—Illinois, Indiana, Kansas, Missouri, Ohio, and Wisconsin, 2003. MMWR Morb Mortal Wkly Rep 2003;52:561–4.

[98] Centers for Disease Control and Prevention. Update: multistate outbreak of monkeypox—Illinois, Indiana, Kansas, Missouri, Ohio, and Wisconsin, 2003. MMWR Morb Mortal Wkly Rep 2003;52:642–6.

[99] Human monkeypox and other poxvirus infections of man. In: Fenner F, Henderson DA, Arita I, et al, editors. Smallpox and its eradication, vol. 29. Geneva: World Health Organization; 1988. p. 1287–319.

[100] Nalca A, Rimoin AW, Bavari S, et al. Reemergence of Monkeypox: prevalence, diagnostics, and countermeasures. Clin Infect Dis 2005;41:1765–71.

[101] Damon IK, Esposito JJ. Poxviruses that infect humans. In: Murray PR, Baron EJ, Jorgensen JH, et al, editors. Manual of clinical microbiology. 8th edition. Washington, DC: ASM Press; 2003. p. 1583–91.

[102] Baker RO, Bray M, Huggins JW. Potential antiviral therapeutics for smallpox, monkeypox and other orthopoxvirus infections. Antiviral Res 2003;57:13–23.

[103] Fine PE, Jezek Z, Grab B, et al. The transmission potential of monkeypox virus in human populations. Int J Epidemiol 1988;17:643–50.

[104] Arita I, Jezek Z, Khodakevich L, et al. Human monkeypox: a newly emerged orthopoxvirus zoonosis in the tropical rain forests of Africa. Am J Trop Med Hyg 1985;34:781–9.

[105] Petro JB, Plasse TR, McNulty JA. Biotechnology: impact on biological warfare and biodefense. Biosecurity and Bioterrorism: Biodefense Strategy, Practice and Science 2003;1:161–8.

ELSEVIER
SAUNDERS

Infect Dis Clin N Am
20 (2006) 443–453

INFECTIOUS
DISEASE CLINICS
OF NORTH AMERICA

Practical Aspects of Implementation of a Bioterrorism Preparedness Program in a Hospital setting

Zakir Hussain A. Shaikh, MD, MPH, CPE[a,b,*]

[a]*Department of Infectious Diseases, Methodist Dallas Medical Center, 1441 North Beckley Avenue, Dallas, TX 75203, USA*
[b]*Infection Control, Methodist Health System, Dallas, TX 75203, USA*

"Plans are nothing; planning is everything."
—General Dwight D. Eisenhower

Response to Hurricane Katrina brought to light the gross inadequacy of the local and federal disaster planning preparedness and the initial public health response [1,2]. This is despite the fact that significant resources have been expended in preparing for just that eventuality, possibly at the cost of other public health initiatives [3]. The disenchantment with current preparedness led the American Medical Association to study the feasibility of developing a federal public health disaster intervention team, which would be better equipped to respond to these disasters. Although this initiative may add to the response of a recognized disaster, it would add little to an individual institution's ability to be better prepared to handle the initial presentation of a biologic disaster or a bioterrorist event.

Success of an institution's preparedness for a bioterrorist event would be determined by its ability to limit exposure of other patients and health care workers before an event is confirmed and a definitive diagnosis is established. The inherent problem with most bioterrorism preparedness plans lies in the initial triggers that would kick the plan into action. Most clues that signal a bioterrorist event rely on unusual clustering of illness with regards to time, place, or person [4,5]. If one waits for an automated or manual surveillance process to raise a warning about a possible clustering, the scenario exists wherein a group of contagious patients already would have

* Department of Infectious Diseases, Methodist Dallas Medical Center, 1441 North Beckley Avenue, Dallas, TX 75203, USA.
E-mail address: zakirshaikh@mhd.com

doi:10.1016/j.idc.2006.03.008

been admitted to the hospital and caused exposure to other patients and health care workers. Although this syndromic surveillance mechanism is useful for its public health implications, it does not provide adequate safeguards for a hospital against the initial untoward biologic exposures.

Most bioterrorism agents are not transmitted from person to person [5,6], and diligent use of standard precautions alone may suffice in limiting the exposure. For other agents, adherence to symptom-based recommendation for use of additional precautions would provide the extra layer of protection. Use of contact precautions while taking care of a patient with skin rash, draining wounds, or diarrheal illness would provide protection against exposure to cutaneous or gastrointestinal anthrax and bubonic plague. Initiation of droplet precautions for patients with flulike illness or symptoms of pneumonia would afford protection against exposure to pneumonic plague. Preparedness for diseases such as smallpox and viral hemorrhagic fevers, in addition to the usual precautions, would require an astute physician's quick thinking based on clinical acumen and a high index of suspicion.

Although it is important to worry about preparedness for novel bioterrorist agents, potential devastation from the naturally occurring possibilities, including pandemic influenza, severe acute respiratory syndrome, and H5N1 avian influenza, is more likely [7]. These real threats, which could be "just a plane ride away," make it imperative to ensure a hospital's continued readiness and ability to identify these cases based on clinical and epidemiologic presentation. This readiness could be achieved by integrating the hospital's day-to-day preparedness in dealing with the threat from naturally occurring biologic agents within the context of preparedness initiative for a less likely bioterrorist event. The success of an institution's bioterrorism preparedness program would be determined by how effectively it handles the implementation of such a conjoined program to maximize the "dual benefit" [8]. For effective implementation of a biologic disaster or bioterrorism preparedness program, multiple practical aspects need to be addressed (Box 1) to achieve the goal of minimizing the morbidity and mortality associated with the event and to provide continued quality care to patients already receiving care in the hospital.

Have a written bioterrorism preparedness plan

A well-written plan is a crucial foundation of an institution's bioterrorism preparedness program. Although several plans are available online [9,10], each institution should customize their plan to meet their unique needs and challenges. A good plan would be one that the users understand, are comfortable with, and can use to gain access to the information they need rapidly. The plan should be a living document of work in progress, with mechanisms for regular and periodic internal reviews to ensure that it stays current. It is vital to ensure continued availability and accessibility of the

Box 1. Practical aspects of implementation of a bioterrorism preparedness program

- Have a written bioterrorism preparedness plan
- Assess the feasibility and viability of the plan
- Disseminate the plan and ensure familiarity by all key stakeholders
- Use elements of daily practice as the backbone of the plan
- Incorporate internal mechanisms for intensified surveillance
- Ensure appropriate internal and external mechanisms of communication
- Test the plan periodically through drills
- Incorporate flexibility and build redundancy for key components of the plan
- Address logistics involving surge capacity
- Improve collaboration with community physicians, area hospitals, and local health departments
- Emphasize community preparedness

plan to all who may need to use it; this may require simultaneous availability of the plan in different forms, including print, electronic media, intranet, and Internet, in the event that one form were to become unavailable during times of crisis.

Although the plan needs to be detailed in establishing authorities and responsibilities for each predefined role, it should not be exhaustive. The objective should be to achieve a right balance of the "strategic" and "operational" planning components, to prevent the plan from being too rigid, and to allow flexibility in decision making under the extraneous circumstance of things going wrong. Because it would be difficult, if not impossible, to predict each unique presentation, the program should allow for measures to address the dynamics caused by uncertainty, so as to "expect the unexpected." Some degree of decentralized operations needs to be built in so that when communications fail, the lower tier leaders could make on-the-spot decisions geared toward achieving the plan's overall goals. The plan should identify all the crucial tasks and roles that must be performed, assign responsibility for accomplishing each of these roles, and ensure that designated individuals have prepared *standard operating procedures* that detail how they carry out their critical tasks. This plan would promote activity-oriented execution at an individual level, while maintaining the result-oriented goal at a higher program level.

The plan should address the physical infrastructure needs of the bioterrorism response plan. The biocontainment area in the emergency department, or the "hot zone," needs to be clearly defined, along with the designated unit within the hospital or the "isolation unit" where the critically ill victims of the biologic disaster would need to be admitted, with the intent of minimizing the exposure to others in the remainder of the facility.

Assess the feasibility and viability of the plan

Although the plan may look good on paper, it is crucial to ensure that it has the potential to work as envisioned. An institution needs to do a critical risk appraisal of the plan, looking beyond to see what can go wrong. The institution needs to test viability of the implied assumptions within the plan as to their "reasonableness." The institution needs to undertake realistic strengths, weaknesses, opportunities, and threats (SWOT) analysis to see if the plan withstands the challenge of different presentation scenarios. A multidisciplinary team should be organized to validate the functionality of the plan and should include key individuals from the emergency department, infection control, disaster management, and physical plant/engineering. This team should use the "tracer methodology" [11] to do a walk-around of the process of registration, triage, emergency department assessment, and admission to the hospital, exercising different scenarios of initial presentation. This process should be more than simply touring the facility; it should include taking the time to understand the physical layouts, patient flow, and security systems. It should be ensured that the waiting areas have proper signage directing patients to use appropriate cough etiquette and have the physical capability to separate patients with respiratory symptoms.

The registration personnel must be included as the first line of defense and educated appropriately to be able to safeguard their own health and to guide patients in following these recommendations. Triage personnel must be trained to recognize a clustering of syndromic presentation, be guided by a predefined threshold, and have the ability to initiate a *biothreat containment alert*. As part of a tiered planning approach with escalating action thresholds, this alert should be executable at a level below the facility's *disaster alert code* to facilitate its rapid implementation, without expending significant resources toward handling the multiple false alarms that possibly may be generated by its lower threshold. The biothreat containment alert should prompt initiation of a separate triage location to avoid contamination of other parts of the emergency department and, similar to a cardiac arrest code, should lead to designated personnel reporting to an assigned location and a "disaster cart" with additional backup medical equipment and supplies being delivered to the "hot zone." A departmental checklist of necessary immediate actions to be taken should be an integral part of this alert. Large-scale events that overwhelm the emergency department biocontainment capacity would require initiation of the full-fledged disaster management protocol, with logistics led in accordance with the Hospital Emergency Incident Command System [12].

The physical plant/engineering staff should ensure that when a biothreat containment alert is called, appropriate plans are in place for a "lockdown" of the potentially contaminated areas, with ability to change the ventilation patterns of these areas to make it a negative pressure zone. The containment area should be physically designated in such a way that it provides an isolated entrance for suspect patients through the decontamination shower, to be used only in the event chemical contamination cannot be ruled out. Structural modifications must be in place to close off the containment area quickly and completely from other parts of the emergency department, with controlled access provided to crucial staff. It also should be ensured that if needed, the designated isolation unit, along with the hallway and elevator leading to it, can be included in "lockdown" zone, to allow the rest of the hospital to remain independently functional.

Disseminate the plan and ensure familiarity by all key stakeholders

After the plan is in place, the institution needs to disseminate to all who might be involved in its implementation, realizing that the main focus of planning is to reduce uncertainty. All key stakeholders need to be trained to acquire mastery and competency of the roles and tasks they are expected to perform and a clear understanding of how they fit into the overall preparedness plan at large. This training helps ground-level employees to make crucial decisions on the run, in the event of communication failure with program leaders and any required last minute plan modification.

The institution needs to ensure that each staff member is familiar with his or her individual and collective responsibility during the disaster response and recognizes the lines of authority while performing those duties. The appropriate medical staff from the emergency department, family practice, internal medicine, infectious disease, and hospitalists' program should be included in the pre-event planning so that they are aware that they may be called on to help and to provide them the opportunity to train in the diagnosis and treatment of bioterrorism agents that have been prioritized in the Centers for Disease Control and Prevention (CDC) categories class A and B [13]. Senior leadership need to be apprised of their expanded roles, responsibilities, and expectations related to bioterrorism and disaster management so that they have the ability to make quick decisions with confidence.

Use elements of daily practice as the backbone of the plan

The plan should incorporate elements of day-to-day practice and emphasize attention to strict infection control measures in routine patient care to control the spread of disease and to limit the loss of life among health care workers, as had occurred with the severe acute respiratory syndrome outbreak in Toronto [14]. Routine infection control practices including hand hygiene should be emphasized for every patient encounter. Standard infection control measures should include practice of respiratory hygiene and cough etiquette in dealing with patients with respiratory symptoms and contact precautions for managing patients with unexplained rashes or draining skin wounds. Adherence to these measures would help to limit exposures for most of the CDC category A bioterrorist agents that have a high potential for being contagious, including pneumonic plague and viral hemorrhagic fevers.

Although the causative agents of bioterrorism may vary, the potential devastating effects may not. This fact should provide a basis to develop a plan to deal with effects common to several agents, rather than developing separate plans for each bioterrorist agent. The plan can be focused on syndromic presentations, with minor adjustments for the probable rapidity and severity as needed. Specific recommendations for managing individual biologic agents with bioterrorism potential should be addressed in an appendix to the main plan.

Incorporate internal mechanisms for intensified surveillance

The bioterrorism preparedness plan should address triage procedures for identifying febrile patients with respiratory symptoms or skin lesions for immediate separation from the common waiting area and rapid medical evaluation. History of foreign travel within 21 days of presentation should be asked of all febrile patients with respiratory symptoms, unexplained skin rash, or other unusual constellation of symptoms. Patients with a positive travel history to areas endemic for diseases of concern or experiencing unusual outbreaks should be isolated from other patients and staff immediately to prevent cross-contamination. Focus on syndromic recognition in the emergency department should lead to initiation of airborne isolation and other appropriate precautions that conform to CDC infection control guidelines [15].

Protocol should be established for immediate notification of emergency department physicians and infection control specialists to determine the need to initiate the biothreat containment alert in the event of multiple patients presenting with similar symptoms. If the hospital uses an electronic medical record, fields incorporating the travel history should be added so that a positive response would generate an automated report of notification to the infection control. This would serve as a backup surveillance mechanism in the event a clustering is not detected on clinical grounds alone.

Ensure appropriate internal and external mechanisms of communication

The institution should be committed to an open, timely, and truthful dialogue with the employees and strive to ensure that the internal communication precedes any form of external communication. This communication would help to build trust, boost employee morale, and prevent a flurry of rumors and false information. Feedback received as a result of addressing employees' questions and concerns may prove vital in anticipating and responding to public and media queries.

Improving the communication flow is probably the biggest challenge in the determination of the programs' eventual success. Just providing the plan would not be enough; there needs to be training, follow-up, and support to encourage use of the appropriate communication channels at horizontal and vertical levels. Strengthening the communication skills and capacity of the staff in the emergency department, especially the registration and the triage personnel, would yield the most benefit in ensuring effective communication of the initial threat at an internal level for timely analysis of the risk potential. One should not expect that sharing and communication between emergency department personnel and the other members of the response team would happen automatically; this communication needs facilitation and encouragement. Communication during a "biothreat containment alert" should use the channels established in the hospitals' disaster response plan to ensure consistency.

The disaster manual should maintain an up-to-date roster of emergency contact information for all key hospital staff (eg, home telephone, fax, beeper, and cell phone) and should have a system in place for notifying, informing, and mobilizing staff, including physicians, nurses, pharmacists, allied health professionals, and other key support staff, in the case of an emergency. The manual also should incorporate current information and a 24-hour response hotline for external contacts, including the local health department, Federal Bureau of Investigation, and CDC.

Test the plan periodically through drills

A variety of methods or tools have been used to train the hospital staff and evaluate the effectiveness of the disaster preparedness plans, including disaster drills, computer simulations, and tabletop exercises [16]. Full-scale disaster drills are time-consuming and expensive, however; one large-scale drill conducted by the US Department of Justice in May 2000 cost $3 million [17]. Despite this, it is still important to participate in city-wide drills and table-top exercises because an important part of the joint emergency planning is to understand how available community resources should be used to respond together to any bioterrorist event. Hospitals must overcome the attitude that they can handle events by themselves and remember that the institutional and public health plans must dovetail to reap maximum benefit of all available resources.

The institution should begin by testing their plan with progressive drills to assess the operations' continuity on a regular basis and to ensure that everyone in the response team knows how to react. Running the "fire drills" tests how well the plan has been laid out and how effectively it has been communicated to the employees. The institution should let employees know they are going to test their familiarity with disaster procedures at random times, then simulate some of the scenarios set out in the plan rather than playing out the entire drill each time, recognizing that normal functioning of the hospital cannot be stopped during the exercise. The idea is to assess individual components of the preparedness plan during different shifts and to prioritize testing of the weakest link. Drills should not be intended as a test in the strictest sense, but rather as an opportunity to identify weakness; build teamwork; improve coordination; and enhance acquired skills, knowledge, and competencies. After completion of the drill, the institution should ensure a proper debriefing session facilitated by trained observers [18], to maximize the learning opportunity, provide for constructive critique, and discuss changes that need to be implemented as a result of the exercise.

Incorporate flexibility and build redundancy for key components of the plan

It is important that bioterrorism preparedness include contingency planning, recognizing the adage that "if something can go wrong, it will." The observation by German strategist Helmut von Moltke that "No plan survives contact with the enemy" mandates this flexibility to afford protection against a tendency to try to stick to a predefined game plan, despite situation dictating otherwise. A detailed checklist for each role, enumerating assigned responsibilities and tasks, should be incorporated as an attachment to the plan to allow for substitute personnel to fill in the role at the last minute. Preparedness for this level of flexibility could be achieved by cross-training individuals for other roles and responsibilities they could be expected to fill in at times of need.

The plan operations and contingency response should incorporate redundancy of key personnel, equipment, and processes to add stability and allow flexibility in handling the unexpected. Such redundancy may be ensured by a forcing function that would prevent an erroneous action from being performed or facilitate performance of a desired action and provide for a safeguard against fatigue failures.

Address logistics involving surge capacity

A large-scale bioterrorist event likely would overwhelm the existing facility capacity rapidly, given that the current health care infrastructure frequently is overwhelmed by the demand for services during normal influenza seasons. This situation underscores the need for addressing issues related to surge capacity, to enable hospitals to expand beyond their normal operations to meet a sudden increase in demand that can be sustained for an extended period. To be adequately prepared, the plan should assume no outside help during the first 72 hours and count on existing staff only. This assumption would imply staff working longer hours and extra shifts and needing arrangements for overnight stay in the hospital. Medical equipment and other hospital supplies, including personal protective gear and pharmaceutical caches, would need to be stocked adequately to cater to the increased demand during this period. Ability to update hospital inventory in a real-time manner would need to be incorporated to allow sufficient notice to address continued additional demands though the strategic national stockpile. The CDC's FluSurge software program [19] could be used to estimate some of the potential increased hospital requirements during a pandemic influenza outbreak and to provide a basis for extrapolating usage in response to other biologic disasters or bioterrorist events.

Protocols should be in place for discharging patients with non–life-threatening conditions, closing the facility to elective surgeries, and prioritizing exposed patients who require hospitalization. Strategies to increase bed capacity should be addressed, including the use of nonconventional beds in the outpatient areas. The role of enhanced hospital security in enforcing and controlling facility access should be emphasized to help deal with emergency department overcrowding during times of panic and enforcing of quarantine measures, if implemented.

The plan should address functionality of the health care team in the event of having fewer patient care staff show up to work and losing crucial administrative personnel. Policies should include criteria for use of emergency and volunteer staffing during such a crisis and address their liability and credentialing issues. Human resources should look into the feasibility of having incentives and provisions for encouraging existing health care workers to continue working in the event of a major biologic disaster and the legality of the staff's right to refuse assignment involving patients infected with agents of bioterrorism. Mechanisms should be in place for early identification of illness and psychosocial issues among employees to allow rapid access to evaluation and treatment and to allay anxiety of the workforce, including concerns for their families' well-being.

Improve collaboration with community physicians, area hospitals, and local health departments

A biologic disaster or bioterrorist event poses unique challenges because it may go unrecognized for days [20], with the possibility of victims presenting to different hospitals or physician practices. This possibility underscores the importance of building alliance with community physicians, who could be the initial gatekeepers funneling patients with unusual illness into the health care system. Educating community physicians about the importance of providing advance notice to the hospital emergency department staff would help with institution of appropriate precautions in a timely manner. Similarly, collaboration and information sharing with other area hospitals, preferably using the existing network of infection control practitioners, could provide the heads-up of a possibility of a suspected exposure to a biologic disaster or bioterrorist agent within the community.

Integration of the institution's goals into the local health department's preparedness initiative could yield significant benefits, especially if there is a two-way flow of information. The health department would obtain information from area hospitals as part of the laboratory or syndromic surveillance system. In return, the hospitals would benefit from the health department's commitment to share information of any ongoing investigation into a suspected case of biologic disaster or bioterrorist agent, in a timely but confidential manner to avoid undue media hype.

Emphasize community preparedness

The effectiveness of disaster preparedness and response depends on the involvement of the local communities. An integral part of the program should be to work with the established communities (eg, business, ethnic, neighborhood, nongovernmental) to educate the public on emergency and disaster procedures and preparedness initiatives. The hospital should partner with the local media in the planning phase so that they can serve the vital role of disseminating key messages to the public and help portray a realistic image to the national media. This platform would enable communication to the public in a consistent and timely way and go a long way in preparing for the "fear factor" and prevent the system from getting overwhelmed by the "worried well."

Summary

In an ideal world, bioterrorism preparedness efforts would leave nothing to chance and include planning for everything. So the question remains, can the medical community practically plan for everything? Although it is true that "forecasting is always difficult, particularly when it's the future we are dealing with," if one has a good plan for dealing with the probable, one might stand a better chance of responding adequately to the improbable. In this context, Eisenhower's dictum could be interpreted to mean that in planning for a bioterrorist threat, original plans would need to be changed to address the dynamics caused by uncertainty, but proper planning with periodic testing would go a long way in minimizing the chaos associated with this change. If after all this preparation the outlook still looks dismal, some consolation can be derived from the quote of a German officer, "the reason the American army does so well in war is because war is chaos and the American army practices chaos on a daily basis."

References

[1] Katrina reveals fatal weaknesses in US public health. Lancet 2005;366:867.

[2] Ready or not? Protecting the public's health from disease, disasters, and bioterrorism. Trust for America's Health December 2005. Available at: http://www.healthyamericans.org/reports/bioterror05/bioterror05ExecSum.pdf. Accessed January 10, 2006.

[3] Dowling KC, Lipton RI. Bioterrorism preparedness expenditures may compromise public health. Am J Public Health 2005;95:1672.

[4] Noah DL, Sovel AL, Ostroff SM, et al. Biological warfare training: infectious disease outbreak differentiation criteria. Milit Med 1998;163:198–201.

[5] Franz DR, Jahrling PB, Friedlander AM, et al. Clinical recognition and management of patients exposed to biological warfare agents. JAMA 1997;278:399–411.

[6] Simon JD. Biological terrorism. JAMA 1997;278:428–30.

[7] Madeline Drexler. Secret agents: the menace of emerging infections. Washington, DC: John Henry Press; 2002.

[8] Guidotti TL. Why do public health practitioners hesitate? Journal of Homeland Security and Emergency Management 2004;1:403.

[9] University of California. Irvine Medical Center's Bioterrorism/WMD Readiness Plan. Available at: http://www.ucihs.uci.edu/emergencymanagement/emergencyMngtProgram/emergOpsPlan/pdfs/bioterrorism.pdf. Accessed January 10, 2006.

[10] East Carolina University Brody School of Medicine's Biological Terrorism Readiness Plan. Available at: http://www.ecu.edu/prospectivehealth/forms/04BioTerReadPlan.pdf. Accessed January 10, 2006.

[11] Tracer methodology: how it can help you improve quality. Healthcare Benchmarks Qual Improv 2004;11:61–3.

[12] Pletz B, Cheu D, Russell P, et al. HEICS III. The Hospital Emergency Incident Command System Update project. Prepared by the San Mateo County Health Services Agency, Emergency Medical Services, under Prevention 2000 Block Grant Contract No. EMS-6040. State of California Emergency Medical Services Authority, San Mateo, California. June 1998. Available at: http://www.emsa.cahwnet.gov/dms2/heics3.htm. Accessed January 10, 2006.

[13] Rotz LD, Khan AS, Lillibridge SR, et al. Public health assessment of potential biological terrorism agents. Emerg Infect Dis 2002;8:225–30.

[14] Booth CM, Matukas LM, Tomlinson GA, et al. Clinical features and short-term outcomes of 144 patients with SARS in the greater Toronto area. JAMA 2003;289:2801–9.

[15] Siegel J, Strausbaugh L, Jackson M, et al. Draft guideline for isolation precautions: preventing transmission of infectious agents in healthcare settings, 2004. Healthcare Infection Control Practices Advisory Committee. Available at: http://www.premierinc.com/all/safety/resources/guidelines/downloads/2004-draft-iso-guideline.pdf. Accessed January 10, 2006.

[16] Cosgrove SE, Jenckes MW, Kohri D, et al. Evaluation of hospital disaster drills: a module-based approach. prepared by Johns Hopkins University Evidence-based Practice Center under Contract No. 290–02–0018. AHRQ Publication No. 04–0032. Rockville (MD): Agency for Healthcare Research and Quality; 2004.

[17] Inglesby TV, Grossman R, O'Toole T. A plague on your city: observations from TOPOFF. Clin Infect Dis 2001;32:436–45.

[18] Klein KR, Brandenburg DC, Atas JG, et al. Use of trained observers as an evaluation tool for a multi-hospital bioterrorism exercise. Prehosp Disast Med 2005;20:159–63.

[19] FluSurge version 2.0. Software to estimate the impact of an influenza pandemic on hospital surge capacity. Centers for Disease Control and Prevention, US Department of Health and Human Services; 2005. Available at: http://www.cdc.gov/flu/flusurge.htm. Accessed January 10, 2006.

[20] Vastag B. Experts urge bioterrorism readiness. JAMA 2001;285:30–2.

ELSEVIER
SAUNDERS

Infect Dis Clin N Am
20 (2006) 455–473

INFECTIOUS
DISEASE CLINICS
OF NORTH AMERICA

Microbial Forensics: Application to Bioterrorism Preparedness and Response

Stephen A. Morse, MSPH, PhD[a,*],
Bruce Budowle, PhD[b]

[a] *Bioterrorism Preparedness and Response Program, Centers for Disease Control and Prevention, 1600 Clifton Road, MS C-12, Atlanta, GA 30333, USA*
[b] *Federal Bureau of Investigation, Laboratory Division, Quantico, VA 22135, USA*

The threat of terrorist or criminal use of pathogenic microorganisms and their toxins is a concern in the United States and internationally [1]. The detection of West Nile virus in New York City in 1999 raised concerns that the emergence of this infectious agent was the consequence of a deliberate act [2]; however, on further investigation, no evidence of bioterrorism was found [3,4]. On October 2, 2001, a previously healthy 63-year-old employee of American Media in Boca Raton, Florida, awoke from sleep with fever, emesis, and confusion [5]. At the emergency department, a lumbar puncture was performed for presumed bacterial meningitis; the examination of the Gram stain of the cerebrospinal fluid revealed many polymorphonuclear white blood cells and many large gram-positive bacilli singly and in chains. On the basis of the cerebrospinal fluid appearance, a diagnosis of anthrax was considered. The clinical laboratory of the medical center presumptively identified the organism as *Bacillus anthracis* within 18 hours after plating; this identification was confirmed by a Laboratory Response Network (LRN) member laboratory [6] within the Florida Department of Health on the following day (October 4). Although the case was reported to local public health authorities when anthrax was first suspected, a public announcement was not made until the final laboratory diagnosis of inhalational anthrax was confirmed [5].

At this point, there was no conclusive evidence that an act of bioterrorism was responsible for this case of inhalational anthrax. A great difficulty that confronts public health and law enforcement personnel is differentiating between a natural infection and one resulting from an intentional attack. Before 2001, the last case of inhalational anthrax in the United States was in

* Corresponding author.
E-mail address: sam1@cdc.gov (S.A. Morse).

0891-5520/06/$ - see front matter. Published by Elsevier Inc.
doi:10.1016/j.idc.2006.03.004

1976 in a home craftsman from California, who died after being infected by endospores that were present on contaminated imported yarn containing goat hair [7]. Since the beginning of the twentieth century, most cases of inhalational anthrax in the United States have resulted from occupational exposure to contaminated animal hides or products.

During the subsequent investigation of the case of anthrax in Florida in 2001, extensive environmental sampling at the patient's home and travel destinations failed to detect the presence of *B anthracis*. Endospores of *B anthracis* were found on the patient's computer keyboard at his workplace, however, and recovered from asymptomatic coworkers [8] and a hospitalized coworker [8,9], suggesting the American Media building as the site where the infection had been acquired. Coworkers had reported that on September 19, 2001, the patient had closely examined an unusual letter containing powder. This together with the finding of *B anthracis* endospores in regional and local postal centers that processed mail destined for the American Media building implicated one or more mailed letters or packages as the probable source of exposure. When letters containing endospores were discovered at the offices of NBC, CBS, ABC, and the New York Post [9] and in the offices of Senator Patrick Lahey [10], bioterrorism became a reality in the United States, and a possible covert attack became an overt bioterrorism event.

The use of the US postal system as a method for disseminating endospores of *B anthracis* set off national panic, and the Federal Bureau of Investigation (FBI) began an investigation. The need to exploit forensic evidence that could assist in identifying the perpetrator of this heinous act thrust the nascent field of microbial forensics into the spotlight. The occurrence of this event created an urgent need for enhanced capabilities that make possible the full and robust forensic exploitation and interpretation of microbial evidence from acts of bioterrorism or biocrimes.

Microbial forensics is a new discipline, dedicated to the characterization, analysis, and interpretation of evidence for attribution purposes from an act of bioterrorism, biocrime, hoax, or inadvertent release of a microorganism or toxin [11]. Attribution is the information obtained regarding the identification or source of a material to the degree it can be ascertained. The goal of attribution is the identification of the individuals involved in carrying out the event, which is necessary for criminal prosecution or for actions that may be taken as a result of national policy decisions [12].

To prepare for the next bioterrorist attack or biocrime and to deter a future event, a strong microbial forensics program is being developed [11–14]. For the purpose of this article, microbial forensics is considered as an evolving subdiscipline of forensic science, which combines several scientific disciplines (eg, molecular biology, microbiology, genomics, bioinformatics, biochemistry) to analyze evidence from a bioterrorism act, biocrime, hoax, or inadvertent release, for the purpose of attribution. This article describes the field of microbial forensics, the challenges to consider, and how this emerging field is integrated into the preparedness and response of the United States to a bioterrorist attack.

Epidemiology and forensics

Epidemiology studies the occurrence, features, and determinants of disease in populations. The same general principles of epidemiologic investigation apply to a bioterrorist attack or crime involving a biologic agent as would apply to any other disease [15]. When an outbreak has occurred or surveillance systems have detected an abnormality, a detailed but expedient epidemiologic investigation has to be performed. Important considerations in the investigation of acute outbreaks of infectious disease include (1) determining that an outbreak has occurred, (2) defining the population at risk, (3) determining the method of spread and reservoir, and (4) characterizing the agent. The use of epidemiologic methods as part of an ongoing investigation of a health problem for which there is suspicion or evidence regarding possible intentional acts or criminal behavior as factors contributing to the health problem has been called *forensic epidemiology* [16]. Forensic epidemiology was instrumental in documenting the true nature of the Sverdlovsk incident of 1979, in which at least 66 people died of anthrax as the result of an accidental release of endospores from a biological weapons facility [17,18].

Forensics and epidemiology should not be thought of as separate disciplines in the context of a crime, but rather should be treated as integrated disciplines [16]. Many of the practices used in epidemiology are similar to those in microbial forensics. A forensic investigation of a case in which the weapon is a pathogen or toxin attempts to determine the identity of the causal agent and its source in much the same manner as an epidemiologic investigation would attempt to identify the causal agent and its source in a disease outbreak. Many of the molecular techniques used to characterize organisms used in an act of bioterrorism, or biocrime, are techniques that have been used for years to trace outbreaks of infectious diseases, which is a practice called *molecular epidemiology*. One distinction between microbial forensics and molecular epidemiology is that data from microbial forensic analyses are not only scrutinized by scientists, but also are evaluated by the legal system.

An epidemiologic investigation may identify numerous indicators that raise the level of suspicion that an outbreak may have been caused intentionally [19], warranting further investigation. These epidemiologic clues include the following:

- A single case of disease caused by an uncommon agent (eg, smallpox, viral hemorrhagic fever, inhalation or cutaneous anthrax, glanders) without adequate epidemiologic explanation

- The presence of an unusual, atypical, or antiquated strain of an agent or antibiotic resistance pattern
- Higher morbidity and mortality in association with a common disease or syndrome or failure of such patients to respond to usual therapy
- Unusual disease presentation, such as inhalation anthrax or pneumonic plague
- Disease with an unusual geographic or seasonal distribution (eg, plague in a nonendemic area, influenza occurring in the Northern Hemisphere in the summer)
- An unexpected increase in the incidence of stable endemic disease, such as tularemia or plague
- Atypical disease transmission through aerosols, food, or water, in a mode suggesting sabotage (ie, no other possible explanation)
- Several unusual or unexplained diseases coexisting in the same patient without any other explanation
- Unusual illness that affects a large, disparate population (eg, respiratory disease in a large heterogeneous population may suggest exposure to an inhaled biologic agent)
- Illness that is unusual (or atypical) for a given population or age group (eg, outbreak of measles-like rash in adults)
- Unusual pattern of death or illness among animals that is unexplained or attributed to an agent of bioterrorism that precedes or accompanies illness or death in humans
- Unusual pattern of death or disease in humans that precedes or accompanies illness or death in animals, which may be unexplained or attributed to an agent of bioterrorism.
- Agents of an unusual illness isolated from temporally or spatially distinct sources that have a similar genotype
- Simultaneous clusters of similar unusual illness in noncontiguous areas, domestic or foreign
- Large numbers of unexplained diseases or deaths
- Large numbers of ill individuals who seek treatment at about the same time (point source with compressed epidemic curve)

Most of the above-listed epidemiologic clues simply suggest an unusual cluster of cases. Epidemiologic investigations have shown that even indicators that are highly specific, such as a single case of disease caused by an uncommon agent, an unusual disease presentation, or a disease with an unusual geographic distribution, may signal a new natural outbreak. This can be illustrated by three examples.

In the first, the community outbreak of individuals with smallpox-like lesions in the Midwest may have indicated the deliberate release of smallpox virus. A thorough integrated epidemiologic and laboratory investigation identified the disease as monkeypox, an exotic disease in the United States.

Although the epidemiologic data did not support this mode of transmission, the appearance of monkeypox, a potential bioterrorism agent [20], could suggest bioterrorism [21]. Second, the outbreak on Martha's Vineyard of primary pneumonic tularemia in 11 patients may have indicated a deliberate aerosol release of *Francisella tularensis* type A. The epidemiologic investigation suggested that infection was associated with lawn mowing and brush cutting, activities that could aerosolize the organism from the environment [22]. Third, the occurrence of plague in a couple visiting New York City in November 2002, was highly unusual and suggested the possibility of bioterrorism because these infections occurred outside the area where plague is endemic in the United States [23]. On initial consultations with medical personnel, the couple reported that they had traveled from Santa Fe County, New Mexico, where routine surveillance conducted by the New Mexico Department of Health had identified *Yersinia pestis* in a dead wood rat and fleas collected several months earlier on their New Mexico property. One day after the patients were evaluated, the New Mexico Department of Health and Centers for Disease Control and Prevention investigated the couple's New Mexico property and a nearby hiking trail where rodents and fleas were collected. The *Y pestis* isolate from one of the patients and isolates from seven flea pools (collected in July and November) were compared by pulsed-field gel electrophoresis and multiple locus variable number tandem repeat assays (MLVA) and shown to be indistinguishable. The MLVA patterns were distinct from other *Y pestis* MLVA patterns from surrounding regions. This finding indicated that the *Y pestis* infection most likely was acquired on their property in New Mexico.

The epidemiologic methods in common between microbial forensics investigations and nonforensic microbial investigations include the identification and characterization of specific disease-associated pathogens or their toxins and determination of their mode of transmission. As in nonforensic investigations, microbial forensics investigators analyze evidence to assist in determining the source of the agent ultimately to determine the individual, method, and location responsible for the contamination event.

Scenarios

The forensic approach to biologic and chemical terrorism differs, based on inherent differences between the two modes of attack. The important distinctions between these forms of terrorism are presented in Table 1. The main distinction between biologic terrorism and chemical terrorism is the time it may take to become aware of the attack (see later). Bioterrorist attacks (or biocrimes) occur as one of two scenarios (ie, overt and covert). In either scenario, biologic agents could be introduced into populations by several routes, including aerosol; contaminated food, water, or medical products; fomites; or release of infected arthropod vectors [25,26]. Because investigators currently lack the ability to conduct real-time monitoring for

Table 1
Important distinctions between biologic and chemical terrorism

	Type of terrorism	
Criterion	Biologic (covert)	Chemical
Speed at which attack results in illness	Delayed—usually days to weeks after attack	Rapid—usually minutes to hours after attack
Distribution of affected patients	Diffuse spread through city or region; major international epidemic in worst-case scenario	Concentrated near point of release
First responders	Emergency department nurses and physicians, infectious disease physicians, infection control practitioners, epidemiologists, public health practitioners, hospital administrators, medical examiners, laboratory experts	Paramedics, police, firefighters, emergency rescue, law enforcement, military personnel
Release site of weapon	Difficult to identify; may not be possible or useful to cordon off area of attack	Quickly discovered; possible or useful to cordon off area of attack
Decontamination of patients and environment	Not necessary or limited in most cases	Crucial in most cases
Medical interventions	Vaccines or antibiotics or both (if available)	Chemical antidotes (if available)
Patient isolation/quarantine	Crucial if highly infectious disease is involved (eg, smallpox); advance hospital planning for isolating large numbers of patients is crucial	After decontamination there is no need

Adapted from Henderson DA. The looming threat of bioterrorism. Science 1999;283:1279–82; with permission. © American Association for the Advancement of Science.

the release of a biologic agent in all parts of the United States, a covert release of a microorganism or toxin in a population likely would go unnoticed for some time, with individuals exposed leaving the attack area before the act of terrorism becomes evident. This differs from the likely scenario in a chemical attack (Table 1) [24], and a biologic attack likely would necessitate an investigation to identify the point source of infection.

Because of the incubation period, the first signs that a microorganism or toxin has been released may not become apparent until hours or weeks later, when individuals become ill and seek medical care. The "first responders" to a covert release of a microorganism or toxin are likely to be the astute clinician, laboratory or public health worker, or medical examiner who recognizes the index case or identifies the responsible agent. This scenario is exemplified by the identification of the index case in the 2001 anthrax attacks [5]. The clinical history and physical examination of a patient are a departure point for epidemiologic investigation. Although public health is the "first responder," the epidemiologic information collected is invaluable in a microbial forensics investigation. A major component of a microbial forensic case is trace-back to a cause and source. In this sense, a search for commonalities and clustering to identify the source of infection is no different from the standard epidemiologic methods used to investigate outbreaks of infectious diseases [27]. The intersections between an epidemiologic and microbial forensic investigation of an outbreak are summarized in Table 2.

Methods

Traditional microbiologic laboratory methods, such as culturing, play an important role in identifying the pathogen, and culture remains the clinical laboratory gold standard method for identifying viable pathogens and for providing a basis for selecting appropriate antimicrobial therapy. Based on the nature of the event, the type of evidence from a covert release is likely to be a culture or clinical specimen from an affected individual or samples (eg, food, water, environmental) collected during the epidemiologic investigation of an outbreak. Because of the length of the incubation period, however, it may be difficult to isolate viable microorganisms or nondegraded protein toxins from nonclinical specimens collected during a subsequent investigation. In addition to culture, analytical methods, such as nucleic acid–based or antibody-based assays, are used to characterize the microbial forensic evidence.

A microbial forensic investigation encompasses many aspects that are beyond those pertaining to public health. These differences are most apparent in an overt event. The most likely responders to an overt release of a microorganism or toxin (including hoaxes) are law enforcement or HAZMAT

Table 2
Opportunities to collect evidence for a microbial forensics investigation during a biologic agent response

Key elements	Opportunity
Rapid detection of outbreak	
Swift agent identification and confirmation	+
Identification of population at risk	+
Determination of how agent is transmitted, including assessment of efficiency of transmission	+
Determination of susceptibility of pathogen to treatment	+
Definition of public, medical, and psychological health implications	
Control and containment of epidemic	
Decontamination of individuals, if necessary	+
Identification of law enforcement implications/assessment of threat	+
Augmentation and surge capacity of local health and medical resources	
Protection of the population through appropriate public health and medical actions	
Dissemination of information to enlist public support	
Assessment of environmental contamination and cleanup/decontamination of biologic agents that persist in the environment	+
Tracking and preventing secondary or additional disease outbreak	

personnel and firefighters because of their terrorism response training. Portable field assays may be used by these responders to assess the threat for public health, safety, and security purposes. Potential bioterrorism samples are transported to an LRN laboratory, where expert analysis is conducted using validated protocols and reagents [6,28]. A major component of this process is to establish and maintain the law enforcement chain of custody as it is with clinical specimens and cultures arising from a covert event. Microbial forensics laboratories may perform detailed characterization assays to identify clues to the origin of a pathogen or toxin or its preparation as a weapon. In addition to microbiologic analyses (eg, culture), the evidence collected from an overt event is likely to be amenable to chemical and physical analyses that may yield information about the methods, means, processes, and locations involved in the preparation and dissemination of the biological weapon. The type of evidence found at the crime scene (in particular for an overt event) might include powders, liquids (eg, water), food, or other environmental samples. In addition, traditional forensic evidence, such as hair, fibers, documents, fingerprints, and human DNA, may be collected and analyzed.

Nucleic acid–based methods

An important goal of microbial forensics is the acquisition of data that can differentiate an isolate or sample from similar samples as precisely as possible. Ideally, for attribution, the forensic scientist attempts to narrow the possible sources of a sample, while excluding most, if not all, other sources. This individualization may not always be achievable. To enhance attribution capabilities, a useful tool of microbial forensics is the use of nucleic acid–based assays that enable association (or elimination) of a pathogen with specific sources on genetic information from the full or partial genome of that pathogen.

The use of nucleic acid–based assays for microbial identification, characterization, and attribution purposes is analogous to its use for human DNA forensic analysis, which is used widely in the forensic arena to associate and exclude DNA-containing biologic evidence with suspected individuals [29,30]. At present (and maybe never), nucleic acid analytical assays used in microbial forensics cannot routinely achieve the level of attribution that is achieved with human DNA forensics. The vast numbers of microorganisms, their complex biologic and ecologic diversities, and their capacity for genetic exchange complicate the analysis and interpretation of bioterrorism and biocrime evidence in ways that do not have an impact on human DNA forensics.

Budowle and colleagues [30] identified many questions that potentially could be addressed through the genetic analysis of forensic samples. Defining the questions to answer provides direction for an investigation. The answers to these questions may provide information that can be used for attribution purposes or provide investigative leads. These questions are as follows:

- What might be deduced concerning the nature and source of the evidentiary sample?
- Is the pathogen detected of endemic origin or introduced?
- Do the genetic markers provide a significant amount of probative information?
- Does the choice of markers allow the effective comparison of samples from known and questioned sources?
- If such a comparison can be made, how definitively and confidently can a conclusion be reached?
- Are the genetic differences too few to conclude that the samples are not from different sources (or lineages)?
- Are these differences sufficiently robust to consider that the samples are from different sources?
- Is it possible that the two samples have a recent common ancestor, or how long ago was there a common ancestor?
- Can any samples be excluded as contaminants or recent sources of the isolate?
- Are there alternative explanations for the results that were obtained?

The degree to which these questions can be addressed depends on the context of the case and the available knowledge of the genetics, genomics, phylogeny, and ecology of the microorganism in question. Genetic markers that may be used for forensic attribution include single nucleotide polymorphisms (SNPs); repetitive sequences, insertions, and deletions (INDELS); mobile genetic elements; pathogenicity islands; virulence and antimicrobial resistance genes; housekeeping genes; structural genes; and whole genomes [30–32]. Many of these markers have been used for the molecular subtyping of pathogens where public health and epidemiologic needs are foremost. Developments in molecular epidemiology will contribute to the analytical toolbox of the microbial forensic scientist. The essential components of a highly precise and robust subtyping system for an infectious agent often are the same for forensic and public health and epidemiologic purposes and include (1) identification of diversity; (2) development of validated and robust molecular typing assays; (3) development of reference population databases; (4) establishment of guidelines for interpretation of analytical results, either qualitative or based on theoretical and probabilistic approaches; and (5) validation of the system with studies of actual disease outbreaks [11,13,30,33].

The genotyping of many of the biothreat agents presents a challenge compared with other infectious disease–causing microorganisms [31]. The genetic relationship between many medically important microorganisms has been determined based on SNPs, presence of known virulence factors, and macrorestriction patterns of the genomic DNA [34–38]. Agents such as *B anthracis* [33,39–43], *F tularensis* [44–49], *Y pestis* [50–54], and *Brucella* spp. [55, 56] are relatively monomorphic, however, and exhibit little molecular variation among isolates from similar geographic areas. The identification and use of rare variants would be significant for obtaining the deepest resolution possible. The ongoing effort to sequence multiple strains of these biothreat agents will facilitate the development of nucleic acid–based assays for attribution purposes (Table 3).

Table 3
Publicly available genome sequences of CDC category A and B agents

Agent	Strain	Accession number[a]	Size (nucleotides)	Reference
Bacteria				
Bacillus anthracis[b]	Ames	NC 003997	5,227,293	[57]
	Ames ancestor	NC 007530	5,227,419	
	Sterne	NC 005945	5,228,663	
Brucella abortus (biovar 1)	9-941	NC 006932	2,124,241 (chr I)	
		NC 006933	1,162,204 (chr II)	
B melitensis	16M	NC 003317	2,117144 (chr I)	[58]
		NC 003318	1,177,787 (chr II)	
B melitensis (biovar 1)	2308	NC 007618	2,121,359 (chr I)	
		NC 007624	1,156,948 (chr II)	
B suis	1330	NC 004310	2,107,794 (chr I)	[59]
		NC 004311	1,207,381 (chr II)	
Burkholderia mallei[c]	ATCC 23344	NC 006348	3,510,148 (chr I)	
		NC 006349	2,325,379 (chr II)	
B pseudomallei[d]	1710b	NC 007434	4,126,292 (chr I)	
		NC 007435	3,181,762 (chr II)	
	K96243	NC 006350	4,074,542 (chr I)	
		NC 006351	3,173,005 (chr II)	
Coxiella burnetii	RSA 493	NC 002971	1,995,281	[60]
Francisella tularensis[e]	Schu 4	NC 006570	1,892,819	[61]
Rickettsia prowazekii	Madrid E	NC 000963	1,111,523	[62]
Yersinia pestis[f]	CO92	NC 003143	4,653,728	[63]
	KIM	NC 004088	4,600,755	[64]
Y pestis biovar *medievalis*	91001	NC 005810	4,595,065	
Viruses				
Ebola	Reston	NC 004161	18,891	[65]
	Zaire	NC 002549	18,959	[66]
Lassa segment S		NC 004296	3402	[67]
Lassa segment L		NC 004297	7279	[68]
Variola major	India 1967	NC 001611	185,578	[69,70]

[a] NC, refseq.

[b] Draft sequences are available for *B anthracis* strains A2012, Australia 94, CNEVA-9066, A1055, Vollum, USA 6153, and Kruger.

[c] Unfinished or draft sequences are available for *B mallei* strains 10229, 10399, FMH, GB8 horse 4, JHU, NCTC 10247, and SAVP 1.

[d] Unfinished or draft sequences are available for *B pseudomallei* strains 1106a, 1106b, 1655, 1710a, 668, Pasteur, and S13.

[e] The sequencing of *F tularensis* subsp. *holarctica* FSC200 and *F tularensis* subsp. *novicida* genomes is in progress.

[f] The sequencing of the genome of *Y pestis* biovar Antiqua strain Angola is in progress.

Keim and coworkers [33] proposed a nested hierarchal strategy for subtyping these agents. Progressive hierarchical resolving assays type genetic markers based on stability. SNPs generally are stable and good for lineage studies, but tend to have low power for individualizing isolates. Variable number tandem repeat loci (including microsatellite loci) are less stable and tend to evolve more rapidly; these loci (similar to human DNA forensic typing) are useful for distinguishing between similarly related samples.

Interpretations of genetic data from a clinical isolate, a laboratory derived strain, or a reference database and its similarity to an evidence sample can be made quantitatively or qualitatively. Quantitative assessments convey the significance of an analytical result and rely on extant diversity data. Because of the lack of diversity data and limited knowledge of worldwide diversity in many cases, there can be a high degree of uncertainty associated with findings of a "matched" sample with some reference sample. Although most scientists are becoming accustomed to statistical assessments of their data, this uncertainty will limit the use of some quantitative interpretations of microbial forensics results. Qualitative assessments also are useful, however. They can provide direction for an investigation or indicate the samples that are dissimilar and could not be recently related to the evidence in question.

A good example of the use of genetic analysis and a qualitative inference from the analysis was the investigative direction it provided during the anthrax attack in 2001. At one time, it was believed that bacterial genomes did not contain repetitive elements. Numerous species do contain VNTR and microsatellite markers, however, that contribute to their diversity [71–74]. Keim and colleagues [75] developed a MLVA (ie, multi-locus VNTR assay) to exploit the variation in VNTR loci to uncover the diversity within *B anthracis* for phylogenetic and evolutionary studies. The analytical process entails amplifying by polymerase chain reaction simultaneously several specified fragments of DNA (ie, loci) that carry repeat elements. The fragments differ because variation at VNTR loci differ in the number of repeats they contain and are distinguishable by size. The length of a fragment is correlated directly to the number of repeats it contains. To distinguish amplified fragments, they are separated electrophoretically, typically by capillary or slab gel electrophoresis, and detected after excitation by a laser. Because of the inherent variation in *B anthracis* at VNTR loci, MLVA is particularly useful in differentiating isolates.

The spores from the mail were determined to be of the Ames strain by using MLVA and were shown to be qualitatively different from all other strains within a reasonably large reference database [33,75]. Because the Ames strain rarely has been observed in nature, the criminal investigation focused on laboratories as being the possible source of the weapon. The qualitative assessment of Ames did not preclude the possibility that the perpetrator obtained the material from nature, but did offer a more likely direction for the investigators to pursue.

The same methodology was used to investigate the unsuccessful *B anthracis* attack on Tokyo in 1993 by the Aum Shinrikyo [76,77]. MLVA genotyping revealed that isolates recovered from the release site were consistent with a veterinary vaccine strain (Sterne 34F2), which is used in Japan for animal prophylaxis against anthrax and is generally regarded as nonpathogenic in immunocompetent humans.

Non-nucleic acid–based methods

DNA (or RNA) typing alone may not enable identification to the level of uniqueness, or at least to a limited number of putative sources. Chemical and physical analyses of microbial forensic evidence may increase the likelihood for attribution. These types of signatures can be obtained only from crimes where the weaponized material or delivery device is found; they have little use in covert attacks in which the biologic agent is derived from the victims. Many of these methods are relatively new and complementary, but they can be combined to identify signatures of sample growth, processing, geographic location, and chronometry. Matching of sample properties can help to establish the relatedness of disparate incidents. Mismatches might have exclusionary power or signify a more complex causal relationship between the events under investigation. Because the results of these analyses can provide information on how, when, or where microorganisms were grown and weaponized, they cannot be performed using organisms isolated from clinical specimens where the growth medium and culture conditions differ from those used by the perpetrator.

Forensic scientists often analyze materials for comparison purposes to eliminate them as potential sources of the evidence. The chemical characterization of a microorganism or its matrix may assist an investigation by providing information regarding the processes used to grow the agent and when or where it was grown. The sourcing application of stable isotope ratios has been used previously to address forensic questions, such as determining the point-of-origin of illicit drugs [78]. Similar to other organisms, microorganisms carry records of aspects of their growth environment, which consists primarily of nutrients and water, in the stable isotope ratios of their organic compounds. Continentally, storm-track trajectories and moisture origins, such as precipitation, create geographic gradients in the oxygen (^{18}O) and hydrogen (^{2}H) ratios, and local waters can have characteristic isotope signatures [79]. Kreuzer-Martin and associates [80] grew *Bacillus subtilis* in media prepared with water of varying ^{18}O and ^{2}H stable isotope ratios. The ^{18}O and ^{2}H stable isotope ratios of the organic matter in spores harvested from these cultures were measured using a mass spectrometer and shown to be linearly related to those of the media water. In addition, the predicted stable isotope ratios of spores produced in nutritionally identical media prepared with local water from five different locations (with different stable isotope ratios) around the United States matched the measured values of the water sources within a 95% confidence interval. Stable isotope ratio analyses may be a powerful tool for tracing the geographic point-of-origin for microbial products, including vegetative cells and spores. Only 30% of the hydrogen atoms in spores originate from the water used in the culture medium, however; the remaining 70% originate from the organic components of the culture medium [81], which may make the interpretation of the data for geographic location far more complex.

The stable isotope ratios (^{13}C, ^{15}N, ^{2}H) of microbiologic culture media vary based on the biologic sources of the medium components, the most important being the C_3 and C_4 plants that are either a direct source of medium components or the base of the food chain for animal or yeast sources [82]. Based on studies with *B subtilis,* Kreuzer-Martin and associates [82] concluded that growth of microorganisms in different media should yield differences in microbe isotope ratios that are readily measurable. The analysis of stable isotope ratios of microbiologic agents and seized culture media could make it possible to rule out specific batches of media as having been used to culture a batch of microorganisms found (eg, in a weapon delivery system). These investigators also developed a model for *B subtilis* relating the hydrogen isotope ratios of culture media, water, and spores, which works well for spores produced during growth in media without glucose [82,83]. These concepts can be extrapolated to other threat agents; however, differences in the physiology and metabolism require that these methods be validated with each microorganism.

Numerous other technologies can be applied to microbial forensics. Schaldach and coworkers [84] used many of these technologies to examine weaponized spore preparations of *Bacillus globigii,* a commonly used surrogate for *B anthracis*. Scanning electron microscopy coupled with energy dispersive x-ray microanalysis was used to determine the elemental composition of single cells or spores. Scanning electron microscopy–energy dispersive x-ray microanalysis detected the presence of silica, a potential additive in the weaponization process of *B anthracis* endospores. Atomic force microscopy, which provides a high-resolution image of the cellular surface, can be used to provide information on molecules adhering to the spores and on modifications to the exosporium caused by mechanical and chemical treatments during the weaponization process. Through the use of particle (proton)-induced x-ray emission and scanning transmission ion microscopy, the distribution of elements can be mapped within regions of a single cell. Raman and surface-enhanced Raman spectroscopy probes molecular bond vibrations and rotations to produce characteristic spectra. This methodology has been used to distinguish between species of spores by probing the first few nanometers of the spore surface. Bioaerosol mass spectrometry has been developed for the rapid identification of individual cells or spores in an aerosol with many background materials in real time and without reagents. The mass spectral signature obtained reflects the intrinsic biologic agent and the matrix material in which it is embedded or coated.

Time-of-flight secondary ion mass spectrometry captures elemental data (to generate chemical maps) and molecular fragments (to generate mass spectra) on a depth-dependent basis (to generate a depth profile). This complementary technology also can detect the signatures of silica and other additives. Accelerator mass spectrometry combines mass spectrometry and nuclear detection to measure the concentration of an isotope in a sample. Accelerator mass spectrometry reduces the entire sample (<1 mg) to carbon before performing the analysis and provides the ^{14}C measurements on the bulk sample. This can be used to determine the age of the material (ie, when the biologic agent was prepared). Finally, mass spectroscopic methods (eg, liquid chromatography/mass spectrometry and matrix assisted laser desorption/ionization time-of-flight) also have been applied to the detection and characterization of toxins [84,85].

National system

The response to bioterrorism and other outbreaks of infectious diseases is predicated on a strong nationwide laboratory system (eg, the LRN) [6]. The LRN is a partnership between the Centers for Disease Control and Prevention, FBI, and Association of Public Health Laboratories. It was designed to link state and local public health laboratories with other advanced-capacity clinical, military, environmental, veterinary, agricultural, water, and food testing laboratories, including those at the federal level. These laboratories use standard protocols, reagents, and state-of-the-art technologies to identify and confirm threat agents. LRN laboratories also maintain the chain-of-custody for specimens and cultures. Training and proficiency testing play an important role in maintaining the readiness and proficiency of LRN personnel.

The same concept of dedicating resources and establishing centers of excellence is required for microbial forensics. The US Department of Homeland Security, in partnership with the FBI, established the National Bioforensics Analysis Center (NBFAC) [11]. The NBFAC serves as the national reference center for analyses of microbiologic related evidence from bioterrorism and biocrimes. It would be difficult, however, for the NBFAC to prepare for and develop analytical procedures for all possible microorganisms or toxins that could be used as a weapon or in a hoax. Thus the FBI will exploit national assets and work within a partner laboratory network consisting of existing government, academic, and private sector entities for the attribution of biological weapons.

Summary

Responding to a bioterrorism attack presents law enforcement with unique challenges, one of which is determining the perpetrator of the crime.

The discipline of microbial forensics has been established to provide an infrastructure for analyzing forensic evidence for attribution and, it is hoped, to serve as a deterrent. The field of microbial forensics did not have to be developed de novo. The foundations for this field were developed from the epidemiologic investigations of emerging and recurring infectious diseases. These two disciplines share a common ground. Ascertaining the identity and physical properties of a deliberately released biologic agent is paramount, in responding to public health and security threats and in identifying the source of the agent. There are still numerous issues relating to bioterrorism preparedness and response that previously have not been considered by public health practitioners and law enforcement officials [16]. Training courses to strengthen the joint effectiveness of public health and law enforcement investigations and ultimately the collection of evidence for microbial forensics are currently being offered [16,86].

To go beyond public health needs and obtain the deepest level of attribution possible or to determine the processes used to develop the biological weapon, there are many tools available to assist the microbial forensic scientist in characterizing evidence. These include biologic, chemical, and physical methods. The field of microbial forensics will continue to mature and likely will focus on the development of faster analytical tools with increased sensitivity of detection, rigorous validation of methods, and development of interpretation guidelines for conveying the significance of an analytical result.

References

[1] Wilkening DA. BCW attack scenarios. In: Drell SD, Soafer AD, Wilson GD, editors. The new terror: facing the threat of biological and chemical weapons. Stanford: Hoover Institution Press; 1999. p. 76–114.

[2] Preston R. West Nile mystery. New Yorker 1999;75:90–107.

[3] Roos R. CDC sees no evidence of bioterrorism in spread of West Nile virus. Available at: http://www.cidrap.umn.edu/cidrap/content/bt/bioprep/news/wnile.html. Accessed December 28, 2005.

[4] Lanciotti RS, Roehrig JT, Deubel V, et al. Origin of the West Nile virus responsible for an outbreak of encephalitis in the Northeastern United States. Science 1999;286:2333–7.

[5] Bush LM, Abrams BH, Beall A, et al. Index case of fatal inhalational anthrax due to bioterrorism in the United States. N Engl J Med 2001;345:1607–10.

[6] Morse SA, Kellogg RB, Perry S, et al. Detecting biothreat agents: the Laboratory Response Network. ASM News 2003;69:433–7.

[7] Suffin SC, Carnes WH, Kaufman AF. Inhalation anthrax in a home craftsman. Hum Pathol 1978;9:594–7.

[8] Traeger MS, Wiersma ST, Rosenstein NE, et al. First case of bioterrorism-related inhalational anthrax in the United States, Palm Beach County, Florida, 2001. Emerg Infect Dis 2002;8:1029–34.

[9] Jernigan JA, Stephens DS, Ashford DA, et al. Bioterrorism-related inhalational anthrax: the first 10 cases reported in the United States. Emerg Infect Dis 2001;7:933–44.

[10] Hsu VP, Lukacs SL, Handzel T, et al. Opening a Bacillus anthracis-containing envelope, Capitol Hill, Washington, D.C.: the public health response. Emerg Infect Dis 2002;8: 1039–43.

[11] Budowle B, Schutzer SE, Einseln A, et al. Building microbial forensics as a response to bioterrorism. Science 2003;301:1852–3.
[12] Murch RS. Microbial forensics: building a national capacity to investigate bioterrorism. Biosecur Bioterror 2003;1:117–22.
[13] Keim P. Microbial forensics: a scientific assessment. Washington, DC: American Society for Microbiology; 2003.
[14] Budowle B, Schutzer SE, Ascher MS, et al. Toward a system of microbial forensics: from sample collection to interpretation of evidence. Appl Environ Microbiol 2005; 71:2209–13.
[15] Flowers LK, Mothershead JL, Blackwell TH. Bioterrorism preparedness: II. the community and emergency medical services systems. Emerg Med Clin N Am 2002;20:457–76.
[16] Goodman RA, Munson JW, Dammers K, et al. Forensic epidemiology: law at the intersection of public health and criminal investigations. J Law Med Ethics 2003;31:684–700.
[17] Meselson M, Guillemin J, Hugh-Jones ME, et al. The Sverdlovsk anthrax outbreak of 1979. Science 1994;266:1202–8.
[18] Jackson PJ, Hugh-Jones ME, Adair DM, et al. PCR analysis of tissue samples from the 1979 Sverdlovsk anthrax victims: the presence of multiple *Bacillus anthracis* strains in different victims. Proc Natl Acad Sci U S A 1998;95:1224–9.
[19] Treadwell TA, Koo D, Kuker K, et al. Epidemiological clues to bioterrorism. Public Health Rep 2003;118:92–8.
[20] McClain DJ. Smallpox. In: Sidell FR, Takafuji ET, Franz DR, editors. Medical aspects of chemical and biological warfare. Washington, DC: Office of the Surgeon General at TMM Publications; 1997. p. 539–59.
[21] Centers for Disease Control and Prevention. Update: multistate outbreak of monkeypox—Illinois, Indiana, Kansas, Missouri, Ohio, and Wisconsin, 2003. MMWR Morb Mortal Wkly Rep 2003;(52):642–6.
[22] Feldman KA, Enscore RE, Lathrop SL, et al. An outbreak of primary pneumonic tularemia on Martha's Vineyard. N Engl J Med 2001;345:1601–6.
[23] Centers for Disease Control and Prevention. Imported plague—New York City, 2002. MMWR Morb Mortal Wkly Rep 2003;52:725–8.
[24] Henderson DA. The looming threat of bioterrorism. Science 1999;283:1279–82.
[25] Eitzen EM Jr, Takafuji ET. Historical overview of biological warfare. In: Sidell FR, Takafuji ET, Franz DR, editors. Medical aspects of chemical and biological warfare. Washington, DC: Office of the Surgeon General at TMM Publications; 1997. p. 415–23.
[26] Eitzen EM Jr. Use of biological weapons. In: Sidell FR, Takafuji ET, Franz DR, editors. Medical aspects of chemical and biological warfare. Washington, DC: Office of the Surgeon General at TMM Publications; 1997. p. 437–50.
[27] Morse SA, Khan AS. Epidemiologic investigation for public health, biodefense, and forensic microbiology. In: Breeze RG, Budowle B, Schutzer SE, editors. Microbial forensics. San Diego: Elsevier Academic Press; 2005. p. 157–71.
[28] Department of U.S. Homeland Security. Biological incident annex: national response plan. Washington, DC: Department of U.S. Homeland Security; 2004. p. Bio-1–8.
[29] National Research Council (US). Committee on DNA forensic science: the evaluation of forensic DNA evidence. Washington, DC: National Academy Press; 1996.
[30] Budowle B, Johnson MD, Fraser CM, et al. Genetic analysis and attribution of microbial forensics evidence. Crit Rev Microbiol 2005;31:233–54.
[31] Lindler LE, Huang X-Z, Chu M, et al. Genetic fingerprinting of biodefense pathogens for epidemiology and forensic investigation. In: Lindler LE, Lebeda FJ, Korch GW, editors. Biological weapons defense: infectious diseases and counterbioterrorism. Totowa: Humana Press; 2005. p. 453–80.
[32] Cooke CL Jr. Forensic genetic analysis of microorganisms: overview of some important technical concepts and selected genetic typing methods. In: Breeze RG, Budowle B, Schutzer SE, editors. Microbial forensics. San Diego: Elsevier Academic Press; 2005. p. 233–49.

[33] Keim P, Van Ert MN, Pearson T, et al. Anthrax molecular epidemiology and forensics: using the appropriate marker for different evolutionary scales. Infect Genet Evol 2004;4:205–13.
[34] Boyd EF, Nelson K, Wang FS, et al. Molecular genetic basis of allelic polymorphism in malic dehydrogenase (mdh) in natural populations of *Escherichia coli* and *Salmonella enterica*. Proc Natl Acad Sci U S A 1994;91:1280–4.
[35] Chun J, Huq A, Colwell RR. Analysis of 16S–23S rRNA intergenic spacer regions of *Vibrio cholerae* and *Vibrio mimicus*. Appl Environ Microbiol 1999;65:2202–8.
[36] Byun R, Elbourne LD, Lan R, et al. Evolutionary relationships of pathogenic clones of *Vibrio cholerae* by sequence analysis of four housekeeping genes. Infect Immun 1999;67: 1116–24.
[37] Garcia-Martinez J, Martinez-Murcia A, Anton AI, et al. Comparison of the small 16S to 23S intergenic spacer region (ISR) of the rRNA operons of some *Escherichia coli* strains of the ECOR collection and *E. coli* K-12. J Bacteriol 1996;178:6374–7.
[38] Perez Luz S, Rodriguez-Valera F, Lan R, et al. Variation of the ribosomal operon 16S–23S gene spacer region in representatives of *Salmonella enterica* subspecies. J Bacteriol 1998;180: 2144–51.
[39] Harrell LJ, Andersen GL, Wilson KH. Genetic variability of *Bacillus anthracis* and related species. J Clin Microbiol 1995;33:1847–50.
[40] Keim P, Kalif A, Schupp J, et al. Molecular evolution and diversity in *Bacillus anthracis* as detected by amplified fragment length polymorphism markers. J Bacteriol 1997;179:818–24.
[41] Jackson PJ, Walthers EA, Kalif AS, et al. Characterization of the variable-number tandem repeats in *vrrA* from different *Bacillus anthracis* isolates. Appl Environ Microbiol 1997;63: 1400–5.
[42] Schupp JM, Klevyiska AM, Zinser G, et al. *vrrB*, a hypervariable open reading frame in *Bacillus anthracis*. J Bacteriol 2000;182:3989–97.
[43] Zwick ME, Mcafee F, Cutler DJ, et al. Microarray-based resequencing of multiple *Bacillus anthracis* isolates. Genome Biol 2004;6:R10.1–13.
[44] de la Puente-Redondo VA, Garcia del Blanco N, Gutierrez-Martin CB, et al. Comparison of different PCR approaches for typing of *Francisella tularensis* strains. J Clin Microbiol 2000; 38:1016–22.
[45] Johansson A, Goransson I, Larsson P, et al. Extensive allelic variation among *Francisella tularensis* strains in a short-sequence tandem repeat region. J Clin Microbiol 2001;39: 3140–6.
[46] Garcia Del Blanco N, Dobson ME, Vela AI, et al. Genotyping of *Francisella tularensis* strains by pulsed-field gel electrophoresis, amplified fragment length polymorphism fingerprinting, and 16S rRNA gene sequencing. J Clin Microbiol 2002;40:2964–72.
[47] Johansson A, Farlow J, Larsson P, et al. Worldwide genetic relationships among *Francisella tularensis* isolates determined by multiple-locus variable-number tandem repeat analysis. J Bacteriol 2004;186:5808–18.
[48] Svensson K, Larsson P, Johansson D, et al. Evolution of subspecies of *Francisella tularensis*. J Bacteriol 2005;187:3903–8.
[49] Farlow J, Wagner DM, Dukerich M, et al. *Francisella tularensis* in the United States. Emerg Infect Dis 2005;11:1835–41.
[50] Adair DM, Worsham PL, Hill KK, et al. Diversity in a variable-number tandem repeat from *Yersinia pestis*. J Clin Microbiol 2000;38:1516–9.
[51] Klevytska AM, Price LB, Schupp JM, et al. Identification and characterization of variable-number tandem repeats in the *Yersinia pestis* genome. J Clin Microbiol 2001;39: 3179–85.
[52] Motin VL, Georgescu AM, Elliott JM, et al. Genetic variability of *Yersinia pestis* isolates as predicted by PCR-based IS*100* genotyping and analysis of structural genes encoding glycerol-3-phosphate dehydrogenase (*glpD*). J Bacteriol 2002;184:1019–27.
[53] Huang X-Z, Chu MC, Engelthaler DM, et al. Genotyping of a homogeneous group of *Yersinia pestis* strains isolated in the United States. J Clin Microbiol 2002;40:1164–73.

[54] Anisimov AP, Lindler LE, Pier GB. Intraspecific diversity of *Yersinia pestis*. Clin Microbiol Rev 17:434–64.
[55] Verger J-M, Grimont F, Grimont PAD, et al. *Brucella* a monospecific genus as shown by deoxyribonucleic acid hybridization. Int J Syst Bacteriol 1985;35:292–5.
[56] Tcherneva E, Rijpens N, Jersek B, et al. Differentiation of *Brucella* species by random amplified polymorphic DNA analysis. J Appl Microbiol 2000;88:69–80.
[57] Read TD, Peterson SN, Tourasse N, et al. The genome sequence of *Bacillus anthracis* Ames and comparison to closely related bacteria. Nature 2003;423:81–6.
[58] DelVecchio VG, Kapatral V, Redkar RJ, et al. The genome sequence of the facultative intracellular pathogen *Brucella melitensis*. Proc Natl Acad Sci U S A 2002;99:443–8.
[59] Paulsen IT, Seshadri R, Nelson KE, et al. The *Brucella suis* genome reveals fundamental similarities between animal and plant pathogens and symbionts. Proc Natl Acad Sci U S A 2002; 99:13148–53.
[60] Seshadri R, Paulsen IT, Eisen JA, et al. Complete genome sequence of the Q-fever pathogen *Coxiella burnetii*. Proc Natl Acad Sci U S A 2003;100:5455–60.
[61] Larsson P, Oylston PC, Chain P, et al. The complete genome sequence of *Francisella tularensis*, the causative agent of tularemia. Nat Genet 2005;37:153–9.
[62] Andersson SGE, Zomorodipour A, Andersson JO, et al. The genome sequence of *Rickettsia prowazekii* and the origin of mitochondria. Nature 1998;396:133–43.
[63] Parkhill J, Wren BW, Thomson NR, et al. Genome sequence of *Yersinia pestis*, the causative agent of plague. Nature 2001;413:523–7.
[64] Deng W, Burland V, Plunkett G III, et al. Genome sequence of *Yersinia pestis* KIM. J Bacteriol 2002;184:4601–11.
[65] Groseth A, Stroher U, Theriault S, et al. Molecular characterization of an isolate from the 1989/90 epizootic of Ebola virus Reston among macaques imported into the United States. Virus Res 2002;87:155–63.
[66] Volchkov VE, Volchkova VA, Chepurnov AA, et al. Characterization of the L gene and 5′ trailer region of Ebola virus. J Gen Virol 1999;80:355–62.
[67] Auperin DD, McCormick JB. Nucleotide sequence of the Lassa virus (Josiah strain) S genome RNA and amino acid comparison of the N and GPC proteins to other arenaviruses. Virology 1989;168:421–5.
[68] Djavani M, Lukashevich IS, Sanchez A, et al. Completion of the Lassa fever virus sequence and identification of a RING finger open reading frame at the L RNA 5′ end. Virology 1997; 235:414–8.
[69] Shchelkunov SN, Blinov VM, Resenchuk SM, et al. Analysis of the nucleotide sequence of 53 kbp from the right terminus of the genome of variola major virus strain India-1967. Virus Res 1994;34:207–36.
[70] Shchelkunov SN, Totmenin AV, Sandakhchiev LS. Analysis of the nucleotide sequence of 23.8 kbp from the left terminus of the genome of variola major virus strain India-1967. Virus Res 1996;40:169–83.
[71] Gilson E, Clement JM, Brutlag D, et al. A family of dispersed repetitive extragenic palindromic DNA sequences in *Escherichia coli*. EMBO J 1984;3:1417–21.
[72] Lupski JR, Weinstock GM. Short, interspersed repetitive DNA sequences in prokaryotic genomes. J Bacteriol 1992;174:4525–9.
[73] Stern MJ, Ames GF, Smith NH, et al. Repetitive extragenic palindromic sequences: a major component of the bacterial genome. Cell 1984;37:1015–26.
[74] Ussery DW, Binnewiesm TT, Goodview-Oliveira R, et al. Genome update: DNA repeats in bacterial genomes. Microbiology 2004;150:3519–21.
[75] Keim P, Price LB, Klevytska AM, et al. Multiple-locus variable-number tandem repeat analysis reveals genetic relationships within *Bacillus anthracis*. J Bacteriol 2000;182:2928–36.
[76] Takahashi H, Keim P, Kaufmann AF, et al. *Bacillus anthracis* incident, Kameido, Tokyo, 1993. Emerg Infect Dis 2004;10:117–20.

[77] Keim P, Smith KL, Keys C, et al. Molecular investigation of the Aum Shinrikyo anthrax release in Kameido. Japan. J Clin Microbiol 2001;39:4566–7.
[78] Ehleringer JR, Casale JF, Lott MJ, et al. Tracing the geographical origin of cocaine. Nature 2000;408:311–2.
[79] Craig H. Isotopic variation in meteoric waters. Science 1961;133:1702–3.
[80] Kreuzer-Martin HW, Lott MJ, Dorigan J, et al. Microbe forensics: oxygen and hydrogen stable isotope ratios in *Bacillus subtilis* cells and spores. Proc Natl Acad Sci U S A 2003; 100:815–9.
[81] Kreuzer-Martin HW, Chesson LA, Lott MJ, et al. Stable isotope ratios as a tool in microbial forensics: Part 1. microbial isotopic composition as a function of growth medium. J Forensic Sci 2004;49:1–7.
[82] Kreuzer-Martin HW, Chesson LA, Lott MJ, et al. Stable isotope ratios as a tool in microbial forensics: Part 2. isotopic variation among different growth media as a tool for sourcing origins of bacterial cells or spores. J Forensic Sci 2004;49:1–7.
[83] Kreuzer-Martin HW, Chesson LA, Lott MJ, et al. Stable isotope ratios as a tool in microbial forensics: Part 3. effect of culturing on agar-containing media. J Forensic Sci 2005;50:1–8.
[84] Schaldach CM, Bench G, DeYoreo JJ, et al. Non-DNA methods for biological signatures. In: Breeze RG, Budowle B, Schutzer SE, editors. Microbial forensics. San Diego: Elsevier Academic Press; 2005. p. 251–94.
[85] Keys CJ, Dare DJ, Sutton H, et al. Compilation of a MALDI-TOF mass spectral database for the rapid screening and characterization of bacteria implicated in human diseases. Infect Genet Evol 2004;4:221–42.
[86] US Department of Justice, Federal Bureau of Investigation, US Army Soldier Biological Chemical Command. Criminal and epidemiological investigation handbook. 2003. Available at: http://www.edgewood.army.mil/downloads/mirp/ECBC_ceih.pdf.

ELSEVIER
SAUNDERS

Infect Dis Clin N Am
20 (2006) 475–483

INFECTIOUS
DISEASE CLINICS
OF NORTH AMERICA

Index

Note: Page numbers of article titles are in **boldface** type.

doi:10.1016/S0891-5520(06)00050-X

W

Y

Changing Your Address?

Make sure your subscription changes too! When you notify us of your new address, you can help make our job easier by including an exact copy of your Clinics label number with your old address (see illustration below.) This number identifies you to our computer system and will speed the processing of your address change. Please be sure this label number accompanies your old address and your corrected address—you can send an old Clinics label with your number on it or just copy it exactly and send it to the address listed below.

We appreciate your help in our attempt to give you continuous coverage. Thank you.

W. B. Saunders Company
SHIPPING AND RECEIVING DEPTS.
151 BENIGNO BLVD.
BELLMAWR, N.J. 08031

SECOND CLASS POSTAGE
PAID AT BELLMAWR, N.J.

This is your copy of the
CLINICS OF NORTH AMERICA

00503570 DOE—J32400 101 NH 8102

JOHN C DOE MD
324 SAMSON ST
BERLIN NH 03570

XP-D11494

JAN ISSUE

Your Clinics Label Number

Copy it exactly or send your label
along with your address to:
Elsevier Periodicals Customer Service
6277 Sea Harbor Drive
Orlando, FL 32887-4800
Call Toll Free 1-800-654-2452

Please allow four to six weeks for delivery of new subscriptions and for processing address changes.